WHY WE EAT WHAT WE EAT

WHY WE EAT WHAT WE EAT

The Psychology of Eating

EDITED BY

ELIZABETH D. CAPALDI

AMERICAN PSYCHOLOGICAL ASSOCIATION

WASHINGTON, DC

First printing July 1996
Second printing August 1997

Published by
American Psychological Association
750 First Stree, NE
Washington, DC 20002

Copies may be ordered from
APA Order Department
P.O. Box 92984
Washington, DC 20090-2984

In the UK and Europe, copies may be order from
American Psychological Association
3 Henrietta Street
Covent Garden, London
WC2E 8LU England

Typeset in Minion by INNODATA, Hanover, MD
Printer: Edwards Brothers, Inc., Ann Arbor, MI
Cover Designer: Minker Design, Bethesda, MD
Technical/Production Editor: Sarah J. Trembath

Library of Congress Cataloging-in-Publication Data
Why we eat what we eat : the psychology of eating / edited by
    Elizabeth D. Capaldi.
        p.   cm.
    Includes bibliographical references and index.
    ISBN 1-55798-366-6 (acid-free paper)
    1. Food habits—Psychological aspect.   2. Nutrition—
Psychological aspects.   3. Food preferences.   I. Capaldi,
Elizabeth D.
TX357.A65   1996
394.1'019—dc20   96-33870
                                                              CIP

British Library Cataloguing-in-Publication Data
A CIP record is available from the British Library.

Printed in the United States of America

This book is dedicated to the memory of Robert C. Bolles, whose untimely death in 1994 prevented him from writing the main theme-setting chapter for this book. His influence is felt throughout all the chapters. He was one of the earliest to point out the significant roles of environment, experience, and incentives in feeding.

Contents

Contributors

Linda M. Bartoshuk, Yale University School of Medicine, New Haven, Connecticut

Gary K. Beauchamp, Monell Chemical Senses Center, Philadelphia, Pennsylvania

Ilene L. Bernstein, University of Washington, Seattle

Leann L. Birch, The Pennsylvania State University, University Park

Robert C. Bolles, University of Washington, Seattle

Elizabeth D. Capaldi, University of Florida, Gainesville

Adam Drewnowski, University of Michigan Medical School, Ann Arbor

Valerie B. Duffy, School of Allied Health Sciences, University of Connecticut, Storrs

Jennifer A. Fisher, The Pennsylvania State University, University Park

Bennett G. Galef, Jr., McMaster University, Hamilton, Ontario, Canada

Marion M. Hetherington, University of Dundee, Scotland, UK

Bai-Han Li, University of Florida, Gainesville

Julie A. Mennella, Monell Chemical Senses Center, Philadelphia, Pennsylvania

Annie Morien, University of Florida, Gainesville

Douglas S. Ramsay, University of Washington, Seattle

Barbara J. Rolls, The Pennsylvania State University, University Park

Neil E. Rowland, University of Florida, Gainesville

Paul Rozin, University of Pennsylvania, Philadelphia

Glenn E. Schafe, University of Washington, Seattle

Randy J. Seeley, University of Washington, Seattle

Stephen C. Woods, University of Washington, Seattle

PART ONE

Introduction and Overview

Introduction

Elizabeth D. Capaldi

E ating is arguably the most fundamental of human activities. Each of us must eat or we die, and we usually have to eat a number of times each day. In some parts of the globe, obtaining food is the major daily activity. Although obtaining food is not that much of a problem for most of us in Western society, our lives still revolve largely around eating and the inevitable results that eating has on our bodies. Concerns over health and nutrition have increased our interest in diet choice, and body appearance is a major focus in our society. Because of the critical role of food in human life, scientists have long investigated both the foods we eat and the eating process itself. Psychologists are certainly no exception. As this book demonstrates, psychologists have contributed by showing how biology interacts with learning and cognitive factors. We do not all react to food in the same way, even at the physiological level, because of our different experiences with foods. Illness following eating a food can produce a long-lasting aversion to that food, whereas eating foods in combination with other, liked foods or eating with people we like can produce long-lasting likes. Understanding how experience changes reactions to food can help improve eating habits; this book outlines what psychology has come to understand about the development of eating behaviors.

EARLY INVESTIGATIONS AND THE HOMEOSTATIC MODEL

Until recently, the study of eating in psychology took place primarily at the physiological level. Early physiological psychologists sought the internal cue that produced eating (hunger cue) and the internal cue that stopped eating (satiety cue). Researchers working at that time proposed a model of eating that was based on homeostatic principles. They defined homeostasis as a stable internal state that the body is motivated to maintain. In the case of eating, this state is the absence of hunger. Once hunger cues are aroused, this model maintained, eating occurs until they are removed, restoring homeostasis. The image associated with this model is of a thermostat: When the house is at the right temperature, no action is needed; when the house becomes too hot, the air conditioner comes on; when the temperature is restored to a comfortable, predetermined level, the air conditioner turns off. Likewise, when the body does not need food, no action is needed. But when food is needed, action is taken to get that food.

In this early model, the consumption of food was taken to be an unlearned response in reaction to the feeling of hunger. The model did allow for some qualities of learning, proposing that the responses leading to food intake were learned. You might learn, therefore, that food is in the refrigerator and you must go to the refrigerator, open it, and get the food in order to eat; however, the role of learning in this model of hunger was not the primary focus of investigation.

THE PRIMACY OF LEARNING

Beginning in the 1950s, but particularly in the 1960s, evidence accumulated that the homeostatic model had fundamental flaws. First, it was recognized that animals eat in anticipation of hunger. In other words, animals do not wait for hunger cues to elicit eating. Second, it was learned that the development of eating patterns and preferences is subject to learning, as are digestive responses. The latter fact was discovered early in the 1900s by Pavlov, but it was not appreciated until much later. Also, learning does not depend on hunger or some other need being reduced, as implied by the homeostatic model. Animals learn responses that result in provision of foods that do not restore homeostasis, for example, learning to respond for saccharin.

Today, the emphasis in the study of eating is on learning and experience and how these interact with biological predispositions to produce behavior. This behavior includes both eating patterns and physiological responses. Pavlov (1927) marked the earliest shift in psychology away from the homeostatic model by showing that animals salivate in response to anticipated food. More recently, all sorts of physiological responses have been shown to occur in anticipation of events, rather than in reaction to events. Indeed, Pavlov began his work by studying stomach secretions, not salivation. He was interested in the different stomach secretions produced by different types of food, more acidic for meat, for example. He realized he had discovered something important when he found the stomach secreted acid *before* the meat arrived, if a signal preceded the meat. The fact that physiological responses are subject to learning is not part of our commonsense mentality. We believe, from lessons learned in grammar school, that digestive responses are the same in all people and that the effect of food on the body is the same as well. Yet physiological research has shown that these responses are heavily affected by the organism's experiences. When one experiences a food that is too rich and is difficult to digest, it may be a matter of a learning history with that food rather than inherent physiology.

A good example of the paradigm change that has occurred is provided by the example of specific hungers. Early researchers hypothesized a "wisdom of the body," whereby internal cues signal a need for food elements, thereby producing a desire for those elements, which in turn causes animals to choose foods containing those elements. We all hope that this is true so that when we crave ice cream we can argue that some critical food element must be present in ice cream. Indeed, some have argued that chocolate craving is produced by craving for potassium (there is no evidence for this idea).

Researchers believed they had found evidence for the "wisdom of the body" in the following experiment (Rozin & Kalat, 1971): Rats became sick on distinctive Diet A, which contained no thiamine. Later, they were given a choice between Diet A and a second distinctive diet, Diet B, which contained thiamine. The rats chose Diet B. These results were interpreted to illustrate that the rats' bodies needed thiamine and guided them to the thiamine-rich diet. Rozin and Kalat, however, showed that what the rats were really doing was avoiding the diet that made them ill, Diet A. Given a choice between Diet A and another distinctive diet, Diet C, which also contained no thiamine, rats chose Diet C. Thus, rats manage to select diets containing the nutrients they need in part by avoiding diets that make them not feel well.

Later research showed that although rats learn to select diets that contain nutrients, they have no sensors for most food elements. They can taste sweet, sour, salt, and bitter, and they innately approach salt and sweet and avoid sour and bitter. These built-in tendencies, which are present in humans as well as rats, go a long way toward guiding animals to appropriate foods. In nature, poisons are bitter; sour fruit is not ripe; sweet fruit is ripe; and a preference for salt will produce ingestion of many needed minerals. Beyond these simple genetically mediated preferences, however, food choice is learned.

Learning about food begins prenatally and continues with breast or bottle feeding in infancy. The foods the mother eats determine the preferences of the child (see chapter 4, this volume). In addition, the eating patterns imposed by parents on their children have lifelong effects (see chapter 5, this volume). Social experience is important, but so are individual experiences. Rats and people learn to avoid foods that make them sick and to approach foods that give them pleasure and make them feel well. The ingestion of particular foods is also a learned behavior, therefore. Throughout life, experience continues to change food preferences: Every eating experience is a learning experience.

IMPLICATIONS OF A LEARNING MODEL FOR EATING

The change in focus in the study of eating behaviors from mechanistic models to ones that depend on learning has significant implications: If eating is a learned behavior, then it can be changed. In other words, learning techniques conceivably can be used to change food preferences. If, for example, you would like to increase your preference for broccoli, you could just eat broccoli repeatedly. Although this should reduce your dislike or increase your liking of broccoli, it may not be a pleasurable way for you to proceed. Two other methods would be more pleasant and effective: You could mix broccoli with sugar or some other preferred food, or you could mix broccoli with other nutritious foods (such as cheese sauce). Many people already do this to enjoy broccoli more. Raw broccoli is served with high-fat dips, and cooked broccoli is served with cheese sauce. What you may not realize is that your preference for plain broccoli will increase as a result of these experiences of broccoli with more preferred foods.

Producing a dislike for a preferred food works on the same principles. Pairing a food with an unpleasurable event—like a disliked taste (bitter or sour), an illness, or an image of something disgusting—can produce a dislike for a food.

The research reviewed in this book offers both hope and direction. To the extent that our eating patterns and preferences are learned, they can be modified. Obesity and weight loss are a national obsession. The most critical element for body weight is fat; fat contains 9 calories per gram, and proteins and carbohydrates contain only 4. There is also evidence that low-fat diets produce less weight gain than equally caloric high-fat diets. To reduce one's preference for fat, one could attempt to produce a mild aversion for it by imagining disgusting images along with fat. Explicitly pairing fat with a bitter or sour taste should also reduce the preference for fat with repeated exposure. But perhaps easiest of all, eating less fat should reduce the preference for fat. Anecdotally, people who switch to skim milk from whole milk ultimately report a dislike for whole milk, considering it too rich. Theoretically, therefore, preferences for more healthful food can be learned.

THIS VOLUME

The main focus of this book is on the role of learning and experience in eating. The book covers the major areas of basic psychological research in this area, including biological, learning, developmental, cognitive, and social perspectives. The focus is on normal eating behavior. Although the principles discussed here must apply to disordered eating as well, we do not focus on anorexia, bulimia, and other eating disorders. An understanding of how the basic psychological processes operate in normal eating is necessary before attempting to understand disordered eating. A consistent picture of eating as a learned and constantly changing behavior emerges from the chapters in this book. The volume also reviews the biological basis of feeding, including genetically mediated differences among people in their ability to taste foods and in other physiological mechanisms that interact with learning to determine feeding.

In 1988 the American Psychological Association brought together a group of researchers who studied the role of taste and experience in eating. That conference resulted in *Taste, Experience, and Feeding* (Capaldi & Powley, 1990), a volume that consisted of chapters by the leading researchers in the area. Much of the work in that volume had just begun in 1988, and we stated at that time our intention of looking again at this area in the future. The present volume is a result of that second look.

The purposes of the volume are to update the earlier volume and to make the work accessible to a wider audience. The first volume was intended for researchers in the area, whereas this book is intended for students, both undergraduate and graduate, as well as dietitians, pediatricians, doctors, and practitioners in the weight-control and food industries. Other educated individuals who want to improve their understanding of their own eating patterns can also benefit from this book, as can parents who desire to do the best job possible in establishing the eating patterns of their children. Each of us can use the information in this book not only to understand our own eating patterns, but also to modify them if desired.

The volume is organized into six sections. Chapter 1 by Ramsay, Seeley, Bolles, and Woods sets the tone for the book by demonstrating the importance of learning even in the physiological responses that underlie eating. Each of the remaining sections discusses a different major set of psychological processes contributing to eating.

Part 2 discusses the basic learning processes affecting eating. Foods that are associated with illness are avoided, a learning process that is rapid and resistant to change. Schafe and Bernstein (chapter 2) review this type of learning, including how chemotherapy and other sources of illness can produce food aversions. Most food preferences are produced by beneficial effects of food: We learn to like foods associated with nutrients and foods that taste good. We also learn to like foods merely by eating them repeatedly. The learning involved in producing conditioned food preferences is reviewed in Capaldi's chapter (chapter 3).

Part 3 deals with the development of eating patterns beginning prenatally. Mennella and Beauchamp (chapter 4) show that infants' food preferences are affected by foods eaten by the mother during pregnancy. Birch and Fisher (chapter 5) examine the various factors in childhood that affect the development of the child's eating patterns, patterns that persist into adulthood.

Part 4 examines the biological basis of eating patterns, beginning with Duffy and Bartoshuk's (chapter 6) review of genetically mediated differences among individuals in sensory reactions to food. Rowland, Li, and Morien's review of the physiological bases of feeding follows (chapter 7). This chapter discusses the search for internal cues that elicit eating and that lead to its cessation. These two chapters describe the two main sources of cues that elicit eating: internal hunger-related cues and sensory aspects of the food.

Part 5 reviews social factors in feeding. Both rats and humans are highly social animals. Galef (chapter 8) reviews social influences on feeding in animals and how animals communicate about food with each other. Much of human eating behavior is also determined by the social context provided by family and peers, an area reviewed by Rozin (chapter 9).

The final section, Part 6, describes eating patterns in normal adults that result from the processes described in the earlier chapters. Hetherington and Rolls (chapter 10) discuss a short-term satiety factor that ensures that we consume a variety of food, and Drewnowski (chapter 11) describes eating patterns characteristic of normal and obese individuals.

CONCLUSION

The study of eating has changed dramatically in the last 50 years. We do not yet understand how the social, developmental, learning, and physiological factors all interact, but we do know that all these factors are important. This information is encouraging because most of these factors are under our control. In the future, in principle at least, we should be able to train our children and ourselves to eat in a manner that we consider desirable.

REFERENCES

Capaldi, E. D., & Powley, T. L. (Eds.). (1990). *Taste, experience and feeding.* Washington, DC: American Psychological Association.

Pavlov, I. P. (1927). *Conditioned Reflexes.* Oxford, England: Oxford University Press.

Rozin, P., & Kalat, J. W. (1971). Specific hungers and poison avoidance as adaptive specializations of learning. *Psychological Review, 78,* 459–486.

Ingestive Homeostasis: The Primacy of Learning

Douglas S. Ramsay, Randy J. Seeley, Robert C. Bolles, and Stephen C. Woods

The realization that the body actively maintains the constancy of its internal environment was stated clearly by Claude Bernard (1878). This process has been termed *homeostasis*, and it refers to the mechanisms responsible for the adjustment of physiological parameters to maintain bodily equilibrium. The teleological argument typically applied to explain the existence of such a control system is that animals capable of maintaining important physiological parameters within a specified range derive some benefit from this ability. Crucial determinants of the internal state of the body are the amount and type of foods that are ingested. Although it is axiomatic that the continued well-being of an animal depends on the consumption of a nutritionally well-balanced diet, the process of ingesting these foodstuffs (i.e., eating, especially in a general omnivore such as the human or the rat) poses a challenge to the homeostatic systems attempting to maintain a physiological equilibrium.

There is a second, less-well-described aspect of the behavior of eating by omnivores. Foods contain salts, sugars, complex carbohydrates, fats,

We (D. S. R., R. J. S., and S. C. W.) would like to acknowledge the contributions of Robert Bolles during the early development of this chapter. His untimely death was a great loss. He will be missed.
Preparation of this chapter was supported by National Institutes of Health Grants DK-17844, DA-07391, DE-00379, and AA-07247.

amino acids, toxins, and so on, all of which must be appropriately processed and disposed of by the body as it selectively gleans the particular nutrients needed to ensure survival (see Rozin & Schulkin, 1991). Few if any natural foodstuffs contain the precise ingredients and in the exact proportions needed by the consumer at any point in time. In addition, although the food-derived necessities of life (i.e., energy sources) are continuously expended, they are not continuously ingested. Hence, even foods that are ideal in a nutritional sense must be taken into the body in boluses and most of the ingredients stored until needed by various organ systems. In other words, eating and the postmeal period are times when excess nutrients (relative to any moment's specific energetic needs) are passed from the digestive system into the circulation and from the circulation in turn into one or another storage organ. The point is that the consumption of complex foods in relatively large amounts at one time (i.e., meals) necessarily disrupts many of the physiological parameters the body has evolved mechanisms to defend. Therefore, although it is true that we eat to survive, the refinement of the behavioral and physiological processes included in the umbrella term *eating* is shaped by a multitude of homeostatic mechanisms that are engaged during ingestion to minimize the meal-related perturbations. The basics of the argument that perturbations caused by meals, especially large meals, have potentially aversive consequences are presented by Woods (1991).

In this chapter we review the common application of homeostatic principles to ingestive behavior, and we conclude that the predominant model, which is based on the principle that when the body becomes depleted in some crucial parameter related to food (e.g., blood glucose or stored fat), eating is initiated (the so-called depletion–repletion model), cannot account for most instances of eating. We then discuss a less understood strategy of homeostatic regulation: learning. As the role of learning in the control of ingestion and its consequences becomes appreciated, novel interpretations of previous findings become apparent. When one considers an animal's ability to learn from its ingestive experience combined with the physiological mechanisms subserving homeostatic regulation, a new and valuable framework for understanding ingestive behavior results. The model we present in this chapter is speculative and intended to stimulate discussion of the role of learning in all aspects of regulatory behavior.

HOMEOSTASIS AND INGESTIVE BEHAVIOR

Negative Feedback Loops

A potential role of negative feedback loops was recognized early in the scientific investigation of food intake. Many models were based on these principles, which can be generically categorized as depletion–repletion models of ingestive behavior (e.g., Friedman & Stricker, 1976; Stricker, 1991). The idea is simple: The well-adapted animal continually monitors the status of its fuel reserves. If the reserves fall below a critical threshold, an error signal is generated, which activates a corrective mechanism (e.g., eating). If the corrective mechanism is successful at replenishing the monitored fuel stores, the error signal ceases and the corrective mechanism is deactivated. This model has often been compared to the functioning of the thermostat in a house. When the house's temperature falls below a critical level, the thermostat detects the perturbation and sends a signal to the furnace. The furnace in turn generates heat and warms the house until such time as the thermostat detects that room temperature is restored and turns off the furnace.

Numerous negative feedback models have been proposed to account for feeding and related behaviors. The two most cited examples are the glucostatic (Mayer, 1953, 1955) and the lipostatic (Kennedy, 1950) models of food-intake regulation. The glucostatic theory postulated that because continuous glucose oxidation is essential for the survival of some tissues (e.g., the brain), some parameter of glucose levels or availability naturally evolved to become a "regulated" variable. Furthermore, this variable should accurately reflect the status of this critical commodity, should be readily detectable, and should be controllable by both behavioral and physiological mechanisms. A drop (or change) in available glucose (e.g., hypoglycemia) provides a stimulus (error signal) that activates a corrective action on the part of the animal to restore blood glucose levels. Mayer postulated that certain regions of the hypothalamus are glucose-sensitive (or, to be more precise, sensitive to their own rate of utilization of glucose) and that changes in glucose use by these tissues activate behavioral and physiological responses. Corrective responses to a decrease of glucose utilization might include increased consumption of available glycogen stores in the liver, the conversion of other compounds to glucose (i.e., gluconeogenesis), and the initiation of a meal. Likewise, the glucostatic theory postulated that as critical parameters associated with glucose availability and utilization increase above some optimal level, an opposing set of responses is activated that might include storing circulating glucose for future use or stopping eating.

Analogously, the lipostatic theory posited that there is an ideal level of stored fuel in the form of fat. Hence, fat stores were hypothesized to be monitored, and a decrease in the reservoir (error signal) was hypothesized to activate a negative feedback loop to replenish fuel stores. The amount eaten was therefore hypothesized to be under the control of error signals indicating too small or too great an amount of energy reserves in the form of lipid. Although there is not agreement as to the nature of the error signal for the regulation of stored fat (see Stallone & Stunkard, 1991), a compelling argument can be made that the pancreatic hormone insulin is such a signal (Schwartz, Figlewicz, Baskin, Woods, & Porte, 1992; Woods, 1995).

More contemporary versions of hypotheses based on the same principles are those of Friedman, Tordoff, and Ramirez (1986) and of Even and Nicolaidis (1985; Even, Coulaud, & Nicolaidis, 1988). Rather than focusing on a single nutrient or energy source such as glucose or stored fat as the sole determinant of the critical error signal, they contended that energy usage, as reflected in some critical organ such as the liver or the brain, is what is important and that it is independent of the actual fuel or fuels being utilized. Such hypotheses recognize and build on the existence of metabolically adaptive organs and systems that can interconvert fuels from one form to another as needed. Bolles (1980) argued that with the evolution of an energy storage system, organs such as the liver were necessary to "convert almost anything available into almost anything needed" (p. 67). The more contemporary versions of negative feedback models of food ingestion take these evolutionary innovations into account. All of these examples, however, are based on the same premise and operate in the same fashion. Perturbations (error signals) in a critical index of fuel status are detected by the organism and activate hard-wired (i.e., innate) negative feedback loops to correct the disruptions and hence keep the animal on its ideal course.

Negative feedback loops such as those described are but one of several strategies by which important parameters can be regulated, and they have significant drawbacks. Foremost among the shortcomings of reliance upon such simple mechanisms is that an error signal must be generated to activate the corrective response. In other words, the animal must experience a perturbation of an important physiological parameter before corrective measures are initiated. Furthermore, if the corrective mechanism cannot be activated immediately (e.g., owing to an unavoidable delay until meal initiation can take place), the severity of the parameter's deviation from defended levels may continue to increase. If the maintenance of homeostatic equilibrium is advantageous, it would seem far better in a teleological sense to protect critical parameters in such a way as to prevent or minimize such disruptions.

Feedforward Regulation

Feedforward regulation is one mechanism that has been suggested to address the limitations encountered with negative feedback loops (Houk, 1988); it does not require a homeostatic disruption, or error signal. In feedforward regulation, a correlate of an impending and imminent perturbation of a regulated parameter reliably precedes the actual perturbation. Houk uses the example of core body temperature as a critical parameter that is homeostatically regulated. When an organism is placed in a cold environment, its surface starts losing heat before the core is impacted. Although skin (surface) temperature is certainly important to the organism, small fluctuations in its level are less vital to life than comparable fluctuations of temperature in "vital" organs. A feedforward system might enable the organism to detect a drop in skin temperature (that precedes an imminent drop in core temperature) and activate corrective warming responses without the organism having experienced a reduction in core temperature. Hence, such a system uses sensors to monitor variables that change before more critical and presumably homeostatically regulated parameters are disrupted and thereby allows activation of corrective responses that reduce or prevent disturbances of the more vital systems.

Feedforward strategies have also been proposed to participate in the regulation of ingestive behavior. For example, it is well known that animals stop eating long before ingested nutrients enter the circulation in large quantities. Hence, "preabsorptive" feedforward signals are often suggested to be major limiters of meal size. They cause the organism to demonstrate "satiety" (i.e., stop eating) well before the meal being consumed can have a major caloric impact within the body. The ingested foodstuffs, therefore, do not need to cause a major perturbation in a regulated system (error signal) to activate a negative feedback loop that turns off the meal. Instead, preabsorptive signals that predict an upcoming homeostatically disruptive event activate corrective responses (stopping the meal in this instance) such that the disruption is dampened. Hormones and other intercellular signals secreted when food begins entering the gut are hypothesized to mediate this feedforward satiety system (e.g., Smith & Gibbs, 1992). The point is that feedforward systems, unlike negative feedback systems, do not depend on the occurrence of an error signal in a critical and homeostatically controlled parameter to accomplish regulation.

A feedforward regulatory strategy offers the advantage of activating corrective responses in advance of an otherwise imminent disruption such that the disruption can be avoided. However, the effective operation of a reflexive, or hard-wired, feedforward mechanism has significant obstacles. Specifically, the feedforward signal must contain sufficient information about the nature and degree of the pending disturbance that the appropriate corrective responses can be activated. In the case of ingestive behavior, this would be a challenging determination. Preabsorptive information about the quantity and quality (e.g., carbohydrate, protein, fat) of the food ingested would need to be encoded by a complex array of specialized peripheral receptors. In addition, there would be no means of adjusting errors in the corrective response elicited by a hard-wired feedforward controller. Opportunistic feeders, like general omnivores, take advantage of an enormous range of different foodstuffs. These animals are capable of adapting to a variety of diets and they adjust their feeding patterns accordingly. It is difficult to imagine such an animal being innately prepared to "decode" accurately the contents of every potential food it might encounter so it could select the appropriate preparatory response. Nonetheless, animals do make accurate anticipatory corrective responses on the basis of preabsorptive aspects of the food being consumed, and these responses serve to defend the homeostatic equilibrium. Appropriate activation of corrective responses on the basis of signals that precede the disturbance has caused Houk (1988) to suggest that "there must be special adaptive mechanisms" (p. 102) involved in feedforward regulation. We argue that, learning is the special adaptive mechanism that allows for regulation in the absence of error signals (see Somjen, 1992).

Learning from ingestive experiences enhances an animal's ability to defend critical parameters and hence effectively maintain homeostasis. Through experience with particular foodstuffs and situations, animals learn to activate appropriate responses in anticipation of upcoming events. Originally neutral stimuli can acquire significance because of the events or contingencies they predict. With learning, these once-neutral stimuli elicit responses that prepare animals to compensate for homeostatically disruptive events that are about to occur. In the ideal situation, the learned response has the correct magnitude and temporal characteristics to prevent or offset the homeostatically disruptive event. Foodstuffs that initially disrupt homeostasis no longer do so (at least to the same potentially dangerous degree) after the animal has learned to compensate for the postingestive consequences of the food. In this regard, eating has marked similarity to the development of drug tolerance (see Woods, 1991; Woods & Strubbe, 1994). Whereas a drug may have a large initial effect on a homeostatically regulated parameter (i.e., an organism is sensitive to or intolerant of a novel drug), repeated experience with a drug's effects can lead to a reduction of the observed effect following drug administration (i.e., drug tolerance develops). Learning plays a major role in the development of tolerance to drugs (Ramsay & Woods, 1996; Siegel, 1989; Siegel, Krank, & Hinson, 1987; Wenger, Tiffany, Bombardier, Nicholls, & Woods, 1981). Likewise, learning plays a critical role in the regulation of ingestive behavior (Weingarten, 1990; Woods, 1995; Woods & Strubbe, 1994).

The regulation of blood glucose provides an excellent example of the role of learning in ingestive behavior. Foods that are high in readily absorbable sugars can cause a large increase in blood sugar. Rising blood glucose levels activate a negative feedback loop that reduces blood glucose through several mechanisms such as the increased release of the pancreatic hormone insulin. Increased circulating insulin permits glucose to leave the blood and enter cells at a higher rate, thereby reducing blood glucose concentrations and ameliorating the perturbation. When a food-related increase of blood glucose can be anticipated by the animal (e.g., by the existence of a sugar-signaling sweet taste), the postprandial increment of blood glucose is substantially attenuated through the release of insulin before the absorption of glucose. This early secreted insulin has been termed *cephalic insulin* because its secretion is mediated by a neural connection from the brain to the pancreas (Powley, 1977; Woods, 1991; Woods & Kulkosky, 1976).

Cephalic insulin is easily modifiable by learning, and a compelling case can be made that all instances of secretion of cephalic insulin are due to learning (e.g., see Woods, 1995; Woods & Kulkosky, 1976). Through learning, cues associated with foods that increase blood glucose (and hence elicit the release of insulin) come to elicit insulin release in the absence of a change of glucose (Woods, 1976, 1977; Woods et al., 1977). Animals provided with food-associated conditioned stimuli but denied access to the food become hypoglycemic owing to the conditioned release of insulin (Woods, 1976; Woods et al., 1977). The converse is also true. If the conditioned stimuli signaling the meal are omitted, hyperglycemia (excessively elevated blood glucose) results, because the conditioned release of cephalic insulin does not occur. For example, when glucose is put directly into the stomach, thus omitting the oropharyngeal predictive cues, less insulin is initially secreted and blood glucose levels become higher than when the same amount of glucose is consumed orally (e.g., Louis-Sylvestre, 1976; Steffens, 1976). Finally, if glucose-predictive cues are present but there is little or no glucose in the food (e.g., saccharin is substituted for glucose), insulin would be secreted and blood glucose would decrease (e.g., Deutsch, 1974). In this instance, a homeostatic disturbance occurs in the opposite direction (i.e., conditioned hypoglycemia; see Woods, 1995).

In contrast to a hard-wired feedforward mechanism, learning provides valuable flexibility to homeostatic regulation. Predictive cues can entrain corrective responses so that they can be elicited before an actual homeostatic disturbance. Yet these cues do not need to be specified in advance (i.e., to be hard-wired). Evolution may have shaped some classes of cues (e.g., tastes and smells) to become more readily associated than others (e.g., sights and sounds) with the postingestive consequences of food (Garcia & Koelling, 1966). Nevertheless, this generic learning strategy allows animals (especially omnivores) to accommodate to changes in their environment that might introduce, alter, or remove traditional food sources. Furthermore, errors in the regulatory response can be adjusted with experience. In sum, if an animal lives in a sufficiently predictable environment, it can learn to avoid homeostatic disturbances by using anticipatory compensatory responses.

Thus, error signals are not generated, and regulation does not depend on negative feedback loops.

It is important to realize that the elicitation of learned responses that circumvent homeostatic disruptions is a special instance of a feedforward system. In this schema, an environmental cue indicates that a particular food is about to enter the system. The taste of the food predicts an upcoming change in a regulated parameter (i.e., it is analogous to the change of skin temperature that would normally precede a change of core temperature). The important difference, from our point of view, is that the taste is not hard-wired to the compensatory response.

ROLE OF NEGATIVE FEEDBACK IN LEARNED RESPONSES

Negative feedback loops provide the basis for the acquisition of learned responses that compensate for and thus prevent homeostatic disturbances. If necessary, they also provide feedback so that learned responses can be adjusted to match changing environmental conditions more appropriately. In other words, if a learned response does not adequately maintain homeostasis, an error signal is necessarily generated. The error signal in turn results in a reflexive adjustment to correct the current perturbation. In addition, it provides feedback to modify the learned response so that the organism is better able to maintain homeostasis in the future.

Negative feedback loops also perform an important protective function. Unpredictable events can occur, and when they do, negative feedback loops are necessarily activated. In addition, some homeostatically disruptive events are of sufficiently great magnitude that they exceed the corrective capability of existing learned regulatory responses. Researchers investigating the mechanisms underlying the control of ingestion often create dramatic error signals (e.g., low blood volume or glucose level—hypovolemia or hypoglycemia, respectively) to study negative feedback loops. Textbooks and review chapters in fact are replete with examples of negative feedback loops that regulate ingestive behaviors. Loss of blood volume is a potent cue to initiate drinking (Stricker & Wolf, 1969); loss of plasma sodium elicits sodium appetite (Rabe, 1975); a large drop in blood sugar or in glucose utilization can initiate eating (Grossman, 1986; Lotter & Woods, 1977; Mackay, Callaway, &

Barnes, 1940; Smith & Epstein, 1969; Ritter & Taylor, 1989); and a forced decrease of body fat can increase food intake (Kennedy, 1950; Woods, Decke, & Vasselli, 1974). However, it is important to realize that the operation of these mechanisms is probably the exception and not the rule. Error signals may occur for a variety of reasons, and in those instances in which the perturbation is unanticipated, negative feedback loops are called into action. In predictable environments, error signals are seldom generated, and negative feedback loops are rarely employed once animals have used learned responses in the defense of homeostasis.

It might be argued that once the learned anticipatory response comes to prevent severe changes in the homeostatic variable being monitored, there would be no more error signal and, consequently, the learned anticipatory response should extinguish. Of course, once the anticipatory response begins to extinguish, the error signal returns and so does the contingency between the cue and the error signal. In this way, negative feedback could be responsible not only for the acquisition of the learned anticipatory response but for the maintenance of the response as well.

Such a strategy requires that error signals not be avoided entirely, but rather that they return periodically and thereby reinstate the contingencies that supported acquisition of the learned anticipatory response originally. If, as we have postulated previously, having to invoke negative feedback circuits in response to error signals is homeostatically undesirable, is it possible to construct a strategy in which the learned anticipatory response can be maintained with little need for homeostatic disturbances (i.e., error signals)? We believe the answer is *yes* and that some forms of learning are better able to maintain a learned response in the absence of error signals. For example, avoidance responding is often cited as an example of learned behavior that persists (i.e., fails to extinguish) to a greater extent than other types of learning (e.g., Bolles, 1967, 1975).

In a prototypical avoidance-learning experiment, animals are placed in an apparatus with two connected chambers (a shuttle box). Presentation of a signal (e.g., a light) in one chamber indicates that seconds later a shock will follow if the animal does not move into the other chamber. With experience, animals learn to avoid shocks by moving quickly into the alternate chamber when the signal is presented (e.g., Solomon & Wynne, 1953). The puzzle of avoidance learning is that once animals have learned to move to the correct chamber, the learned response is maintained even though the animal rarely receives any further shock. In essence, the animal performs a learned response without receiving error signals (i.e., shocks). Such learned avoidance responses are remarkably resistant to extinction. Should the animal make an infrequent error, however, the shock serves to reinforce the learned avoidance response.

Shock is a powerfully aversive stimulus and thus easily supports avoidance learning in an experimental setting. It is less clear what aspect of ingestive behavior might be similarly aversive such that it would support an analogous form of avoidance learning. Avoidance learning is the basis for the so-called eating paradox (Woods, 1991). Although food is a necessary commodity, the disruptive homeostatic consequences of eating large meals are apparently aversive. Large meals, like shock, support the acquisition of avoidance responses such as the secretion of cephalic insulin. Once a corrective response is learned, changes to homeostatic variables are minimized and error signals are effectively avoided. These anticipatory responses would be highly resistant to extinction, and as long as they continued to be made, error signals would continue to be avoided. With such a strategy, as long as the environmental conditions remain relatively constant, disturbances in homeostatically regulated variables would be infrequent and homeostatic regulation would proceed with little need for negative feedback loops.

REINTERPRETATION OF DEPLETION–REPLETION MODELS OF INGESTIVE BEHAVIOR

Our contention is that under normal conditions, most ingestive behavior is regulated by learned responses that have been acquired to defend homeostatic parameters as efficiently as possible given environmental limitations (Woods & Strubbe, 1994). Furthermore, the regulation of ingestive behavior occurs with little reliance on negative feedback loops. This "learning" view of the regulation of ingestive behavior leads to alternate interpretations of existing data as discussed subsequently.

When a reliable change in a regulated variable is observed before a meal, it is traditionally interpreted as being an error signal correlated with the depletion of a critical metabolic fuel. The subsequent meal is typically viewed as being elicited by a negative feedback loop that was activated by the error signal. However, these premeal changes may also be viewed as learned anticipatory responses that protect homeostatically regulated parameters from the challenge of the impending meal. For example, Campfield and Smith (1991) observed declines in blood glucose that are reliably followed by meal initiation. One interpretation of such data is that these declines in blood glucose cause the animal to eat. From a learning perspective, these declines in blood glucose could be a learned response that ameliorates the rise in blood glucose that would otherwise accompany the upcoming meal. Indeed, it seems reasonable that when meals are predictable, learned responses should be acquired to defend regulated variables and that these responses should occur in anticipation of the homeostatic challenge (i.e., before the meal).

A second example can be found in changes of metabolic rate that accompany ingestion. Analogous to the decline in blood glucose that precedes a meal, metabolic rate also declines before eating. Once again, a negative feedback interpretation might be that the decline of metabolic rate provides an error signal that is a correlate of diminishing metabolic fuels (e.g., Even & Nicolaidis, 1985). This signal reflexively activates eating to replenish the depleted fuels. As a result of food ingestion, metabolic rate rises. Again, a learning perspective offers an alternate interpretation. Processing of ingested food results in the homeostatic disturbance of metabolic rate (i.e., the rate is elevated). Animals might therefore be expected to learn to lower metabolic rate in anticipation of an upcoming meal and thereby circumvent extreme postprandial increases of metabolism. Consequently, the observed decline in metabolic rate before a meal may not be a signal to eat but rather the reflection of a learned response that ameliorates the hypermetabolic effects of meals.

CLINICAL IMPLICATIONS

To the degree that individuals rely on learned responses to make appropriate food-related responses, errors can and do occur. The two obvious types of meal-related errors are failing to make an anticipatory response and making the correct anticipatory response but at an inappropriate time. As discussed previously, feedforward mechanisms are based on the individual's monitoring certain predictive stimuli and making neurally mediated responses (e.g., secreting cephalic insulin to prepare for and minimize imminent hyperglycemia, or curtailing the eating process to circumvent the need for the body to cope with too many ingested calories at once). When these responses cannot be made, one should consume small meals to be safe. When the nerve between the brain and the pancreas is compromised such that cephalic insulin cannot be secreted, animals and humans eat smaller meals (see Woods, 1991). Consistent with this fact is the finding of Collier and colleagues that individuals of every species studied, when given a choice, prefer to eat their food each day as a large number of small meals (Collier, 1986; Collier, Johnson, Hill, & Kaufman, 1986) and that they eat larger meals only when each small meal has excessive costs associated with procuring it and then only after they have had sufficient opportunity to adapt to eating larger meals. It is reasonable to assume that the adaptation process involves learning to secrete insulin cephalically (and many other responses) to process the food that must be consumed at one time. Humans can adopt an incredibly wide array of eating styles on the basis of lifestyle and opportunities, ranging from one or fewer meals each day to multiple meals plus snacks. The flexibility to accommodate to diverse eating schedules is afforded by the learned neural control that can be exerted over key metabolic processes (see Dworkin, 1993).

Rats easily learn to secrete cephalic insulin in anticipation of meals, especially meals high in carbohydrates (Woods, 1976, 1977, 1995; Woods et al., 1977). It is therefore reasonable to assume that individual humans with a history of consuming large amounts of sweet, sugar-laden foods likewise secrete cephalic insulin (as well as make other adaptations) in response to meal-related stimuli. If their diet were to change or they were to encounter the same stimuli in the absence of their normal food (e.g., if they encountered an artificial sweetener for the first time), they would be expected to secrete cephalic insulin inappropriately. This is exactly what happens in the clinical syndrome called *reactive hypoglycemia*. When individuals with reactive hypoglycemia begin eating, they secrete so much cephalic insulin that their blood glucose does not rise (as usually happens during a meal) but decreases, often to clinically low levels. The treatment is to adopt a lifestyle of eating numerous small meals (preferably low in sugar) as opposed to a few larger ones each day (see review in Woods, 1991). The point is that reliance on learned metabolic responses to help in the homeostatic control of critical body parameters is appropriate only as long as the environment is stable (or at least highly predictable).

CONCLUSION

The strategy of negative feedback has been the primary focus of research on homeostasis. Consequently, considerable effort has been invested in the search for the error signals that drive corrective negative feedback loops. In contrast, the current thesis suggests that most regulation occurs in the absence of error signals. Learning provides a flexible and dynamic feedforward mechanism by which perturbations in homeostatically regulated variables can be prevented, especially in predictable environments. This learning strategy is an improvement over negative feedback because regulation can be achieved with fewer fluctuations in the regulated variable. An important corollary of this position is that learned responses can and do anticipate events that challenge homeostasis. For researchers investigating regulation through negative feedback loops, such learned responses may be mistakenly interpreted as error signals. The distinction between error signals and preparatory learned responses is crucial if a more complete understanding of homeostatic regulation is to be achieved. In the study of food-intake regulation, one should recognize that ingestive behavior is a psychobiological process uniting physiology and the psychology of learning.

REFERENCES

Bernard, C. (1878). *Leçons sur les phénomènes de la vie communs aux animaux et aux végétaux*. Paris: J. B. Baillière.

Bolles, R. C. (1967). *Theory of motivation*. New York: Harper & Row.

Bolles, R. C. (1975). *Learning theory*. New York: Holt.

Bolles, R. C. (1980). Some functionalistic thoughts about regulation. In F. M. Toates & T. R. Halliday (Eds.), *Analysis of motivational processes* (pp. 63–75). London: Academic Press.

Campfield, L. A., & Smith, F. J. (1991). Systemic factors in the control of food intake: Evidence for patterns as signals. In E. M. Stricker (Ed.), *Handbook of behavioral neurobiology: Neurobiology of food and Fluid intake* (pp. 183–206). New York: Plenum Press.

Collier, G. (1986). The dialogue between the house economist and the resident physiologist. *Nutrition and Behavior, 3,* 9–26.

Collier, G., Johnson, D. F., Hill, W. L., & Kaufman, L. W. (1986). The economics of the law of effect. *Journal of the Experimental Analysis of Behavior, 48,* 113–136.

Deutsch, R. (1974). Conditioned hypoglycemia: A mechanism for saccharin-induced sensitivity to insulin in the rat. *Journal of Comparative and Physiological Psychology, 86,* 350–358.

Dworkin, B. R. (1993). *Learning and physiological regulation.* Chicago: University of Chicago Press.

Even, P., Coulaud, H., & Nicolaidis, S. (1988). Integrated metabolic control of food intake after 2-deoxy-D-glucose and nicotinic acid injection. *American Journal of Physiology, 255,* R82–R89.

Even, P., & Nicolaidis, S. (1985). Spontaneous and 2-DG-induced metabolic changes and feeding: The ischymetric hypothesis. *Brain Research Bulletin, 15,* 429–435.

Friedman, M. I., & Stricker, E. M. (1976). The physiological psychology of hunger: A physiological perspective. *Psychological Review, 83,* 409–431.

Friedman, M. I., Tordoff, M. G., & Ramirez, I. (1986). Integrated metabolic control of food intake. *Brain Research Bulletin, 17,* 855–859.

Garcia, J., & Koelling, R. E. (1966). Relation of cue to consequence in avoidance learning. *Psychonomic Science, 4,* 123–124.

Grossman, S. P. (1986). The role of glucose, insulin and glucagon in the regulation of food intake and body weight. *Neuroscience & Biobehavioral Reviews, 10,* 295–315.

Houk, J. C. (1988). Control strategies in physiological systems. *FASEB Journal, 2,* 97–107.

Kennedy, G. C. (1950). The hypothalamic control of food intake in rats. *Proceedings of the Royal Society of London, 137B,* 535–548.

Lotter, E. C., & Woods, S. C. (1977). Injections of insulin and changes of body weight. *Physiology & Behavior, 17,* 575–580.

Louis-Sylvestre, J. (1976). Preabsorptive insulin release and hypoglycemia in rats. *American Journal of Physiology, 230,* 56–60.

Mackay, E. M., Callaway, J. W., & Barnes, R. F. (1940). Hyperalimentation in normal animals produced by protamine insulin. *Journal of Nutrition, 20,* 59–66.

Mayer, J. (1953). Glucostatic mechanisms of regulation of food intake. *New England Journal of Medicine, 249,* 13–16.

Mayer J. (1955). Regulation of energy intake and body weight: The theory and the lipostatic hypothesis. *Annals of the New York Academy of Sciences, 63,* 15–43.

Powley, T. L. (1977). The ventromedial hypothalamic syndrome, satiety, and a cephalic phase hypothesis. *Psychological Review, 84,* 89–126.

Rabe, E. F. (1975). Relationship between absolute body-fluid deficits and fluid intake in the rat. *Journal of Comparative and Physiological Psychology, 80,* 468–477.

Ramsay, D. S., & Woods, S. C. (1996). Biological consequences of a drug administration: Implications for acute and chronic tolerance. Manuscript submitted for publication.

Ritter, S., & Taylor, J. S. (1989). Capsaicin abolishes lipoprivic but not glucoprivic feeding in rats. *American Journal of Physiology, 256,* R1232–R1239.

Rozin, P. N., & Schulkin, J. (1991). Food selection. In E. M. Stricker (Ed.), *Handbook of behavioral neurobiology: Neurobiology of food and fluid intake* (pp. 297–328). New York: Plenum Press.

Schwartz, M. W., Figlewicz, D. P., Baskin, D. G., Woods, S. C., & Porte D., Jr. (1992). Insulin in the brain: A hormonal regulator of energy balance. *Endocrine Reviews, 13,* 387–414.

Siegel, S. (1989). Pharmacological conditioning of drug effects. In A. J. Goudie & M. W. Emmet-Oglesby (Eds.), *Psychoactive drugs: Tolerance and sensitization* pp. 115–180. Clifton NJ: Humana Press.

Siegel, S., Krank, M. D., & Hinson, R. E. (1987). Anticipation of pharmacological and nonpharmacological events: Classical conditioning and addictive behaviors. *Journal of Drug Issues, 17,* 83–110.

Smith, G. P., & Epstein, A. N. (1969). Increased feeding in response to decreased glucose utilization in the rat and monkey. *American Journal of Physiology, 265,* R1423–R1429.

Smith, G. P., & Gibbs, J. (1992). The development and proof of the CC hypothesis of satiety. In C. T. Dourish, S. J. Cooper, S. D. Iversen, & L. L. Iversen (Eds.), *Multiple cholecystokinin receptors in the CNS* (pp. 166–182). Oxford, England: Oxford University Press.

Solomon, R. L., & Wynne, L. (1953). Traumatic avoidance learning: Acquisition in normal dogs. *Psychological Monographs, 67,* (No. 4).

Somjen, G. G. (1992). The missing error signal: Regulation beyond negative feedback. *News in Physiological Sciences, 7,* 184–185.

Stallone, D. D., & Stunkard, A. J. (1991). The regulation of body weight: Evidence and clinical implications. *Annals of Behavioral Medicine, 13,* 220–230.

Steffens, A. B. (1976). Influence of the oral cavity on insulin release in the rat. *American Journal of Physiology, 230,* 1411–1415.

Stricker, E. M. (1991). Homeostatic origins of ingestive behavior. In E. M. Stricker (Ed.), *Handbook of behavioral neurobiology: Neurobiology of food and fluid intake (pp. 45–60).* New York: Plenum Press.

Stricker, E. M., & Wolf, G. (1969). Behavioral control of intravascular fluid volume: Thirst and sodium appetite. In P. J. Morgan (Ed.), *Neural regulation of food and water intake. Annals of the New York Academy of Sciences, 157,* 533–567.

Weingarten, H. P. (1990). Learning, homeostasis, and the control of feeding behavior. In E. D. Capaldi & T. L. Powley (Eds.), *Taste, experience, and feeding* (pp. 14–27). Washington, DC: American Psychological Association.

Wenger, J. R., Tiffany, T. M., Bombardier, C., Nicholls, K., & Woods, S. C. (1981). Ethanol tolerance in the rat is learned. *Science, 213,* 575–577.

Woods, S. C. (1976). Conditioned hypoglycemia. *Journal of Comparative and Physiological Psychology, 90,* 1164–1168.

Woods, S. C. (1977). Conditioned insulin secretion. In Y. Katsuk, M. Sato, S. I. Takagi, & Y. Oomura (Eds.), *Food intake and the chemical senses* (pp. 331–342). Tokyo: University of Tokyo Press.

Woods, S. C. (1991). The eating paradox: How we tolerate food. *Psychological Review, 98,* 488–505.

Woods, S. C. (1995). Insulin and the brain: A mutual dependency. *Progress in Psychobiology, 16,* 53–81.

Woods, S. C., Decke, E., & Vasselli, J. R. (1974). Metabolic hormones and regulation of body weight. *Psychological Review, 81,* 26–43.

Woods, S. C., & Kulkosky, P. J. (1976). Classically conditioned changes of blood glucose level. *Psychosomatic Medicine, 38,* 201–219.

Woods, S. C., & Strubbe, J. H. (1994). The psychobiology of meals. *Psychonomic Bulletin and Review, 1,* 144–155.

Woods, S. C., Vasselli, J. R., Kaestner, E., Szakmary, G. A., Milburn, P., & Vitiello, M. V., (1977). Conditioned insulin secretion and meal feeding in rats. *Journal of Comparative and Physiological Psychology, 91,* 128–133.

PART TWO

How Learning Affects Food Preferences

Taste Aversion Learning

Glenn E. Schafe and Ilene L. Bernstein

When animals or humans eat a particular food before receiving a drug or radiation treatment that induces gastrointestinal discomfort, they subsequently avoid that food (Bernstein, 1991; Garcia, Hankins, & Rusiniak, 1974). This response, termed a *learned taste aversion,* occurs because symptoms induced by the toxic treatment become associated with the food, producing a learned distaste for that food. Taste aversion learning is remarkably robust, with aversions frequently acquired after only one conditioning trial. The hallmark feature of taste aversion learning is the striking change that occurs in the response to a taste. Before conditioning, a palatable taste, such as a sweet drink, is preferred to water by rats and generates positive ingestive responses. After aversion conditioning, the same taste is avoided and elicits reactions of disgust and illness (Grill & Norgren, 1978; Meachum & Bernstein, 1990). An extensive research literature has been generated over the past 30 years directed at understanding this unusual type of learning. In this chapter we review this work with a particular focus on usual and unusual characteristics of learned taste aversions and the possible adaptive significance of this learning as a means of avoiding toxins and selecting a nutritious diet. We also briefly review the neural pathways implicated in learned taste aversions and the potential clinical relevance of this learning.

THEORETICAL ISSUES

Classical Conditioning Model

Primarily as the result of procedural similarities, taste aversion learning has traditionally been considered a variant of classical, or Pavlovian, condition-

Preparation of this chapter supported in part by NIH Grant DC00248.

ing. In the laboratory, learned taste aversions are commonly established by the presentation of a novel taste solution (the conditioned stimulus; CS) followed by administration of a drug (the unconditioned stimulus; US) that produces transient gastrointestinal illness or vomiting (the unconditioned response; UR) (Garcia, Ervin, & Koelling, 1966; Garcia & Koelling, 1966; Garcia et al., 1974). In addition to a group exposed to the pairing of key stimuli, traditional Pavlovian control groups establish the associative nature of the subsequent *avoidance* of the CS (the conditioned response; CR). These control groups receive the taste stimulus (CS) alone, the drug (US) alone, or CS–US exposure in an unpaired fashion. The following three principles are among those that taste aversion shares with traditional Pavlovian conditioning.

Generalization

In the Pavlovian literature, *generalization* is defined as the elicitation of a conditioned response to stimuli that are similar but not identical to the initial training CS. This principle of generalization holds true for taste aversion learning as well. A learned aversion to a particular CS taste generalizes to a second CS to a degree that is proportional to the similarity between the two tastes. The generalization gradients of taste aversions, furthermore, are comparable to traditional classically conditioned responses (Garcia et al., 1974; Riley & Clarke, 1977). The tendency for learned aversions to generalize to tastes on the basis of perceptual similarity has provided a useful methodology for assessing taste perception in rats and hamsters (Nowlis, Frank, & Pfaffman, 1980; Tapper & Halpern, 1968). Learned taste aversions provide a convenient methodology for assessing taste perception in animals.

Extinction

Extinction refers to the weakening of a previously established conditioned response owing to repeated, nonreinforced exposures to the conditioned stimulus. Learned taste aversions have traditionally been considered exceedingly resistant to extinction. Although it is not unusual to find anecdotal reports of conditioned aversions in humans that have persisted for decades (e.g., Garb & Stunkard, 1974), this unusual "resistance to extinction" may stem from procedural features of the paradigm rather than the inherent strength of the learned response. Unlike most classical conditioning protocols, in which exposure to the CS is not under the control of the experimental subject, the conditioned response in a taste aversion experiment is, by definition, avoidance of the taste CS. By avoiding contact with the taste CS, the subject manages to avoid repeated nonreinforced exposure to it, and therefore there is little opportunity for extinction. Experimentally, the extinction of learned taste aversions may be hastened by forced exposure to the taste CS, either by making it the only solution available or by direct infusion into the oral cavity. Under these conditions, extinction occurs at a rate that is comparable to that of other classical conditioning paradigms (Spector, Smith, & Hollander, 1981, 1983).

Latent Inhibition

An important predictor of the ease of conditioning using Pavlovian procedures is the novelty of the conditioned stimulus. Prior exposure to the CS attenuates subsequent conditioning, a phenomenon known as *latent inhibition*. This principle of CS novelty appears to be particularly important in the establishment of learned taste aversions. It is well documented in the taste aversion literature that learning occurs rapidly when the target flavor is novel, whereas aversions to more familiar flavors are less readily established (Kalat & Rozin, 1973; Revusky & Bedarf, 1967).

Unusual Features of Taste Aversion Learning

Although taste aversion learning shares a number of fundamental features with traditional Pavlovian learning, it is unusual in several important respects, including rapid acquisition, tolerance of long delays between presentation of CS and US, and a property known as *selective associability.*

Single-Trial Learning

In traditional Pavlovian paradigms, conditioned responding typically develops gradually over the course of many CS–US pairings. The conditioned nictitating membrane response, for example, may require as many as a thousand CS–US pairings. Robust and long-lasting aversions to novel tastes, however, are commonly established after a single taste–illness pairing (Garcia et al., 1974; Riley & Clarke, 1977). Although one-trial learning is not unique in the learning literature, in the framework of classical conditioning it is quite unusual.

Long-Delay Learning

An even more unusual feature of taste aversion learning, which has set it apart from all other classical conditioning paradigms, is successful learning despite long CS–US intervals. Traditional Pavlovian conditioning appears to rely heavily on the principle of contiguity, or the temporal pairing of two stimuli. Typically, CS–US intervals on the order of 1 or 2 seconds produce optimal learning, and delays of only a few seconds significantly retard acquisition of conditioned responses (Mackintosh, 1974). In contrast, in a typical taste aversion learning experiment, a CS–US interval of a half-hour or more is common, and several authors have reported successful conditioning with delays as long as 4–12 hours (Garcia et al., 1974; Smith & Roll, 1967).

Although many publications attest to the fact that taste aversions can be acquired after lengthy CS–US intervals, there has been little attention paid to whether extremely brief intervals can support this type of learning. This omission stems from the nature of typical taste aversion paradigms, in which CS exposure occurs during a drinking period that is rarely less than 10 minutes and is followed by intraperitoneal injection of the US drug. With such a design, the shortest possible interval between initial exposure to the CS taste and onset of drug symptoms would be about 15 minutes. Genuinely brief intervals, of the type more typical of other learning paradigms (e.g., 2–10 sec), have not previously been explored. This issue was recently addressed in our laboratory through strict control of the timing of CS delivery into the oral cavity and US delivery into the circulation using chronically indwelling intraoral cannulas and jugular catheters. We wanted to determine whether very brief CS–US intervals could support single-trial taste aversion learning and how the strength of conditioning would compare to that found with delay intervals more typical of taste aversion studies. We found that a very brief CS–US interval (10 sec), closer to that which supports "optimal" acquisition in other Pavlovian learning paradigms, failed to support acquisition of a taste aversion (Schafe, Sollars, & Bernstein, 1995). These surprising findings further underscore the unusual temporal parameters of taste aversion learning. They suggest that close temporal contiguity between exposure to the CS taste and the US drug is neither *necessary nor sufficient* for taste aversion acquisition.

34

Selective Associability

An initially surprising feature of taste aversion learning was the fact that its acquisition is dependent on the pairing of a specific cue (i.e., a taste) with a specific consequence (i.e., nausea). Garcia's early experimental work (Garcia & Koelling, 1966) provided an excellent example of this principle and is worth describing in some detail. Rats were given access to a flavored solution in drinking tubes that were wired such that when the rats drank, their licks would produce an audiovisual stimulus (a light and a click). Following ingestion of the "bright-noisy-sweet water" CS, half of the animals received a lithium chloride (LiCl) US, a drug that produces transient gastro-intestinal illness, and half received electric footshock, a US commonly used in Pavlovian experiments. Following recovery, animals were given access to either the flavored solution alone, without any audiovisual cues, or the audiovisual stimulus alone, without any taste. Results indicated that both groups suppressed their intake of the target solution, but the conditions under which suppression was noted depended on the US. Animals that received LiCl suppressed their consumption *only* when the CS solution was a taste, whereas animals that received footshock suppressed *only* when the CS solution was accompanied by audiovisual stimuli. This finding indicates that taste is more readily associated with gastrointestinal illness, whereas auditory and visual cues are more readily associated with pain. These results stood in sharp contrast to the traditional learning theories of the time, which tended to assume that the choice of CS modality was of relatively minor importance in determining associative consequences.

An Evolutionary Perspective

Although Garcia's initial reports of taste aversion learning proved difficult to reconcile with traditional models of associative learning, they were far less surprising when reconsidered in light of their adaptive context. As an omnivore, the rat in its natural environment is an opportunistic forager, taking advantage of nutrient sources as they become available. This strategy necessitates a willingness to try new food sources, some of which may be toxic. Fortunately, many toxins are readily identifiable by a bitter taste, and rats and members of other omnivorous species unconditionally avoid such foods. In many cases, however, a potential toxin is not identifiable by a distinctive taste quality, and other strategies have evolved to cope with this problem. Rats, for example, are notoriously neophobic when encountering new food sources, sampling only small quantities on first exposure (Rozin & Kalat, 1971). If the consequences of ingestion are not aversive and, especially in the case of calorically dense foods, if they are positive (Mehiel & Bolles, 1988a, 1988b), the animal will subsequently increase its intake substantially. If, on the other hand, the food is toxic, cautious sampling may lead to transient illness rather than death, and the animal will subsequently avoid that food. In the rat and other omnivorous species, therefore, both associative and nonassociative mechanisms have evolved that function in concert to guide appetitive behavior.

Within this adaptive context, the unusual features of taste aversion learning, such as one-trial acquisition, tolerance of long interstimulus intervals, and selective associability, become easy to understand. Rapid acquisition, for example, is essential for this associative mechanism to be an effective survival strategy. If it required many conditioning trials with a potentially deadly toxin to learn to avoid consuming the poison, an animal would be dead long before it had an opportunity to take advantage of its learning. Similarly, the associative mechanism underlying taste aversion acquisition must be able to tolerate long interstimulus intervals, because the physiological consequences of ingestion are frequently delayed. The fact that a form of learning has evolved that differs so markedly in its temporal parameters from nearly every other form of associative learning could be viewed as striking evidence of the strong adaptive pressure of toxin avoidance.

Garcia, Lasiter, and Bermudez-Rattoni (1985) have cast the unusual features of taste aversion learning into a more general theory of defensive learning. In their model, they make a distinction between what is called the "gut-defense" system, which has evolved under the selection pressures of plants and animals that employ toxins to fend off foragers and predators, and the "skin-defense" system, which has evolved under the natural selective pressures of predation. In the former system, taste is most readily associated with gastrointestinal illness, whereas in the latter system, exteroceptive stimuli (e.g., lights, sounds) are most readily associated with peripheral injury (e.g., electric footshock). Natural selection appears to have "prepared" organisms with their own associative predisposition. It is interesting that the sensory modalities that associate most readily with illness appear to be species-specific. In the quail, for example, visual rather than gustatory cues are particularly important in food selection. Wilcoxin, Dragoin, & Kral (1971) found that quail that consumed blue (visual), sour (taste) water before being made ill subsequently avoided blue water but not sour water.

Selective pressure to develop the ability to learn to avoid ingesting toxic substances has apparently affected a broad range of species, from the garden slug *Limax* (Sahley, Gelperin, & Rudy, 1981) to primates, including humans (Bernstein, 1978; Garb & Stunkard, 1974). That relatively simple invertebrates are able to acquire taste aversions implies that relatively primitive neural networks can mediate this learning.

Stimuli and Responses in Taste Averson Learning

One of the major difficulties in taste aversion research has been to precisely define the characteristics of the effective unconditioned and conditioned stimuli. This section reviews these difficulties and addresses the issue of whether taste aversion learning, like other Pavlovian paradigms, is characterized by the development of a conditioned response.

Unconditioned Stimulus

Diverse nature of US drugs   There has been considerable controversy in the conditioned taste aversion literature concerning the characteristics of effective unconditioned stimuli. The early studies of Garcia and his colleagues (Garcia et al., 1966; Garcia & Koelling, 1966) typically employed treatments that were known to produce gastrointestinal distress and vomiting in humans (ionizing radiation, apomorphine, and lithium chloride). At that time it was suspected that the primary aversive event, toxicity or nausea, was a necessary condition for the learning to occur. It soon became apparent, however, that neither toxicity nor gastrointestinal distress was necessary for taste aversion learning to occur. One surprising finding was that agents such as amphetamine and its derivatives, which are chemically dissimilar to emetics and produce qualitatively different behavioral responses, were capable of supporting taste aversion learning (see Gamzu, Vincent, & Boff, 1985, for a review). Paradoxically, drugs of abuse such as morphine and ethanol were also found to be capable of establishing learned taste aversions at the same doses that are typically operantly self-administered. This is true even when experimental conditions are such that the drugs are administered in the same manner and at the same dose in both paradigms (Hunt & Amit, 1987).

A special role for nausea? The diverse nature of pharmacological agents that are effective in supporting taste aversion learning appears to indicate that there is no one specific characteristic that they have in common. Garcia (1989), however, has argued that nausea plays a special role in taste aversion acquisition, and there is some compelling evidence in the literature to support this idea. After conditioning with emetic agents such as lithium chloride (LiCl) or apomorphine, for example, both rats and humans display a qualitatively different behavioral response to the CS taste. Unlike those conditioned with nonemetic agents such as amphetamine (Parker, Hills, & Jensen, 1984; Zalaquett & Parker, 1989) or lactose (Pelchat Grill, Rozin, & Jacobs 1983), taste aversions that have been established with emetic agents are accompanied by facial or oromotor reactions indicative of distaste and disgust, a phenomenon known as a "hedonic shift." Data from humans demonstrate this point well. Pelchat and Rozin (1982) surveyed human participants who suffered from food allergies. When their allergic symptoms included nausea, they reported not only avoiding the food but also disliking the taste. In contrast, when the allergic response included symptoms such as mouth sores or hives, participants avoided the food but reported no change in the food's hedonic rating. In other words, these persons avoided eating the food because it caused unpleasant symptoms, not because they found it distasteful. Thus, Pelchat and Rozin argued that nausea not only is sufficient for the establishment of a taste aversion but also is necessary for the development of hedonic shifts or distaste toward foods. Garcia has argued that it is this shift in the hedonic or incentive value of a taste that, by definition, constitutes a genuine learned taste aversion.

Conditioned Stimulus

Taste has occupied a prominent position in the taste aversion literature, primarily because other potential sensory stimuli, such as olfactory cues, have generally proved less effective in the establishment of conditioned aversions after association with toxic drug treatments. Palmerino, Rusiniak, and Garcia (1980), for example, exposed rats to either a saccharin-flavored solution or an almond odor (presented on filter-paper disks on the spout of a water bottle) before injection with LiCl. Following conditioning, robust aversions were displayed to the taste, whereas little-to-no avoidance of the odor was noted. Because odors are such an important part of the flavor characteristics of foods and fluids, it is somewhat surprising that they seem to support such weak aversion conditioning.

Under certain conditions, olfactory cues can become effective in aversion conditioning. Palmerino, Rusiniak, and Garcia (1980), for example, have shown that whereas an odor alone is typically ineffective at establishing a learned aversion, an odor that has been presented in combination with a *taste* is highly effective. Rusiniak, Hankins, Garcia, and Brett (1979), for example, paired either a saccharin flavor alone, an almond odor alone, or a saccharin–almond compound with LiCl administration. Following conditioning, both the taste and the odor were presented separately in a series of one-bottle intake tests. Results showed the strongest evidence of conditioning to the odor that was presented with a taste during conditioning.

This phenomenon, commonly referred to as *taste–odor potentiation*, is somewhat unexpected from the viewpoint of traditional learning theory. Typically, when two stimuli are presented in combination, the more powerful or salient stimulus of the compound tends to acquire most of the associative strength, a phenomenon known as *overshadowing*. Taste–odor potentiation represents a completely opposite effect, in which the weaker odor stimulus becomes quite salient when presented with a taste but not when presented on its own.

Garcia and colleagues (1985) have placed this phenomenon in an adaptive context by noting that in many mammalian species olfactory stimuli are of potential importance to both the skin-defense system (signaling, for example, a nearby predator) and the gut-defense system (signaling the characteristics of a food source). The presence of a taste, along with an odor, signals the importance of the odor to gut-defense and is said to "gate" the odor cue into the gut-defense system, making it readily accessible for association with toxicosis. Of course, reliance on odor cues has the advantage of permitting an animal to avoid completely ingestion of a toxic substance, whereas reliance on taste cues alone requires at least some sampling.

Conditioned Response

The nature of the conditioned response in the taste aversion paradigm has been subjected to numerous interpretations. Operationally, it has been considered to be the avoidance of the CS taste following conditioning, a "response" that is theoretically linked, yet certainly bears little resemblance, to the unconditioned effects of the US drug.

Relatively little attention has been paid to the question of whether exposure to the taste CS provokes other types of responses, particularly responses that are similar to those elicited by the US drug. As we have already indicated, in most testing situations, whether one-bottle or two-bottle, complete avoidance of the aversive taste CS is possible. This is contrasted with standard classical conditioning paradigms in which exposure to CSs such as tones and lights do not depend on a response by the subject but, instead, are presented on a schedule determined by the experimenter. What would happen if exposure to an aversive taste CS could not be avoided? Meachum and Bernstein (1990) examined this question by employing involuntary, intraoral delivery of a taste CS followed by careful behavioral observations. Although the rat is a nonemetic species and hence unable to vomit, a characteristic behavioral response to the administration of the emetic agent LiCl has been reported (Parker et al., 1984). The animal becomes lethargic and adopts a prostrate, often asymmetrical posture. This response, called "lying-on-belly" (LOB), is easily distinguished from other reductions in motor activity such as freezing and may represent a behavioral index of malaise. It is interesting that this same response was seen by Meachum and Bernstein (1990) in animals reexposed to a taste that had previously been paired with LiCl.

The fact that responses such as LOB are seen both in response to treatment with LiCl and following involuntary reexposure to a CS taste paired with LiCl suggests that emetic mechanisms that underlie the response to the US drug are reinstated following CS reexposure. When viewed in this manner, taste aversion learning appears more compatible with traditional Pavlovian paradigms. Treatment with an emetic drug (the US), for example, leads to physiological and behavioral indices of malaise (the UR). Following reexposure to a taste (the CS) that has previously been paired with an emetic drug, a similar behavioral response, perhaps indicative of "conditioned illness," occurs (the CR). The data of Meachum and Bernstein are consistent with an earlier report by Gustafson, Garcia, Hankins, and Rusiniak (1974), who found that the coyote, which, unlike the rat, vomits in response to LiCl treatment, displayed a classically conditioned response of retching on reexposure to a CS taste. The data also provided an interesting parallel to the evidence that nausea can be classically conditioned in humans (Carey & Burish, 1988; Morrow & Morrell, 1982; Nesse, Carli, Curtis, & Kleinman, 1980). In addition to the usual adverse side effects of chemotherapy, for example, many cancer patients experience symptoms of nausea and vomiting in *anticipation* of pharmacological treatment. These symptoms, known as "pretreatment nausea and vomiting," have been shown to be triggered by stimuli previously associated with chemotherapeutic treatment. For example, one recent study indicated that exposure to a beverage that was previously paired with chemotherapy could trigger symptoms of nausea (Bovbjerg et al., 1992).

Whether or not a "conditioned illness" reaction of this type is responsible for taste "avoidance" has been the subject of some debate (e.g., see Coil, Hankins, Jenden, & Garcia, 1978; Goudie, 1979; Grant, 1987). The conclusion of many of these discussions is that the induction of illness is most likely *not* a necessary condition for the expression of a learned taste aversion, especially if the animal has the option to completely avoid consumption of the CS taste.

NEURAL SUBSTRATES

A number of considerations suggest that taste aversion learning is a relatively primitive type of learning that could be mediated by simple neural circuits. Brain stem and pontine nuclei, such as the nucleus of the solitary tract (NST) and the pontine parabrachial nucleus (PBN), are sites of convergence of taste and visceral information that might be sufficient for the establishment of these associations (Garcia et al., 1974; Hermann & Rogers, 1985). There is also the rather startling observation that taste aversion associations are not blocked by general anesthesia. Several laboratories have reported that rats acquire taste aversions even when they are completely anesthetized during and after the administration of the US (Bermudez-Rattoni, Forthman, Sanchez, Perez, & Garcia, 1988; Roll & Smith, 1972). It appears, however, that rats do need to be conscious at the time of CS presentation; because exposure to saccharin while animals are under general anesthesia does not result in the acquisition of a taste aversion. These results imply that higher order neural functions may be involved in taste processing but that illness processing and integration may be accomplished when neural activity is severely compromised by anesthetic drugs. Taken together, these observations have directed considerable experimental attention to the hindbrain.

As the first gustatory and visceral relay of the caudal brain stem, the NST occupies a strategic position for potential convergence and integration of taste and visceral information. However, the importance of the NST in taste aversion learning has been difficult to evaluate because its role in cardiovascular and other vital functions makes lesion studies problematic. Animals with lesions restricted to the rostral (or gustatory) portion of the NST are able to acquire taste aversions (Flynn, Grill, Schulkin, & Norgren, 1991); however, electrophysiological and molecular marker techniques indicate that neurons within NST alter their response properties following acquisition of a taste aversion (Chang & Scott, 1984; Houpt, Philopena, Wessel, Joh, & Smith, 1994; Swank & Bernstein, 1994; Swank, Schafe, & Bernstein, 1995).

The parabrachial nucleus serves as the second gustatory and visceral relay of the caudal brain stem, receiving a dense projection from the NST (Norgren & Leonard, 1971) as well as reciprocal innervation from forebrain regions involved in both gustatory and autonomic functioning (Norgren, 1985). Unlike that of the NST, the role of the PBN has been well documented, and evidence indicates that it plays a critical role in taste aversion acquisition. PBN lesions render animals incapable of acquiring taste aversions, and this deficit appears to be due to a selective disruption of a mechanism responsible for taste–illness associations (Reilly, Grigson, & Norgren, 1993; Spector, Norgren, & Grill, 1992). It is interesting that, with the exception of the PBN, no other brain region has been demonstrated unambiguously to be *necessary* for taste aversion acquisition.

Despite the fact that circuitry intrinsic to the brain stem might appear to be sufficient for the establishment of taste–illness associations, work with chronic decerebrate rats suggests otherwise (Grill & Norgren, 1978). These rats have been reported to be unable to acquire taste aversions despite multiple conditioning trials. This failure appears to be due not to an inability to detect and respond to the taste or the illness-inducing agent, but rather to a deficit in associative ability.

The failure of the chronic decerebrate rat either to acquire or to express taste aversions indicates that forebrain involvement is necessary for the formation of taste–illness associations. Much of the work in this area has concentrated on lesioning structures within central gustatory pathways, as well as other regions, such as the hippocampus and basolateral amygdala, that are known to be important for other types of learning. Unlike lesions of the pontine PBN, which completely eliminate evidence of taste aversion learning, lesions in forebrain structures have less clear-cut effects. Lesions to structures like the hippocampus and lateral hypothalamus are without effect on taste aversion learning. Lesions to the basolateral nucleus of the amygdala and insular (gustatory) neocortex appear to attenuate but not eliminate taste aversion learning (Chambers, 1990; Kiefer & Orr, 1992; Simbayi, Boakes, & Burton, 1986; Yamamoto & Fujimoto, 1991). Although the decerebrate-rat experiments point to forebrain input as critical to taste aversion learning, the nature and source of that input remain unclear.

CLINICAL IMPLICATIONS

Occurrence in Humans

Although taste aversion learning may be a relatively primitive form of learning, there is extensive evidence that humans acquire these aversions readily and that aversion conditioning in humans shares many features with this conditioning in lower organisms. Garb and Stunkard (1974) surveyed nearly 700 persons, Logue and her colleagues (Logue, Ophir, & Strauss, 1981) over 500 college students, and Midkiff and Bernstein (1985) over 1,000 college students. The surveys generally agreed that about half of the respondents reported having experienced a learned food aversion after ingestion of a specific food was followed by gastrointestinal upset. Acquisition generally occurred in a single trial, often with delays of minutes or hours interposed between tasting the food and becoming ill. Aversions were more likely to develop to less familiar and less preferred foods.

College students in these surveys often report a prevalence of aversions to specific alcoholic beverages, which likely stems from the fact that students frequently begin to consume (and overconsume) alcohol in their college years. These aversions represent a situation in which the symptoms of nausea and vomiting were actually caused by the ingestant. To what extent this kind of avoidance learning plays a role in learning to moderate one's drinking patterns is an interesting question that has not been directly addressed.

Food Aversions and Illness

The powerful and robust nature of food aversion conditioning suggests that there may be clinical situations in which this kind of learning significantly affects food acceptability and nutrient intake. Under most circumstances, the development of aversions to one or even a number of foods would not appear to jeopardize a person's nutritional status, because humans normally have a range of food options and can respond to the development of food aversions by selecting nonaversive alternatives. However, Bernstein and Borson (1986) noted conditions in which the food intake of physically and emotionally ill patients could be affected by food aversion learning. In some disorders, ingestion of food produces discomfort, which may act as a US for the development of food aversions. In others, chronic malaise may become associated with eating simply because the malaise is so pervasive. Because food aversions develop rapidly and are subject to generalization, long-lasting symptoms could provide a foundation for aversions to a broad range of foods. Individuals with finicky appetites or narrow preference ranges before the development of illness could be particularly vulnerable to these problems. Such people may not be willing or able to make alternative, nonaversive food choices and, instead, may progressively reduce their food intake. Patients who might be most vulnerable include children, whose menus are typically limited and who tend to avoid new flavors (Birch & Marlin, 1982); older adults, whose diet choices may be narrow owing to mechanical problems with eating or altered taste sensitivity; and patients whose diet is limited to foods of a single ethnic group.

In this way, learned food aversions could play an etiologic role in clinical instances of appetite and weight loss. Symptoms cited by patients as reasons for their diminished food intake reveal commonalities among a variety of anorexia syndromes. Patients with cancer and those with depression with clinically significant weight loss frequently report that foods have altered in their taste quality and that they no longer taste good. Early satiety or bloating is reported by patients with anorexia nervosa as well as those with cancer and depressive illness. Although direct evidence linking food aversion learning with anorexia nervosa and depression is lacking, clear evidence is available implicating food aversions in the syndrome of cancer anorexia. The appetite and weight loss widely experienced by cancer patients has a wide range of causes, some of which stem directly from the disease and some of which are clearly side effects of cancer treatment.

Several lines of evidence have pointed to food aversion learning as a factor in cancer anorexia. Early reports noted the similarity between cancer treatments, such as emetic chemotherapy and radiation, and the USs in typical taste aversion studies (Bernstein, 1978; Bernstein & Webster, 1980). Controlled experiments demonstrated that learned food aversions develop in pediatric and adult cancer patients receiving gastrointestinally toxic (emetic) chemotherapy and that these aversions tend to be directed at specific foods consumed before treatments. Methods were assessed for preventing the development of food aversions in association with cancer treatments. Candy (coconut or rootbeer Lifesavers) was used as a scapegoat or interference stimulus. When taken between the consumption of a meal and the adminis-tration of chemotherapy, the candy was found to have a significant protective effect; children were twice as likely to eat some portion of their test meal at the time of assessment if they had received the scapegoat at conditioning (Broberg & Bernstein, 1987). Thus, exposure to a strongly flavored candy before chemotherapy appears to be a simple and effective way to reduce the impact of chemotherapy on preference for normal menu items.

A far broader extension of this work has been the discovery that food aversions are involved in the anorexia that stems from the disease itself. Rats with experimental tumors were found to develop a profound distaste for the specific, novel diet they were eating while the tumor was growing (Bernstein & Sigmundi, 1980; Bernstein, Treneer, Goehler, & Murowchick, 1985). They apparently associated the taste of their diet with tumor-induced malaise, and this aversion contributed to their reduced appetite. When a new food was introduced, they showed a dramatic, but temporary, reversal of their anorexia. Evidence that food aversion learning plays a role in tumor anorexia in animals is strong. The extent to which such aversions arise in patients with cancer and contribute to their appetite and weight loss remains to be determined.

CONCLUSION

Research on taste aversion learning began with an almost serendipitous observation in an animal laboratory (Garcia & Koelling, 1966). The intense interest and controversy this discovery generated led to an enormous research literature (Riley & Clarke, 1977) and a behavioral paradigm that is extremely well characterized. Despite extensive research interest in taste aversion learning, the paradigm has not been adopted widely as a model for studying neural mechanisms of learning, although we believe that a number of features of taste aversion learning recommend it as such a model. Learned taste aversions are simple, potent, and readily acquired, suggesting that the neural substrates are likely to be detectable with appropriate methodologies.

At a more practical level, relatively little is known about the extent to which taste aversion learning plays a role in human food intake and food choice, either in healthy individuals or those suffering chronic illness. Obstacles to this research include the difficulty of accurately assessing food intake in healthy humans, as well as in those who are ill.

REFERENCES

Bermudez-Rattoni, F., Forthman, D. L., Sanchez, M. A., Perez, J. L., & Garcia, J. (1988). Odor and taste aversions conditioned in anesthetized rats. *Behavioral Neuroscience, 102*, 726–732.

Bernstein, I. L. (1978). Learned taste aversions in children receiving chemotherapy. *Science, 200*, 1302–1303.

Bernstein, I. L. (1991). Flavor aversion. In T. V. Getchell, R. L. Doty, L. M. Bartoshuk, & J. B. Snow (Eds.), *Smell and taste in health and disease* (pp. 417–428). New York: Raven Press.

Bernstein, I. L., & Borson, S. (1986). Learned food aversion: A component of anorexia syndromes. *Psychological Review, 93*, 462–472.

Bernstein, I. L., & Sigmundi, R. A. (1980). Tumor anorexia: A learned food aversion? *Science, 209*, 416–418.

Bernstein, I. L., Treneer, C. M., Goehler, L. E., & Murowchick, E. (1985). Tumor growth in rats: Conditioned suppression of food intake and preference. *Behavioral Neuroscience, 88*, 818–830.

Bernstein, I. L., & Webster, M. M. (1980). Learned taste aversions in humans. *Physiology and Behavior, 25,* 363–366.

Birch, L. L. & Marlin, D. W. (1982). I don't like it; I never tried it: Effects of exposure on two-year old children's food preferences. *Appetite 3,* 353–360.

Bovbjerg, D. H., Redd, W. H., Jacobsen, P. B., Manne, S. L., Taylor, K. L., Surbone, A., Crown, J. P., Norton, L., Gilewski, T. A., Hudis, C. A., Reichman, B. S., Kaufman, R. J., Currie, V. E., & Hakes, T. B. (1992). An experimental analysis of classically conditioned nausea during cancer chemotherapy. *Psychosomatic Medicine, 54,* 623–637.

Broberg, D. J., & Bernstein, I. L. (1987). Candy as a scapegoat in the prevention of food aversions in children receiving chemotherapy. *Cancer, 60,* 2344–2347.

Carey, M. P., & Burish, T. G. (1988). Etiology and treatment of the psychological side effects associated with cancer chemotherapy: A critical review and discussion. *Psychological Bulletin, 104,* 307–325.

Chambers, K. C. (1990). A neural model for conditioned taste aversions. *Annual Review of Neuroscience, 13,* 373–385.

Chang, F. T., & Scott, T. R. (1984). Conditioned taste aversions modify neural responses in the rat nucleus tractus solitarius. *Journal of Neuroscience, 4,* 1850–1862.

Coil, J. D., Hankins, W. G., Jenden, D. J., & Garcia, J. (1978). The attenuation of a specific cue-to-consequence association by antiemetic agents. *Psychopharmacology, 56,* 21–25.

Flynn, F. W., Grill, H. J., Schulkin, J., & Norgren, R. (1991). Central gustatory lesions: II. Effects on sodium appetite, taste aversion learning and feeding behaviors. *Behavioral Neuroscience, 105,* 944–954.

Gamzu, E., Vincent, G., & Boff, E. (1985). A pharmacological perspective of drugs used in establishing conditioned food aversions. *Annals of the New York Academy of Sciences, 443,* 231–249.

Garb, J. L., & Stunkard, A. J. (1974). Taste aversions in man. *American Journal of Psychiatry, 131,* 1204–1207.

Garcia, J. (1989). Food for Tolman: Cognition and cathexis in concert. In T. Archer & L. G. Nelson (Eds.), *Aversion, Avoidance, and Anxiety,* (pp. 45–85). Hillsdale, NJ: Erlbaum.

Garcia, J., Ervin, R. R., & Koelling, R. A. (1966). Learning with prolonged delay of reinforcement. *Psychonomic Science, 5,* 121–122.

Garcia, J., Hankins, W. G., & Rusiniak, K. W. (1974). Behavioral regulation of the *milieu interne* in man and rat. *Science, 185*, 824–831.

Garcia, J., & Koelling, R. A. (1966). Relation of cue to consequence in avoidance learning. *Psychonomic Science, 4*, 123–124.

Garcia, J., Lasiter, P. S., & Bermudez-Rattoni, F. (1985). A general theory of aversion learning. *Annals of the New York Academy of Sciences, 443*, 8–21.

Goudie, A. J. (1979). Aversive stimulus properties of drugs. *Neuropharmacology, 18*, 971–979.

Grant, V. L. (1987). Do conditioned taste aversions result from activation of emetic mechanisms? *Psychopharmacology, 93*, 405–415.

Grill, H. J., & Norgren, R. (1978). Chronically decerebrate rats demonstrate satiation but not bait shyness. *Science, 201*, 267–269.

Gustafson, C. R., Garcia, J., Hankins, W. G., & Rusiniak, K. W. (1974). Coyote predation control by aversive conditioning. *Science, 184*, 581–583.

Hermann, G. E., & Rogers, R. C. (1985). Convergence of vagal and gustatory afferent input within the parabrachial nucleus of the rat. *Journal of the Autonomic Nervous System, 13*, 1–17.

Houpt, T. A., Philopena, J. M., Wessel, T. C., Joh, T. H., & Smith, G. P. (1994). Increased c-fos expression in nucleus of the solitary tract correlated with conditioned taste aversion to sucrose in rats. *Neuroscience Letters, 172*, 1–5.

Hunt, T., & Amit, Z. (1987). Conditioned taste aversion induced by self-administered drugs: Paradox revisited. *Neuroscience & Biobehavioral Reviews, 11*, 107–130.

Kalat, J. W., & Rozin, P. (1973). "Learned safety" as a mechanism in long-delay taste aversion learning in rats. *Journal of Comparative and Physiological Psychology, 83*, 198–207.

Kiefer, S. W., & Orr, M. R. (1992). Taste avoidance, but not aversion, learning in rats lacking gustatory cortex. *Behavioral Neuroscience, 106*, 140–146.

Logue, A. W., Ophir, I., & Strauss, K. E. (1981). The acquisition of taste aversions in humans. *Behavioral Research and Therapy, 19*, 319–333.

Mackintosh, N. J. (1974). *The psychology of animal learning.* New York: Academic.

Meachum, C. L., & Bernstein, I. L. (1990). Conditioned responses to a taste conditioned stimulus paired with lithium chloride administration. *Behavioral Neuroscience, 104*, 711–715.

Mehiel, R., & Bolles, R. C. (1988a). Hedonic shift learning based on calories. *Bulletin of the Psychonomic Society, 26*, 459–462.

Mehiel, R., & Bolles, R. C. (1988b). Learned flavor preferences based on calories are independent of initial hedonic value. *Animal Learning & Behavior, 16,* 383–387.

Midkiff, E. E., & Bernstein, I. L. (1985). Targets of learned food aversions in humans. *Physiology and Behavior, 34,* 839–841.

Morrow, G. R., & Morrell, B. S. (1982). Behavioral treatment for the anticipatory vomiting induced by cancer chemotherapy. *New England Journal of Medicine, 307,* 1476–1480.

Nesse, R., Carli, T., Curtis, G. C., & Kleinman, P. D. (1980). Pretreatment nausea in cancer chemotherapy: A conditioned response? *Psychosomatic Medicine, 42,* 33–36.

Norgren, R. (1985). Taste and the autonomic nervous system. *Chemical Senses, 10,* 143–161.

Norgren, R., & Leonard, C. M. (1971). Taste pathways in rat brainstem. *Science, 173,* 1136–1139.

Nowlis, G. H., Frank, M. E., & Pfaffman, C. (1980). Specificity of acquired aversions to taste qualities in hamsters and rats. *Journal of Comparative and Physiological Psychology 94,* 932–942.

Palmerino, C. C., Rusiniak, K. W., & Garcia, J. (1980). Flavor illness aversions: The peculiar role of odor and taste in memory for poison. *Science, 208,* 753–755.

Parker, L. A., Hills, K., & Jensen, K. (1984). Behavioral CRs elicited by a lithium- or an amphetamine-paired contextual test chamber. *Learning and Motivation, 12,* 307–315.

Parker, L. A., & MacLeod, K. B. (1991). Chin rub CRs may reflect conditioned sickness elicited by a lithium-paired sucrose solution. *Pharmacology, Biochemistry and Behavior, 40,* 983–986.

Pelchat, M., Grill, H. J., Rozin, P., & Jacobs, J. (1983). Quality of acquired responses to tastes by rattus norvegicus depends upon type of associated discomfort. *Journal of Comparative and Physiological Psychology, 97,* 140–153.

Pelchat, M. L., & Rozin, P. (1982). The special role of nausea in the acquisition of food dislikes by humans. *Appetite, 3,* 341–351.

Reilly, S., Grigson, P. S., & Norgren, R. (1993). Parabrachial nucleus lesions and conditioned taste aversion: Evidence supporting an associative deficit. *Behavioral Neuroscience, 107,* 1005–1017.

Revusky, S. H., & Bedarf, E. W. (1967). Association of illness with prior ingestion of novel foods. *Science, 155,* 219–220.

Riley, A. L., & Clarke, C. M. (1977). Conditioned taste aversions: A bibliography.

In L. M. Barker, M. R. Best, & M. Domjan, (Eds.), *Learning mechanisms in food selection*. Waco, TX: Baylor University Press.

Roll, D. L., & Smith, J. C. (1972). Conditioned taste aversion in anesthetized rats. In M. E. P. Seligman & J. L. Hager (Eds.), *Biological boundaries of learning* (pp. 98–102). New York: Appleton-Century-Crofts.

Rozin, P., & Kalat, J. W. (1971). Specific hungers and poison avoidance as adaptive specializations of learning. *Psychological Review, 78*, 459–486.

Rusiniak, K. W., Hankins, W. G., Garcia, J., & Brett, L. P. (1979). Flavor illness aversions: Potentiation of odor by taste in rats. *Behavioral & Neural Biology, 25*, 1–17.

Sahley, C. L., Gelperin, A., & Rudy, J. (1981). One-trial associative learning modifies food odor preferences of a terrestrial mollusc. *Proceedings of the National Academy of Sciences, 78*, 640–642.

Schafe, G. E., Sollars, S. I., & Bernstein, I. L. (1995). The CS-US interval in taste aversion learning: A brief look. *Behavioral Neuroscience, 109*, 799–802.

Simbayi, L. C., Boakes, R. A., & Burton, M. J. (1986). Effects of basolateral amygdala lesions on taste aversion produced by lactose and lithium chloride in the rat. *Behavioral Neuroscience, 100*, 455–465.

Smith, J. C., & Roll, D. L. (1967). Trace conditioning with x-rays as an aversive stimulus. *Psychonomic Science, 9*, 11–12.

Spector, A. C., Norgren, R., & Grill H. J. (1992). Parabrachial gustatory lesions impair taste aversion learning in rats. *Behavioral Neuroscience, 106*, 147–161.

Spector, A. C., Smith, J. C., & Hollander, G. R. (1981). A comparison of dependent measures used to quantify radiation-induced taste aversion. *Physiology and Behavior, 27*, 887–901.

Spector, A. C., Smith, J. C., & Hollander, G. R. (1983). The effect of post-conditioning CS experience on recovery from radiation-induced taste aversion. *Physiology and Behavior, 30*, 647–649.

Swank, M. W., & Bernstein, I. L. (1994). C-fos induction in response to a conditioned stimulus after single trial taste aversion learning. *Brain Research, 636*, 202–208.

Swank, M. W., Schafe, G. E., & Bernstein, I. L. (1995). C-fos induction in response to taste stimuli previously paired with amphetamine or LiCl during taste aversion learning. *Brain Research 673*, 251–261.

Tapper, D. N., & Halpern, B. P. (1968). Taste stimuli: A behavioral categorization. *Science, 161*, 708–710.

Wilcoxin, H. C., Dragoin, W. B., & Kral, P. (1971). Illness-induced aversions in rat and quail: Relative salience of visual and gustatory cues. *Science, 171,* 826–828.

Yamamoto, T. (1993). Neural mechanisms of taste aversion learning. *Neuroscience Research, 16,* 181–185.

Yamamoto, T., & Fujimoto, Y. (1991). Brain mechanisms of taste aversion learning in the rat. *Brain Research Bulletin, 27,* 403–406.

Zalaquett, C. P., & Parker, L. A. (1989). Further evidence that CTAs produced by lithium and amphetamine are qualitatively different. *Learning & Motivation, 20,* 413–427.

Conditioned Food Preferences

Elizabeth D. Capaldi

This chapter reviews the various ways animals, including humans, form preferences for foods through experience and how these preferences might be changed. As will be seen, in omnivores such as rats and people, most food preferences are produced by experience. This fact is counterintuitive because individuals appear to have such pronounced likes and dislikes on their first encounter with a food; yet few of these preferences are built in. Exposure to food with no consequences increases liking; however, if there are consequences of consuming food (getting sick, feeling full), these consequences determine preference. The taste and other sensory qualities of food also contribute to preference. The taste of food produces liking and disliking that appear to be genetically mediated, whereas, the other sensory characteristics of food (odor, temperature, texture, appearance) appear to produce their effect through learning.

Most of the work in this area has been done with animals because their experience can be precisely controlled. The principles derived from the animal work have been validated with humans, however, and human experiments are also described in this chapter.

There are four known ways to increase preference for a food: *mere exposure*, the *medicine effect, flavor–flavor learning*, and *flavor–nutrient learning*. In *mere exposure*, consuming a food repeatedly increases preference for that food. As mentioned in chapter 4, human infants prefer the odor and taste of foods consumed by their mothers. This process continues throughout life and is believed to have a biological basis. Because foods that are consumed without ill effects are known to be safe, consuming familiar, safe foods is one way to avoid potentially poisonous novel foods.

As reviewed by Schafe and Bernstein (chapter 2, this volume), people and animals avoid foods that make them ill. There is some evidence also that foods associated with recovery from illness come to be preferred, although the *medicine effect* is minor compared to the following two ways of increasing preferences.

In *flavor–flavor learning*, pairing a food with an already liked taste of food increases preference for that food. Likewise, pairing a food with a disliked taste of food decreases preference for that food. This is a powerful, quick way to change preference. *Flavor–nutrient learning* involves pairing a taste or flavor with nutrients (calories) to increase liking for that food.

Because chapters 4, 8, and 9 in this volume describe the effects of exposure to foods on liking and chapter 2 describes taste aversion in learning, this chapter focuses on the latter three methods.

METHODS OF INCREASING FOOD PREFERENCES

Medicine Effect

If rats experience two flavors conditionally paired with one injection of apomorphine (which produces illness), with the first flavor presented just before malaise occurs and the second just before recuperation, preference for the first flavor will decrease and preference for the second will increase (Green & Garcia, 1971). The increased preference for the flavor associated with recuperation is an example of the medicine effect. As another example, if a rat is made thiamine-deficient, a flavor that is associated with a diet that leads to recovery from the deficit will be preferred later (Zahorik & Maier, 1972). The medicine effect probably accounts for a small proportion of human food preferences; most preferred foods have not been associated with recovery from illness. Also, there have been some failures to find the medicine effect in humans (Pliner, Rozin, Cooper, & Woody, 1985).

Likewise, although they are robust and long lasting, taste aversions do not seem to account for a large proportion of human food preferences. Because a majority of people do not have any taste aversions (Garb & Stunkard, 1974), other processes must produce food likes and dislikes. A learning process that can produce both food likes and dislikes is flavor–flavor learning.

Flavor–Flavor Learning

Rats, like people, have a genetically mediated preference for sweetness. When rats were given an arbitrary flavor (cinnamon), mixed with a highly preferred concentration of saccharin, and a second flavor (wintergreen), mixed with a lower, less preferred concentration of saccharin, later they preferred cinnamon to wintergreen, even though neither was sweetened at that point (Holman, 1975). The flavor became preferred as a result of being associated with sweetness. Because half the rats had cinnamon paired with the high concentration of saccharin, and wintergreen paired with the low, and half had the reverse pairings, it is clear that the results were not due to an inherent preference for one flavor over the other. The preference for the flavor associated with the sweeter concentrarion was due to an association between the flavor and saccharin's sweet taste.

In this type of learning, the flavor becomes associated with the pleasantness of the experience with saccharin. We do not know exactly how this happens, but it appears that the flavor associated with sweetness becomes more liked itself. This type of learning is long lasting. Indeed, the flavor associated with sweetness continues to be liked unless some other, explicit learning experience counteracts the initial experience (Capaldi, Myers, Campbell, & Sheffer, 1983). In humans this type of learning may account for how some initially disliked flavors come to be liked, such as coffee. Most people first drink coffee with sugar and cream and only later come to like the bitter taste of black coffee. Pairing the bitter taste of coffee with the sweet taste of sugar increases the preference for the taste of coffee (postingestive effects of sugar and cream also increase preference, as is discussed subsequently). Zellner, Rozin, Aron, and Kulish (1983) showed that humans given unfamiliar teas, some sweetened and some unsweetened, showed an increased preference for the tea that had been sweetened, even when it was subsequently given unsweetened.

In these studies of flavor–flavor learning, the flavors were mixed in solution together. Flavor–flavor learning is also possible if there is a short delay between the ingestion of the two flavors. Lavin (1976) gave rats two distinct flavors to drink in succession and subsequently gave them a toxic substance following consumption of the second flavor given alone. A taste aversion was shown to *both* flavors, demonstrating that an association had been formed between the two flavors given initially. This association was formed only if the flavors were separated by 9 seconds or less. (No one has successfully demonstrated flavor–flavor learning at a delay longer than 9 seconds.) Lyn and Capaldi (1994) replicated this finding using a positive reinforcer (sucrose) for conditioning rather than aversion conditioning. After two flavors were consumed in succession, one was paired with sucrose. Later, preference for both flavors increased.

Mixing a sweetener, or any preferred flavor or food, in with another food is a powerful way to produce liking. Despite this fact, only about one third of parents surveyed reported that they use this method either sometimes or often to affect children's food preferences (Casey & Rozin, 1989). This may be because parents do not realize that preference will transfer from the liked flavor to the food. There also may be a prejudice against use of sweeteners, particularly sugar, to affect food preferences. However, because the preference for sweet is built in, there seems no reason not to take advantage of this liking to increase liking for foods that are healthful.

My research group showed that mixing vegetables with sugar produced a greater reaction of pleasantness to the vegetable when it was later given unsweetened. Figure 1 shows the results of one such study. Each college-student participant received both cauliflower and broccoli, each three times. For half of the students, the cauliflower was sweetened with sugar and the broccoli was unsweetened; for the other half, the broccoli was sweetened and the cauliflower unsweetened. Later, when tested with unsweetened broccoli and unsweetened cauliflower, students rated the previously sweetened vegetable as more pleasant than the vegetable that had never been sweetened.

Flavor–flavor learning can also produce dislikes. Mixing a flavor with bitter-tasting quinine produces a later dislike for the flavor (Capaldi & Hunter, 1994).

Flavor–Nutrient Learning

Flavor–calorie for flavor–nutrient learning can occur under the same conditions as flavor–flavor learning. When a flavor is mixed with a substance such as sugar that has calories and tastes good, the flavor will be associated with the sweet taste and with the calories.

If, for example, one flavor is given in solution with 8% sucrose and a

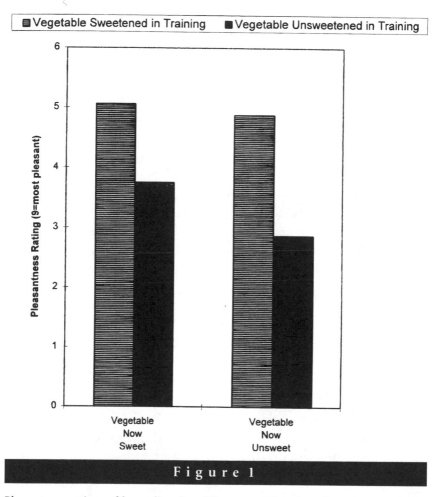

Figure 1

Pleasantness ratings of broccoli and cauliflower as a function of previous experience with the sweetened vegetable.

second flavor with 1% sucrose, preference for the first flavor will increase relative to the second on the basis of either flavor–flavor learning (sucrose tastes sweet) or flavor–nutrient learning (sucrose contains calories). Flavor–flavor learning is demonstrated by Holman's study, described previously, in which preference increased for the flavor associated with the higher concentration of saccharin. This is flavor–flavor learning, not flavor–nutrient learning, because no nutrients are involved when saccharin is used. Demonstrating flavor–nutrient learning that is independent of flavor–flavor learning is more difficult because most highly caloric substances also taste good, and nutritious foods rarely taste really bad.

Testing Flavor–Nutrient Learning

Three methods have been used to test flavor–nutrient learning separately from flavor–flavor learning. First, because flavor–flavor learning is not possible at a delay, showing conditioned flavor preferences with a delay between flavor and consequence illustrates flavor–nutrient learning as a process that is separate from flavor–flavor learning. Capaldi, Campbell, Sheffer, and Bradford (1987a) showed that rats preferred a flavor given in saccharin (the cue) 30 minutes before lab chow (the consequent) to a flavor given in saccharin that preceded nothing. Capaldi et al. (1987a) also showed flavor preferences at a 30-minute delay using dextrose or polycose (a form of hydrolyzed corn starch) or high-fat wet mash as reinforcing consequences.

In *flavor–nutrient* preference conditioning, therefore, preference increases for a flavor that is given before a nutrient is given. This is an important phenomenon because in normal eating there is a delay between tasting the flavor of food and digesting the nutrients in the food. The phenomenon of flavor–nutrient learning shows that preference for the flavor of nutrient-loaded food can increase despite this built-in delay. Animals can thus learn to consume foods that contain nutrients. There is also a downside to this: We are built to learn preferences for flavors associated with high-calorie foods, something that can make weight control difficult.

Bolles and colleagues used a second method to demonstrate flavor–nutrient learning that was independent of flavor–flavor learning. Mehiel and Bolles (1988) gave rats different Kool-aid flavors mixed with substances differing in taste but equal in calories and measured preference among the flavors. Preference for a flavor associated with ethanol (a caloric substance with a taste disliked by rats) was as great as preference for a flavor associated with corn oil or sucrose (caloric substances with tastes liked by rats) that had the same number of calories as the ethanol. These findings suggest that flavor–nutrient learning occurs and that it is more powerful than flavor–flavor learning, at least in rats.

A third method to show flavor–nutrient learning that is independent of flavor–flavor learning is to bypass the oral cavity to deliver nutrients contingent on a flavor. Booth, Lovett, and McSherry (1972) showed that the normal preference for the sweeter of two solutions could be reversed by associating the less sweet solution with the postingestive consequences of 10% glucose. More recently, Sclafani (1990) showed that intragastric infusion of nutrients contingent on rats' licking a tube containing a particular flavor increased preference for that flavor. Thus, even if delivery of the consequent solution bypasses the oral cavity, the solution can produce a conditioned preference. There have been some failures to find a conditioned preference using this technique (e.g., Revusky, Smith, & Chalmers, 1971), however, and in some cases significant aversions have been produced with intragastric fat infusions (e.g., Deutsch, Molina, & Puerto, 1976). Under certain conditions, intragastric infusions can have aversive consequences that interfere with any reinforcing effects.

These findings show that preference for a flavor increases if the flavor is associated with nutritional consequences in normal eating. We call this effect *flavor–nutrient learning* because it seems that animals can discriminate among the postingestive effects of different macronutrients. For example, preference for a flavor previously paired with an intragastric infusion of protein is suppressed by an intragastric protein load but not by a carbohydrate load (Baker, Booth, Duggan, & Gibson, 1987). And intragastric loads of carbohydrate are more effective than intragastric loads of fat in conditioning flavor preferences (Sclafani, 1990). For our purposes, however, the main point is that foods can condition flavor preferences and that conditioning occurs with a delay between a cue flavor and a nutritional consequence only if the consequent contains calories.

Because flavor–flavor learning and flavor–nutrient learning both can occur when a flavor is mixed in a food, whereas only flavor–nutrient learning occurs with a delay, conditioned flavor preferences should be larger when a cue flavor is mixed in a food rather than given before the food; this is indeed the case. Sclafani (1990) reported that larger conditioned flavor preferences were produced by mixing flavors in with solutions than by delayed conditioning of flavors.

The lesson to be learned from these studies is that to change preference for a food, one should mix it with an already preferred food. However, parents rarely use this method; instead, they use the less effective method of following a less preferred food with something that is preferred.

In everyday life, flavor–calorie learning produces preferences for foods that have more calories. Bolles, Hayward, and Crandall (1981) showed that caloric density was more important than number of calories. Preference was greater for a flavor associated with 2 g of a 4-calorie food than for a flavor associated with 4 g of a 2-calorie food. The choice in this study might be equivalent to the choice between a flavor associated with 20 g of nonfat cottage cheese and a flavor associated with a calorically equivalent 2 g of high-fat cheese. Rats, like people, prefer their calories in a dense form, probably as a result of flavor–flavor learning. Foods that are high in density of calories tend to be high in fat. Protein and carbohydrate both have 4 calories per gram, whereas fat has 9 calories per gram. Thus, foods with a high density of calories tend to be high in fat and to be rated as highly palatable.

Also, in everyday life, people tend to eat more than one food at a time. I have already shown that preference increases for food eaten close in time to preferred foods. Thus, eating a vegetable close to a preferred meat increases preference for the vegetable. Also, in meals we often eat foods in sequence, or courses, rather than all mixed together, and typically the last item in a meal is a dessert. This tendency leads to the interesting question of what gets associated with the calories in the meal. If a salad is eaten first and dessert last, will the salad become more preferred as the result of the calories in the dessert? The answer to this question is unfortunately *no,* as is seen in the following discussion of the dessert effect.

Dessert Effect

If rats are given a meal, for example, potatoes, followed by a dessert, such as sucrose, an apparently paradoxical effect occurs. The preference for potatoes *decreases* as a result of being followed by sucrose (Capaldi, Campbell, Sheffer, & Bradford, 1987b). Capaldi et al. (1987b) compared two groups of rats, both of which received a lunch each day; on half the days for all rats, the lunch was rice, and on the other half of the days, the lunch was potatoes. One group of rats had dessert (sucrose) following potatoes and nothing following rice; the other group of rats received the reverse: sucrose following rice and nothing following potatoes. In testing, the rats were given dishes of potatoes and rice side by side, and the amount consumed of each in a free choice was measured. Figure 2 shows the preference for potatoes over rice when sucrose followed potatoes versus when sucrose

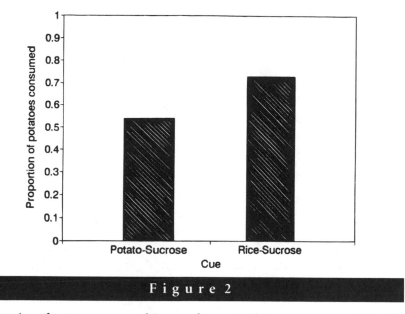

Figure 2

Proportion of potatoes consumed in a preference test between potatoes and rice for animals that experienced sucrose following potatoes (left bar) and for animals that experienced sucrose following rice (right bar).

followed rice. As can be seen, the proportion of potatoes consumed in the test was lower for rats that had sucrose following potatoes than for rats that had nothing following potatoes (and sucrose following rice). Why? Capaldi et al. (1987b) used an interval of 5 minutes between the potatoes and sucrose, too long for flavor–flavor learning to occur. Yet sucrose does contain calories; on the basis of flavor–nutrient learning, therefore, the preference for potatoes should increase when potatoes are followed by sucrose, not decrease.

A closer analysis of flavor–nutrient learning suggests one possible reason for the dessert effect. Postingestive effects of consumption take some time. A flavor that follows a meal may be more closely associated in time with the postingestive consequences of the meal than is the flavor of the meal itself. Boakes and Lubart (1988) showed that a flavor of saccharin that followed ingestion of glucose was preferred to a flavor of saccharin that occurred alone. They suggested that what appears to be backward conditioning (glucose reinforcer precedes saccharin flavor cue) is really forward conditioning (saccharin flavor cue precedes reinforcer–postingestive consequences of glucose). Consistent with this hypothesis, they showed that a flavor of saccharin that followed glucose by 60 minutes was not preferred to a flavor of saccharin that occurred alone. After 60 minutes, the postingestive effects of glucose would dissipate.

Capaldi et al.'s (1987b) dessert effect may have occurred, therefore, because when sucrose followed potatoes, the flavor of sucrose was more closely associated with the postingestive consequences of potatoes than was the flavor of potatoes. For the group that received rice alone and sucrose following potatoes, the flavor of rice was associated with the postingestive consequences of rice, whereas the flavor of potatoes was not associated with the postingestive consequences of potatoes; therefore, rice was preferred to potatoes.

This analysis implies that our habit of eating dessert at the end of a meal increases preference for the sweet taste of the dessert because the postingestive consequences of the meal are more closely associated with the flavor of the dessert than with the flavor of the meal.

In general, a flavor consumed later in a meal is more strongly associated with the postingestive consequences of a meal than a flavor consumed earlier in the meal. To test this statement, one might give two flavors sequentially in a meal and later test preference between the two flavors. However, there is a complicating factor in comparing preference for a flavor given early in a meal to a flavor given later in the meal. Hunger decreases during a meal, and hunger also affects food preferences, as is discussed later.

Elizalde and Sclafani (1988) showed that associations between the flavor of a nutritional reinforcer and its own postingestive effects can interfere with forming an association between a cue flavor and those postingestive effects. They used polycose as a reinforcer. One group was preexposed to polycose plus acarbose, a drug that blocks digestion of starch. The other group was not preexposed. Subsequently, both groups were given flavor conditioning with polycose following a cue flavor at a delay. The group that was preexposed to acarbose plus polycose formed a larger conditioned preference than the other group. Presumably, the preexposed group had learned in Phase 1 that the flavor of polycose was not associated with nutritional benefit; therefore, in Phase 2 the flavor of polycose did not block learning about the flavor cue.

Studies of flavor–nutrient learning show that preference is increased most for the flavor that is most closely associated with nutritional consequences. This suggests that our habit of eating dessert at the end of the meal will increase preference more for the dessert than for the preceding foods. Preference for the flavor of the reinforcer or a flavor following it may be increased, whereas preference for the preceding cue flavor is not increased. Rewarding a child for eating spinach with a dessert will not increase preference for spinach, therefore; rather, it will increase preference for the dessert. Another set of effects, *contrast effects*, also suggest that rewarding children for eating a disliked food is ineffective.

Contrast Effects in Flavor Preference Learning

The effectiveness of a reinforcer is reduced if it is closely accompanied by a preferred reinforcer, a phenomenon termed *negative contrast* (see Mackintosh, 1974). Contrast effects have been demonstrated in consuming behavior. Flaherty and Checke (1982) showed that consumption of saccharin was reduced if saccharin was followed by sucrose. They called this effect *anticipatory negative contrast*. Consumption of saccharin is reduced in anticipation of the following preferred sucrose. Note that the anticipatory contrast effect discovered by Flaherty is analogous to our dessert effect, except that we measured later preference for potatoes that preceded sucrose, whereas Flaherty and his colleagues measured current consumption of saccharin that preceded sucrose. Perhaps preference for potatoes is reduced by sucrose following because sucrose is preferred to potatoes. Contrast or comparison effects may account for the dessert effect.

If the preceding is true, then following a food by a preferred caloric food may produce two opposing effects: The preferred food may increase preference for the first food (flavor–nutrient learning), and the preferred food may reduce current consumption of the first food because of contrast or comparison effects and may also reduce preference for that food (dessert effect). Thus, the final preference for a flavor may depend on the algebraic sum of the increase in preference produced by flavor–nutrient learning and the decrease in preference produced by contrast.

My group initially suggested that preference conditioning and negative anticipatory contrast may operate simultaneously and produce opposing effects on intake to account for some paradoxical findings in preference learning (Capaldi, Sheffer, & Pulley, 1989). For example, a higher concentra-

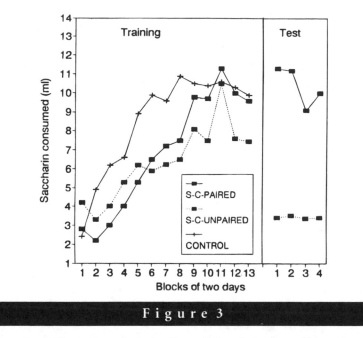

Figure 3

Consumption of flavored saccharin by Group S-C and the control group in training, and for Group S-C in test. For Group S-C, one flavor of saccharin preceded chocolate milk in training (paired); the other flavor occurred alone (unpaired). In testing a choice was given between the two flavors.

tion of sucrose used as a reinforcer sometimes produces less of a conditioned preference than a lower concentration. This may be because a higher concentration of sucrose also results in a stronger negative contrast effect that reduces the net conditioned preference.

In a subsequent series of experiments, my group measured both reinforcement and contrast simultaneously (Capaldi & Sheffer, 1992). In one experiment, rats received one flavor of saccharin preceding chocolate milk and a second flavor of saccharin alone. Consumption during training was measured, as well as subsequent preference between the two flavors of saccharin. Figure 3 shows consumption during training and flavor preference in a later test. As Figure 3 shows, rats that received saccharin preceding chocolate milk (Group S-C) suppressed consumption of saccharin compared to a control group that received only saccharin (anticipatory negative contrast). These same rats preferred the flavor of saccharin that preceded chocolate milk to the flavor that occurred alone in a later test of conditioned flavor preferences. Thus, contrast (decreased consumption) and reinforcement (increased preference) can indeed occur simultaneously.

An interesting aspect of the results is that, in training, consumption of the two different flavors of saccharin did not differ significantly, although the tendency was for rats to consume more of the flavor that preceded chocolate milk. Lucas and Timberlake (1992) also recently reported that rats consumed more of a flavor of saccharin that preceded sucrose than of a flavor that occurred alone. When a within-subject comparison is made between two flavors, therefore, one of which precedes a reinforcer and one of which does not, the data are clear in showing preference for the flavor preceding the reinforcer (flavor–nutrient learning). This is so despite the fact that consumption of both flavors is suppressed compared to that of a control group that does not receive the preferred reward.

Summarizing, I have thus far discussed two reasons that following a food by a more liked food may not increase preference for the first food. First, the food that is eaten closer in time to postingestive consequences is more strongly associated with those consequences than an earlier occurring cue flavor. This includes the flavor of the reinforcer itself and flavors that occur after the delivery of the reinforcer. Second, a comparison, or contrast, process can reduce the value of a cue flavor that precedes a more preferred reinforcer. This could explain why only 7% of parents reported that giving children a reward for eating a food increased preference for it (Casey & Rozin, 1989).

HUNGER AND FOOD PREFERENCES

My father told me his advice to his son on hearing his grandchild would not drink his milk: Take him outside and let him play in the sun; when he gets thirsty, he'll drink. My father's commonsense approach will get the child to drink milk, but what might not be so obvious is that this experience also will increase preference for milk. One way to induce an animal to eat is to deprive it of food. Consuming a food when deprived increases later preference for that food.

Revusky and Garcia (1970) and Revusky (1967) originally suggested that a food consumed when hungry would become preferred as a result of the taste of food being paired with the long-delayed consequences of consumption. Revusky (1967) showed that a flavor consumed under high deprivation was preferred later to a flavor consumed under low deprivation even when the rats were tested under low deprivation. However, my colleagues and I showed in a series of studies (Capaldi & Myers, 1982; Capaldi, Myers, Campbell, & Sheffer, 1983) that Revusky's findings were due in part to his using a 24-hour deprivation schedule in which the flavor given under high deprivation occurred immediately before the daily feeding and the flavor given under low deprivation occurred immediately after feeding. When this is done, the flavor given before feeding (high deprivation) can be associated with the following daily meal. (In Revusky's study, the flavor given after feeding, under low deprivation, was probably not associated with the postingestive effects of the meal because it followed the meal by 1 1/2 hours). Thus, Revusky's (1967) results may show that a flavor associated with a following meal is preferred to a flavor not associated with a meal (another example of flavor–nutrient learning), rather than having anything to do with the effects of deprivation level. It is important to give the flavors under different deprivation levels while not simultaneously associating the flavors differentially with the daily meal.

In another series of studies (Capaldi, Sheffer, & Owens, 1991), my associates and I showed that rats preferred a flavor that was experienced under high deprivation to one that was experienced under low deprivation when the flavors were given separately from feeding in *unsweetened* food. In the first experiment in this series, six different groups of rats were run in a factorial design combining amount of food used to deliver flavors (1 g or 16 g of wet mash) with three different combinations of high and low deprivation: 2 and 26 hours, 2 and 43 hours and 24 and 43 hours. One flavor of wet mash was given under the higher deprivation and one under the lower deprivation condition. Subsequently, preference between the flavors was measured. Figure 4 shows the results of this experiment: There was a clear preference for the flavor of food given under high deprivation whether testing was done under high or low deprivation.

In previous work using the same procedures, my group found that if flavors were delivered in saccharin or sucrose solutions, preference was for the flavor received under the *lower* deprivation level (Capaldi & Myers, 1982; Capaldi et al., 1983). This cross-study comparison suggested that there might be something aversive about sweetness under high deprivation. Accordingly,

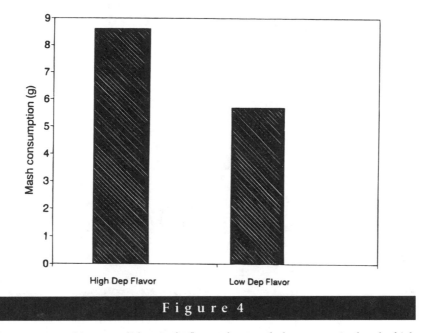

F i g u r e 4

Grams consumed in a two-dish test of a flavor of wet mash that was received under high deprivation versus a flavor that was received under low deprivation. From *Animal Learning and Behavior, 19.* © 1991 by Psychonomic Society Publications. Reprinted with permission.

we ran an additional experiment using the same procedures, except sweetened or unsweetened food delivered the flavors. In this experiment, the low deprivation was 2 hours and the high deprivation was 43 hours. There were four groups in a factorial design combining amount of food used to deliver the flavor (1 vs. 20 g of wet mash) with whether or not the mash was sweetened. Figure 5 shows the results: Rats preferred the flavor experienced under the higher deprivation condition when unsweetened food was used to deliver the flavors, but using sweetened food eliminated this preference.

Apparently there is something aversive or unpleasant about sweetness when food deprivation is high. This may explain why sweet foods are typically eaten at the end of the meal under low food deprivation rather than at the beginning of the meal. Other anecdotal data also indicate that sweetness is not pleasant under very high food deprivation. When food deprivation is extreme, preference for food elements other than sweet seems to increase. Lepkovsky (1977) reported that during World War II, American soldiers in a German prison camp were subsisting on a ration that was 200

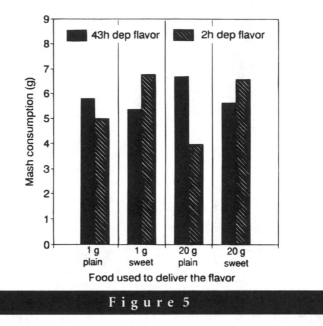

Figure 5

Grams consumed in a two-dish test of a flavor of wet mash that was received under high deprivation versus a flavor that was received under low deprivation. Groups differed in the amount of wet mash received in training and in whether or not the mash was sweetened. From *Animal Learning and Behavior, 19.* © 1991 by Psychonomic Society Publications. Reprinted with permission.

calories short of basal needs. They were ultimately saved by Red Cross food parcels. Trading of the food parcels produced a point value for each food that pretty much reflected the nutritional composition of the food. The two top items were powdered milk at 150 points and meat at 120 points. No points at all were listed for jam, sugar, or chocolate bars. Also in this connection, it is interesting to note that highly sweetened main dishes are uncommon in human cuisines. These anecdotal data are consistent with our animal work showing that the reinforcing effect of food as measured by conditioned food preferences is increased by food deprivation only if unsweetened food is used.

Although the reinforcing effect of sweet food does not increase with increasing deprivation, its palatability may increase. Cabanac (1971) reported that humans' ratings of the pleasantness of sweet solutions were higher immediately preceding a glucose load than they were following one. He postulated that the pleasantness of stimuli is related to their usefulness to the body, a phenomenon he termed *alliesthesia*. Cabanac's phenomenon may be related to the fact that high deprivation was defined as the state prior to a glucose load, and low deprivation, the state after the glucose load. Rats prefer flavors given shortly before a meal to those given after a meal (Capaldi & Myers, 1982; Revusky, 1967), but they do not prefer flavors given in sweetened solutions under high deprivation to those given under low deprivation when the flavors are not associated with meals.

In our studies, my colleagues and I have measured reinforcing effectiveness, not palatability. Palatability is only one aspect of reinforcing effectiveness. Our data show that the reinforcing effectiveness of sweet solutions or foods is not increased by deprivation intervals of from 2 to 48 hours. Accordingly, in addition to any presumed palatability increase, there must also be aversive effects of consuming sweet solutions and food under high deprivation, effects that reduce the reinforcing effectiveness of sweetness.

I have shown thus far that preference for a flavor increases as a result of being consumed when the animal is food-deprived. A more dramatic demonstration that the reward or incentive value of the food is increased is provided by the following finding reported by Capaldi, Davidson and Myers (1981): After rats had consumed food when food-deprived, the pellets served as reinforcers when the rats were satiated. One group of rats (Group P) was given a total of 40 Noyes pellets (0.045 g each) when hungry, the other Group (Group A) received no pellets but were on the same deprivation schedule as Group P—1 week of receiving only 13 grams to eat each day. After this, both groups were fed all they wanted for 12 days until they had regained all the lost weight. They were then run in a differential conditioning problem while satiated, in which the pellets were placed in one color alley (black or white) and no reinforcer was given in the other color alley. Group P learned to run faster in the alley containing the pellets than in the other alley, whereas Group A did not. Experiencing the Noyes pellets when hungry was sufficient to make them a reinforcer under the satiation.

This experiment showed that pellets become a conditioned reinforcer as a result of having been consumed under food deprivation; it can be viewed as an example of flavor-nutrient learning. The taste of pellets was paired with the postingestive effects of eating the pellets. Most people are aware that food they have eaten when hungry is pleasant to eat even when they are not hungry. This experiment suggests that this is a learned effect.

Capaldi and Myers (1978) showed that once rats had eaten pellets when hungry, they would continue to eat them when satiated. The strength of the eating response was dependent on the similarity of the cues present in training and testing. Eating when satiated was more strongly elicited if the same reward magnitude was used in satiation than if a different one was used (Capaldi & Myers, 1978). Eating in satiated testing was also more strongly elicited following training with partial reward than following training with consistent reward. Perhaps the most interesting aspect of conditioned eating is that it is stimulus-bound. An animal trained to eat pellets when hungry in a straight alley runway can be satiated on pellets in its home cage, and it will resume eating pellets when placed again in the runway. The conditioning situation is sufficient to reelicit eating that has ceased because of satiation (Capaldi & Myers, 1978). Weingarten (1983) reported the same phenomenon later, using a specific punctate stimulus as a cue. Rats that had been given food every day following a specific conditioned stimulus resumed eating when satiated on presentation of the stimulus. This finding supports the suggestion of some diet plans that one eat only in one place. Conditioned eating will be restricted to that one place, and one will have less of a learned urge to eat in other places.

Summarizing, another way to produce a learned food preference is to give the food to a hungry organism. This learned increase in preference transfers to the satiated state and is highly resistant to extinction.

CHARACTERISTICS OF FOOD PREFERENCE LEARNING

As reviewed by Schafe and Bernstein (chapter 2, this volume), taste aversion learning occurs rapidly; is resistant to extinction; and may occur despite long delays between taste and sickness. The data reviewed here show that flavor preferences that are based on positive systemic consequences are also possible. These preferences also are established rapidly, are resistant to extinction, and are possible with long delays between flavors and consequences.

Rapidity of Learning

In the earliest studies of flavor preference conditioning using positive consequences, a fairly large number of conditioning trials were used. Holman

(1975), for example, used 20 pairings of flavors in his original study showing flavor–flavor learning. More recent studies have used fewer pairings successfully. Capaldi et al. (1983) used only six pairings (three under high deprivation and three under low deprivation) and found a highly significant preference for the flavor given in a sweet solution under low deprivation. Mehiel and Bolles (1988) used only four pairings of sucrose with a flavor and showed a significant flavor preference. Boakes, Rossi-Arnand, and Garcia-Hoz (1987) found conditioning to be maximally strong following only two pairings in flavor–flavor learning, whereas learning was slower in flavor–nutrient learning at a delay.

The number of trials necessary to produce conditioned flavor preferences has not been systematically investigated in the different flavor conditioning paradigms. However, the data available suggest that conditioning is rapid, especially in flavor–flavor learning. In flavor–nutrient learning, enough studies have used small numbers of pairings (fewer than 10) to lead to the conclusion that a large number of conditioning trials is not necessary to obtain effects.

Resistance to Extinction

Conditioned flavor preferences are surprisingly resistant to extinction. Figure 6 shows data from an experiment by Capaldi et al. (1983) in which rats received one flavored sweet solution under high deprivation and another under low deprivation. This conditioning produces a preference for the flavor given under low deprivation. As Figure 6 shows, this preference persisted over 28 days of testing with no sign of diminution.

Why are flavor preferences so persistent? Consider the data from the Capaldi et al. (1983) experiment shown in Figure 6. In testing, the rats were given both flavors side by side in a two-bottle test; the preferred flavor was consumed more than the nonpreferred. If anything, this behavior should increase preference for the already preferred flavor (because preference increases with exposure; thus, test performance may produce an increase in the previously learned preference. Additionally, the initial difference in preferences is not explicitly counteracted by the experiences given in testing. Both flavors in testing are given under common test circumstances. In the Capaldi et al. (1983) experiment, one flavor was experienced under high deprivation in training and the other under low deprivation. In testing,

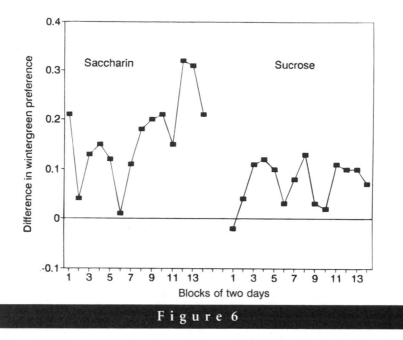

Figure 6

Preference for wintergreen when it was consumed under low deprivation in training minus preference for wintergreen when it was consumed under high deprivation in training. Shown are data over 28 days of two-bottle testing (wintergreen vs. cinnamon) for rats trained with saccharin solution and rats trained with sucrose solution.

both flavors were experienced under both deprivation levels. The initial difference in affective value for the two flavors may be maintained under the common, new experience. (The fact that conditioned flavor preferences are so persistent suggests that affective conditioning is involved, an issue that is discussed subsequently.)

Consistent with this idea, conditioned flavor preferences can be eliminated quickly by reversal training. Capaldi et al. (1983) reversed the contingencies experienced by the animals, thereby reversing affective conditioning; this rapidly reversed the preference.

Delay

Conditioned flavor preferences can be formed with a considerable delay between flavor and consequence. Capaldi et al. (1987a) used a 30-minute delay between presentation of flavors and consequences and obtained significant flavor preferences; Capaldi and Sheffer (1992) found significant conditioned flavor preferences with a 5-hour delay between flavors and reinforcer. Not all investigators have obtained this result, however (see Simbayi, Boakes, & Burton, 1986), and there are good reasons to expect difficulty in obtaining conditioned flavor preferences after a delay. The reinforcer for long-delay learning seems to be some aspect of the postingestive consequences of consuming caloric food (recall that flavor–flavor learning is not possible with a delay). If a flavor precedes consumption of a caloric food at a delay, the flavor of the caloric food itself is more closely paired in time with the postingestive consequences of the food than is the cue flavor. Indeed, as I discussed earlier, a flavor that occurs after a food is given may be more strongly associated with the postingestive consequences of the food than with the flavor of the food itself.

One reason flavor preference learning at a delay can be difficult to demonstrate, therefore, is that the flavor of the reinforcing food can be associated with its own nutritional consequences, blocking conditioning of the flavor cue to those consequences.

LEARNING PROCESSES INVOLVED IN FLAVOR PREFERENCE LEARNING

Theorists have most commonly considered flavor preference learning to be a case of classical conditioning. In taste aversion learning, the flavor is considered the conditioned stimulus (CS) and sickness the unconditioned stimulus (US). In flavor preference experiments that are based on positive consequences, the flavor is the CS and either another flavor (in flavor–flavor learning) or postingestive consequences (in flavor–nutrient learning) is considered the US. Flavor–flavor learning does not easily fit the CS–US framework, however, and the question can be raised whether this is the best way to view flavor–nutrient learning.

Flavor–Flavor Learning

Flavor–flavor learning does not require that a CS be paired with a US. Flavor–flavor learning also occurs when a flavor US is associated with another flavor US (i.e., one of the flavors does not need to be neutral before conditioning). Rescorla and Cunningham (1978) showed that flavor–flavor learning occurred when solutions were given of sucrose plus hydrochloric acid or quinine and of sodium chloride plus hydrochloric acid or quinine. All of these flavors can be used as USs. Flavor–flavor learning seems to occur whenever two flavors are given together, whether the flavors are neutral or not. Also, flavor–flavor learning is not possible with a delay of longer than 9 seconds between the two flavors and is optimal when the flavors are given in solution together. In classical conditioning, which involves the association between a CS and a US, it is optimal to have the CS precede the US.

Rescorla and Cunningham (1978) and Durlach and Rescorla (1980) have suggested that flavor–flavor learning involves formation of within-compound associations, a type of learning that can occur whenever two stimuli are presented in compound. This is a more neutral description that seems preferred to the arbitrary designation of one flavor as a US and the other as a CS and of learning as involving an association between a CS and a US. Although flavor–flavor learning often involves a neutral flavor and a flavor that could be used as a US, neither flavor seems to be functioning as a US. Rather, the two flavors become associated with each other as a result of being experienced together. It is true that no one seems to have investigated flavor–flavor learning when two neutral flavors are paired, but there is no reason to believe that flavor–flavor learning would not occur under these conditions, inasmuch as two neutral external stimuli become associated when experienced in compound.

The basic result of flavor–flavor learning is that any affective tone of one of the flavors transfers to the other flavor. This is so whether the affective tone of one of the flavors is inherent (as when sucrose or quinine is used) or the affective tone of one of the flavors has been learned (as when one of the flavors has been paired with illness). Pairing a flavor with saccharin increases preference for the flavor (Holman, 1975); pairing a flavor with quinine or with a flavor that has been associated with illness decreases preference for the flavor (Fanselow & Birk, 1982; Lavin, 1976). Pairing a flavor with another flavor that has been associated with calories increases preference for that flavor (Lyn & Capaldi, 1994).

Flavor–Nutrient Learning

Flavor–nutrient learning, in contrast to flavor–flavor learning, requires that the reinforcer associated with the cue contain nutrients (i.e., a US is necessary). A cue flavor becomes associated with some aspect of the postingestive consequences of food containing calories. One hypothesis is that flavor–nutrient learning is a form of operant conditioning. Eating can be viewed as an operant response that is reinforced by the nutritional consequences of eating. The flavor in conditioned flavor preference experiments can then be viewed as a discriminative stimulus.

In most of the studies discussed previously, consumption of food was used as a measure of the increased preference for it. Data from these studies, therefore, conceivably can be interpreted in terms of operant conditioning of consumption. Capaldi et al.'s (1981) study of resistance to satiation used a different measure of "preference": reinforcement of a preceding instrumental response. This measure is a more powerful measure of conditioned preference than is consumption because results cannot be interpreted in terms of conditioning of consumption as an operant response. There is a considerable amount of evidence that instrumental responses learned under high food deprivation are made more persistently and vigorously when tested under low hunger than are responses learned under low hunger. For example, rats trained to run a straight alley under high food deprivation run more rapidly in a low deprivation test than rats trained under low deprivation, even if they are tested with no food present; therefore, conditioned reinforcing value of the food cannot be responsible for the effect (Capaldi & Hovancik, 1973). My colleagues and I suggested that instrumental responses learned under high deprivation are more strongly conditioned than those learned under low deprivation. If this is so, learning to eat a particular food under high deprivation may produce greater consumption of the food later because of a stronger conditioned eating response (when consumption is viewed as an instrumental response).

Capaldi et al.'s (1981) experiment using pellets to reinforce a new response in testing cannot be interpreted in this manner. In that experiment, the reinforcer previously consumed under high deprivation was used to reinforce a new response (running the alley) as a measure of reinforcing value or preference. Because the running response was not made in high deprivation training, its greater strength for rats trained under high deprivation cannot be attributed to stronger conditioning under high deprivation. This experiment thus shows clearly that the reinforcing value of the pellets was increased by the conditioning history. This experiment provides particularly strong evidence that the reinforcing effectiveness of food can be changed by the conditioning history and evidence against the hypothesis that learned consumption differences are responsible for the effect.

In flavor–nutrient conditioning, the mechanism appears to be transfer of affect from the nutrient to the flavor rather than a cognitive expectancy of receiving calories being conditioned to the flavors. If a cognitive expectancy of receiving nutrients were formed when a flavor is paired with nutrients, the conditioned flavor preference should extinguish when the nutrients no longer follow. Although conditioned flavor preferences of course do ultimately extinguish, they are highly resistant to extinction. This great resistance to extinction implies that the affect elicited by the flavor has changed as a result of the initial pairing.

IMPLICATIONS OF CONDITIONED FOOD PREFERENCES

The fact that individual differences in taste preferences can be related to differences in experience with foods is of tremendous practical importance. Individual persons differing in weight also differ in their taste preferences, particularly for fat. Obese persons show a greater preference for fat than normal-weight persons, whereas persons with anorexia show less (Drewnowski, 1988). These differences in preferences may be produced by experience, and perhaps some of the methods that we know change food preferences could be used to change an individual's preference for fat. Some work has been done on this issue in the case of salt.

Recall that mere familiarity is an important determinant of food preference. Exposure to particular intensities of flavors also affects preferences. People on a low-salt diet ultimately show preferences for lower intensities of salt in soup and on crackers. This change in preference takes longer to occur than one might think: 2–4 months. The preference change is a sensory phenomenon. People given 10 grams of extra sodium per day in the form of salt on their food show an increase in the level of salt preferred in soup or crackers; people given 10 grams of extra sodium per day in the form of a salt tablet show no change in preference. It is tasting the salt that causes the preference changes, not simply ingesting the salt (Beauchamp, 1987) Would exposure to a low-fat diet reduce the preferred level of fat, as exposure to a low-salt diet reduces the preferred level of salt? If results with fat were similar to those with salt, one would expect that any change in preference would take months to develop. Knowledge that the taste of food will improve after months on a diet could motivate adherence to the diet. Another way to reduce the preference for fat would be to pair it with already disliked tastes (flavor–flavor learning), a method that has not yet been tried.

Consider what most of us do instead. We eat foods that are in essence sweet–fat combinations, as pointed out by Drewnowski (e.g., 1991): brownies, ice cream, chocolate chip cookies. Each time we eat a brownie we are giving ourselves a learning trial pairing fat with sweet, increasing preference for fat by flavor–flavor learning. Likewise, salt on French fries or meat will increase preference for the fat and other components of these foods owing to flavor–flavor learning. We eat our dessert at the end of the meal, or alone, increasing preference for the fat and other components in the dessert by flavor–nutrient learning.

REFERENCES

Baker, B. J., Booth, D. A., Duggan, J. P., & Gibson, E. L. (1987). Protein appetite demonstrated: Learned specificity of protein-cue preference to protein need in adult rats. *Nutrition Research, 7*, 481–487.

Beauchamp, G. K. (1987). The human preference for excess salt. *American Scientist, 75*, 27–33.

Boakes, R. A., & Lubart, T. (1988). Enhanced preference for a flavor following reversed flavor-glucose pairing. *Quarterly Journal of Experimental Psychology; 40B*, 49–62.

Boakes, R. A., Rossi-Arnaud, C., & Garcia-Hoz, V. (1987). Early experience and reinforcer quality in delayed flavour-food learning in the rat. *Appetite, 9*, 191–206.

Bolles, R. C., Hayward, L., & Crandell, C. (1981). Conditioned taste preferences based on caloric density. *Journal of Experimental Psychology: Animal Behavior Processes, 7*, 59–69.

Booth, D. A., Lovett, D., & McSherry, G. M. (1972). Postingestive modulation of the sweetness preference gradient. *Journal of Comparative and Physiological Psychology, 78*, 485–512.

Cabanac, M. (1971). Physiological role of pleasure. *Science, 173*, 1103–1107.

Capaldi, E. D., Campbell, D. H., and Sheffer, J. D., & Bradford, J. P. (1987a). Non-reinforcing effects of giving "desserts" in rats. *Appetite, 9,* 99–112.

Capaldi, E. D., Campbell, D. H., Sheffer, J. D., & Bradford, J. P. (1987b). Conditioned flavor preferences based on delayed caloric consequences. *Journal of Experimental Psychology: Animal Behavior Processes, 13,* 150–155.

Capaldi, E. D., Davidson, T. L., & Myers, D. E. (1981) Resistance to satiation: Reinforcing effects of food and eating under satiation. *Learning and Motivation, 12,* 171–195.

Capaldi, E. D., & Hovancik, J. R. (1973). Effects of previous body weight level on rats' straight alley performance. *Journal of Experimental Psychology, 97,* 93–97.

Capaldi, E. D., & Hunter, M. J. (1994). Taste and odor in conditioned flavor preference learning. *Animal Learning & Behavior, 22,* 355–365.

Capaldi, E. D., & Myers, D. E. (1978). Resistance to satiation of consummatory and instrumental performance. *Learning and Motivation, 9,* 197–201.

Capaldi, E. D., & Myers, D. E. (1982). Taste preferences as a function of food deprivation during original taste exposure. *Animal Learning & Behavior, 10,* 211–219.

Capaldi, E. D., Myers, D. E., Campbell, D. H., & Sheffer, J. D. (1983). Conditioned flavor preferences based on hunger level during original flavor exposure. *Animal Learning & Behavior, 11,* 107–115.

Capaldi, E. D., & Sheffer, J. D. (1992). Contrast and reinforcement in consumption. *Learning and Motivation, 23,* 63–79.

Capaldi, E. D., Sheffer, J. D., & Owens, J. (1991) Food deprivation and conditioned flavor preferences based on sweetened and unsweetened foods. *Animal Learning & Behavior, 19,* 361–368.

Capaldi, E. D., Sheffer, J. D., & Pulley, R. J. (1989). Contrast effects in flavor preference learning. *Quarterly Journal of Experimental Psychology, 41B(3),* 307–323.

Casey, R., & Rozin, P. (1989). Changing children's food preferences: Parents opinions. *Appetite, 12,* 171–182.

Deutsch, J. A., Molina, F., & Puerto, A. (1976). Conditioned taste aversion caused by palatable nontoxic nutrients. *Behavioral Biology, 16,* 161–174.

Drewnowski, A. (1988). Obesity and taste preferences for sweetness and fat. In G. A. Bray, J. LeBlanc, S. Inoue, and M. Suzuki (Eds.), *Diet and obesity* (pp. 153–161). Tokyo/Basel: Japan Scientific Societies Press/S. Karger.

Drewnowski, A. (1991). Obesity and eating disorders: Cognitive aspects of food preference and food aversion. *Bulletin of the Psychonomic Society, 29*, 261–264.

Durlach, P. J., & Rescorla, R. A. (1980). Potentiation rather than overshadowing in flavor-aversion learning: An analysis in terms of within-compound associations. *Journal of Experimental Psychology: Animal Behavior Processes, 6*, 175–187.

Elizalde, G., & Sclafani, A. (1988). Starch-based conditioned flavor preferences in rats: Influence of taste, calories and CS-US delay. *Appetite, 11*, 179–200.

Fanselow, M., & Birk, J. (1982). Flavor–flavor associations induce hedonic shifts in taste preference. *Animal Learning & Behavior, 10*, 223–228.

Flaherty, C. F., & Checke, S. (1982). Anticipation of incentive gain. *Animal Learning & Behavior, 10*, 177–182.

Garb, J. L., & Stunkard, A. J. (1974). Taste aversions in man. *American Journal of Psychiatry, 131*, 1204–1207.

Green, K. F., & Garcia, J. (1971). Recuperation from illness: Flavor enhancement in rats. *Science, 193*, 749–759.

Holman, E. W. (1975). Immediate and delayed reinforcers for flavor preferences in rats. *Animal Learning & Behavior, 6*, 91–100.

Lavin, M. J. (1976). The establishment of flavor–flavor associations using a sensory preconditioning training procedure. *Learning and Motivation, 7*, 173–183.

Lepkovsky, S. (1977). The role of the chemical senses in nutrition. In M. R. Kare & O. Maller (Eds.), *The Chemical Senses and Nutrition* (pp. 413–428). New York: Academic Press.

Lucas, G. A., & Timberlake, W. (1992). Negative anticipatory contrast and preference conditioning: Flavor cues support preference conditioning while environmental cues support contrast. *Journal of Experimental Psychology: Animal Behavior Processes, 18*, 34–40.

Lyn, S. A., & Capaldi, E. D. (1994). Robust conditioned flavor preferences with a sensory preconditioning procedure. *Psychonomic Bulletin & Review, 1*, 491–493.

Mackintosh, N. J. (1974). *The psychology of animal learning.* New York: Academic.

Mehiel, R., & Bolles, R. C. (1988). Learned flavor preferences based on calories are independent of initial hedonic value. *Animal Learning & Behavior, 16*, 383–387.

Pliner, P. Rozin, P., Cooper, M., & Woody, G. (1985). Role of specific postingestive effects and medicinal context in the acquisition of liking for tastes. *Appetite, 6*, 243–252.

Rescorla, R. A., & Cunningham, C. L. (1978). Within-compound flavor associations. *Journal of Experimental Psychology: Animal Behavior Processes, 4*, 267–275.

Revusky, S. H. (1967). Hunger level during food consumption: Effects on subsequent preference. *Psychonomic Science, 7,* 109–110.

Revusky, S., & Garcia, J. (1970). Learned associations over long delays. In G. H. Bower (Ed.), *The psychology of learning and motivation: Advances in research and theory,* (Vol. 4; pp. 1–84). New York: Academic Press.

Revusky, S. H., Smith, M. H., Jr., & Chalmers, D. V. (1971). Flavor preferences: Effects of ingestion-contingent intravenous saline or glucose. *Physiology & Behavior, 6,* 341–343.

Sclafani, A. (1990). Nutritionally based learned flavor preferences in rats. In E. D. Capaldi & T. L. Powley (Eds.), *Taste, experience and feeding* (pp. 139–156). Washington, DC: American Psychological Association.

Simbayi, L. C., Boakes, R. A., & Burton, M. J. (1986). Can rats learn to associate a flavour with the delayed delivery of food? *Appetite, 7,* 41–53.

Weingarten, H. (1983). Conditioned cues elicit eating in sated rats: A role for learning in meal initiation. *Science, 220,* 431–433.

Zahorik, D. M., & Maier, S. F. (1972). Appetitive conditioning with recovery from thiamine deficiency as the unconditional stimulus. In M. E. P. Seligman L & J. L. Hager (Eds.), *Biological boundaries of learning.* New York: Appleton-Century-Crofts.

Zellner, D. A., Rozin, P., Aron, M., & Kulish, D. (1983). Conditioned enhancement of human's liking for flavors paired with sweetness. *Learning & Motivation, 14,* 338–350.

PART THREE

How Tastes Are Developed

4

The Early Development of Human Flavor Preferences

Julie A. Mennella and Gary K. Beauchamp

T he chemical senses, that is, the senses of taste, smell, and chemical irritation, together convey information about the overall flavor of a food. These senses not only function in the human infant, but also change during development, probably as a function of both physical maturation and response to the environment. This chapter focuses on the development of taste and smell perception as it relates to the feeding behavior of infants and young children. We review the literature that suggests that the fetus and newborn infant have functioning chemosensory systems and that their feeding and expressive behaviors are modulated by taste and smell stimuli. Although these sensory systems are operable early in development, the human fetus and newborn infant are not merely miniature adults; their sensory systems mature postnatally and are likely influenced by experiences in ways not yet fully understood.

TASTE AND SMELL PERCEPTION IN THE HUMAN FETUS AND PREMATURE INFANT

Taste

The sensation of taste, or gustation, occurs when chemicals stimulate taste receptors on the tongue and other parts of the oropharynx. These receptors,

This research was supported in part by grants from the National Institute on Alcohol Abuse and Alcoholism (AA09523) and the National Institute on Deafness and Other Communication Disorders (DC00882) of the National Institutes of Health.

localized in the taste buds, are innervated by portions of the facial (VIIth), glossopharyngeal (IXth), and vagal (Xth) cranial nerves. Taste stimuli are often separated into a small number of "primary" tastes: sweet, salty, bitter, sour, and perhaps savory, that is, the taste of certain amino acids and ribonucleotides (also known as *umami taste*).

Taste cells first appear in the human fetus early in gestation, and morphologically mature cells appear at about 14 weeks (Bradley, 1972). Chemicals present in the amniotic fluid may stimulate the fetal taste receptors when the fetus begins to swallow episodically at about the 12th week of gestation (Conel, 1939; Liley, 1972; Pritchard, 1965). The chemical composition of the amniotic fluid varies over the course of gestation, particularly as the fetus begins to urinate. By term, the human fetus has swallowed significant amounts of amniotic fluid (200–760 ml daily) and has been exposed to a variety of substances including glucose, fructose, lactic acid, pyruvic acid, citric acid, fatty acids, phospholipids, creatinine, urea, uric acid, amino acids, proteins, and salts (Liley, 1972). Differential fetal swallowing following the injection of sweet or bitter substances into the amniotic fluid (DeSnoo, 1937; Liley, 1972) suggests that the fetus shows a preference for sweet and a rejection of bitter; these observations are inconclusive because of the methodological limitations in measuring fetal responses, however.

Studies on taste sensation in the preterm infant suggest that the preference for sweet taste is evidenced before birth. When preterm infants who had been fed exclusively by gastric tube were presented intraorally with small amounts of either glucose solutions or water, they exhibited more nonnutritive sucking in response to the glucose than to the water (Tatzer, Schubert, Timischl, & Simbruner, 1985). Because premature infants are at risk for aspirating fluids owing to an immature suck–swallow coordination, a method was developed that did not necessitate the delivery of any fluids while administering a taste (Maone, Mattes, Bernbaum, & Beauchamp, 1990). Rather, the taste substance was embedded in a nipple-shaped gelatin medium that released small amounts of the substance when it was mouthed or sucked. Infants born preterm and tested between 33 and 40 weeks postconception produced more frequent, stronger sucking responses when sucking on the sucrose-sweetened nipple compared with a latex nipple, thus indicating that responses to sweet tastes are evident prenatally (see Figure 1).

Newborn Infants' Suckling

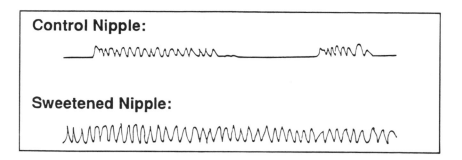

Premature Infants' Suckling

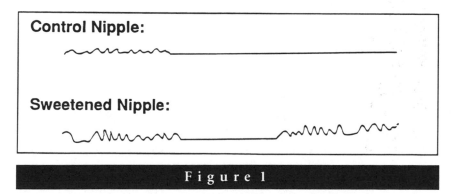

Figure 1

Sucking curves generated by a term (top two traces) and a preterm (bottom two traces) infant. Each trace represents 30 sec from a 2.5-min trial. Term infant: top, latex nipple; bottom, sucrose-flavored gelatin nipple. Preterm infant: top, latex nipple; bottom, sucrose-flavored gelatin nipple. The sweetened nipple elicited more sucking in both term and preterm infants. (Redrawn from Maone et al., 1990.)

Role of Prenatal Taste Experiences in Modifying Later Behaviors

Although the sense of taste is functional *in utero*, it is not known whether variations in experience during this period can affect later perceptions and preferences in humans. However, there are suggestive animal studies. Hill and colleagues (Hill & Mistretta, 1990; Hill & Prezekop, 1988) demonstrated that rat pups born to mothers that were severely depleted of sodium during pregnancy have altered sensitivity to salt. Specifically, the development of normal salt-receptive elements that mature in the rat postnatally is disrupted by maternal sodium depletion. Moreover, offspring of mother rats that were treated during pregnancy with a chemical that exaggerates sodium appetite and induces hormonal responses similar to those elicited by vomiting showed elevated salt appetite as young adults (Nicholaides, Galaverna, & Meltzer, 1990). Some human data are consistent with these experiments in rodents (e.g., Crystal & Bernstein, 1994), but more work is needed to validate the possibility that human individual differences in the avidity for salt are influenced by events during gestation. In view of the role of excess salt intake in blood pressure elevations, this remains an important area of research. For the other taste qualities, there are few nonhuman or human data to suggest that experience in utero influences later taste-mediated behaviors. As is discussed later in the chapter, it may be that, relative to olfaction, experience impacts less on taste sensitivity and preferences.

Olfaction

The sensation of smell, or olfaction, occurs when chemicals stimulate the olfactory receptors in the nasal cavity (see Figure 2). These receptors are located on the cilia of the neurons of cranial nerve I. Unlike the sense of taste, there may be many different classes of odor stimuli, perhaps hundreds or thousands. A family of genes that may code for a large number of receptor proteins that detect odorous compounds has been identified recently (Buck & Axel, 1991). Sensory information from the olfactory receptor neurons are projected to the main olfactory bulbs, from there to the amygdala, and then to selected diencephalic areas, many of which are involved in modulating feeding behaviors.

Odors can reach the olfactory receptors in two ways; they can either

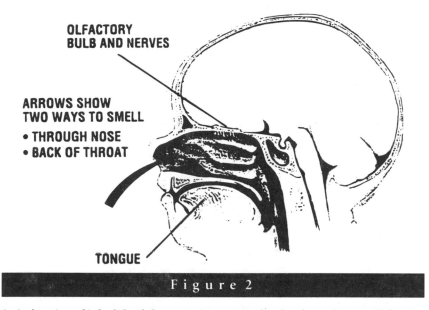

OLFACTORY
BULB AND NERVES

ARROWS SHOW
TWO WAYS TO SMELL
• THROUGH NOSE
• BACK OF THROAT

TONGUE

Figure 2

Sagittal section of infant's head demonstrating retronasal and orthonasal routes of olfaction. From *Pediatric Basics,* 65. © 1993 Gerber Products Company. Reprinted with permission.

enter the nares during inhalation (orthonasal route) or travel from the back of the nasopharynx toward the roof of the nasal cavity (retronasal route) during suckling in infants and chewing and swallowing in older children and adults (see Figure 2). Retronasal olfaction contributes significantly to the perception of flavor (Rozin, 1982). For example, holding one's nose while eating interrupts retronasal olfaction and thereby eliminates many of the subtleties of food, leaving only the taste components (sweet, salty, sour, bitter, and savory) remaining. Another example of the importance of olfaction in flavor perception is the loss of the ability to discriminate common foods when olfactory receptors are blocked by a head cold.

Although the olfactory system is well developed before birth (Arey, 1930; Bossey, 1980; Nakashima, Kimmelman, & Snow, 1985), it is not known whether the human fetus responds to olfactory stimuli. However, recent reports indicate that the environment in which the fetus lives, the amnion, can indeed be odorous. The odor of amniotic fluid not only indicates certain disease states (Mace, Goodman, Centerwall, & Chinnock, 1976) but also reflects the types of foods eaten by the pregnant mother (Hauser, Chitayat, Berbs, Braver, & Mulbauer, 1985).

In a recent study, amniotic fluid samples were obtained from 10 pregnant women who were undergoing routine amniocentesis (Mennella, Johnson, & Beauchamp, 1995). Approximately 45 minutes before the procedure, 5 of the women ingested placebo capsules, and the remaining 5 ingested capsules containing the essential oil of garlic. Randomly selected pairs of samples, one from a woman who ingested garlic and the other from a woman who ingested placebo capsules, were then evaluated by a panel of adults who were trained in sensory procedures. The odor of the amniotic fluid obtained from 4 of the 5 women who had ingested the garlic capsules was judged to be stronger or more like garlic than the paired samples collected from the women who consumed placebo capsules (see Figure 3). Thus, garlic ingestion by pregnant women significantly altered the odor of their amniotic fluid.

Because the normal fetus has open airway passages that are bathed in amniotic fluid (Schaffer, 1910) and swallows significant amounts of amniotic fluid during the latter stages of gestation, inhaling more than twice the volume it swallows (Duenholter & Pritchard, 1976; Pritchard, 1965), the fetus may be exposed to a unique olfactory environment before birth (see Schaal, Orgeur, & Rognon, 1995).

Role of Prenatal Olfactory Experiences in Modifying Later Behaviors

Studies of rodents have revealed that experiences in utero can result in olfactory preferences (see reviews by: Smotherman & Robinson, 1988; Schaal & Orgeur, 1992). For example, rat pups, born by Cesarean section, preferred their mother's fluid to that of an unrelated rat when tested immediately after birth, thus indicating this odor preference is acquired prenatally (Hepper, 1987). Moreover, the fetus can acquire information about the dietary choices of the mother as evidenced by the finding that offspring of mothers who had eaten garlic during pregnancy exhibited a preference for garlic when compared to offspring of mothers not exposed to garlic (Hepper, 1988).

Whether similar mechanisms operate in humans remains unknown, although it has been demonstrated that the human fetus can respond to a wide variety of sensory stimuli that occur naturally in its environment. For example, the fetus responds to extrauterine auditory stimuli as indicated

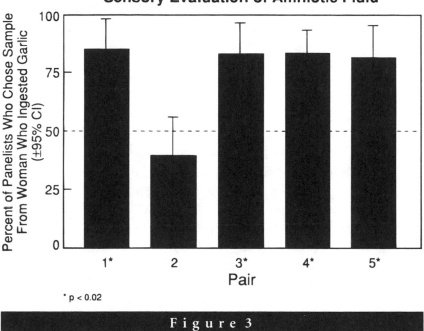

Sensory Evaluation of Amniotic Fluid

* p < 0.02

	Figure 3

Percentage of panelists who chose amniotic fluid sample obtained from pregnant woman who ingested garlic capsules as smelling stronger or more like garlic than sample obtained from woman who ingested placebo capsules. According to a forced-choice paradigm, panelists were presented individually with pairs of amniotic fluid samples, one of the pair obtained from a woman who ingested garlic capsules and the other from a woman who ingested placebo capsules. Panelists were asked to indicate which of the pair smelled "more like garlic" or "stronger." A value of 50% would be expected if there were no difference in the odor of the samples and hence the panelists responded at random. (Data represent mean ±95% CI.)

by changes in heart rate (Fifer & Moon, 1988) and blinks when a bright light source is applied to the mother's lower abdomen (Birnholtz, 1988). That prenatal sensory experiences can subsequently affect the behavior of the newborn is best illustrated by the finding that human newborns exhibit a preference for a specific voice, melody, or passage experienced prenatally (De Casper & Spence, 1986) and that they can discriminate between human voices (De Casper & Fifer, 1980; De Casper & Prescott, 1984). Research is needed to explore the olfactory memories and capabilities of the human fetus.

TASTE AND SMELL PERCEPTION DURING HUMAN INFANCY

Taste

In some of the earliest investigations of human taste development, facial expressions, suggestive of contentment and liking or discomfort and rejection, were used to assess the newborn's responsiveness to taste stimuli. During the first few hours of life, infants display relatively consistent, quality-specific facial expressions when the sweet taste of sugars (facial relaxation, sucking movements), the sour taste of concentrated citric acid (facial grimaces), and the bitter taste of concentrated quinine and urea (tongue protrusions, facial grimaces) are presented into the oral cavity (Ganchrow, Steiner, & Munif, 1983; Rosenstein & Oster, 1990; Steiner, 1977). No distinct facial response is evidenced for salt taste (Rosenstein & Oster, 1990; Steiner, 1977).

The most frequently used method to study taste preferences involves comparing how much the infant consumes of a taste solution and the diluent solution during brief presentations; these intake studies generally use weaker concentrations of taste stimuli than the studies on facial expressions mentioned previously. If the infant ingests more of the taste solution than the diluent, one can infer that (a) the infant can detect the taste, and with less certainty, (b) the infant prefers or likes the tastant more than the diluent. In most studies, the diluent was water; however, slightly sweetened water has been used as the diluent for testing the infant's response to sour and bitter tastes. Consistent with the finding for premature infants, newborn infants exhibit a strong acceptance of sweet-tasting sugars. They respond even to dilute sweet solutions and can differentiate varying degrees of sweetness (Desor, Maller, & Turner, 1977). In contrast, newborns reject the sour taste of citric acid, whereas they are apparently indifferent to the taste of low-to-moderate concentrations of salt and the bitter taste of urea (Desor, Maller, & Andrews, 1975). Finally, as was the case for premature infants, the study of the newborn infant's sucking patterns has been used as an alternative to the measurement of intake. Such studies also indicate that sweet stimuli enhance suckling and thus are positive, whereas salt taste is negative in that it suppresses sucking relative to the infant's response to the diluent alone (Crook, 1978).

Although each measure has its limitations, the convergence of research findings supports the conclusion that newborns are quite sensitive to and prefer sweet taste, whereas they reject substances having a strong sour taste. Conclusions regarding the newborn's responses to bitter and salty tastes are more problematic. Newborns respond with highly negative facial expressions to concentrated quinine and urea, but they do not reject moderate concentrations of urea (Desor, Maller, & Andrews, 1975). The reasons for this differential response remain unclear. Perhaps the newborn can detect bitter substances but the ability to reject a substance or modulate intake requires further maturation. Further studies using a variety of bitter stimuli and additional behavioral measures could resolve this question. Additionally, bitter-tasting chemicals may interact with one or more of several different transduction pathways (Spielman, Huque, Nagai, Whitney, & Brand, 1994). The newborn infant may be differentially sensitive to bitter compounds owing to different rates of maturation of these transductive sequences. With regard to salt perception, studies measuring intake and facial expressions suggest that the newborn infant is indifferent to and may not detect salt; however, salt does appear to suppress some parameters of sucking in newborns. Here, too, more research is needed to clarify the newborn's response to salt. No studies suggest that the taste of salt is attractive to the newborn infant.

Babies beyond the neonatal period have been particularly neglected in studies of taste development. Nonetheless, a few findings suggest that changes in taste responses occur during this time in development. Studies conducted in Mexico focused on the responses of well-nourished and malnourished infants, aged 2–24 months, to determine whether the protein–calorie status of the infants affected their taste preferences (Vasquez, Pearson, & Beauchamp, 1982). At all ages, both the well-nourished and malnourished infants preferred the sucrose but rejected the bitter (urea) and sour (citric acid) stimuli. The infants under the age of 1 year preferred the salty solutions to water, whereas those older than 1 year were indifferent to the salt.

The infant's salt preference is of considerable interest. Recall that newborn infants were indifferent to or rejected salt relative to plain water. The suggestion of a developmental shift in salt acceptability has been supported in more recent studies of children in the United States, in which preferential ingestion of salt water relative to plain water first emerged at approximately 4 months of age (Beauchamp, Cowart, & Moran, 1986). Additionally, studies that measured the infant's patterning of suckling as well as intake demonstrated age-related changes in the response to salt that were consistent with an increased sensitivity occurring at 3–6 months of age (Beauchamp, Cowart, Mennella, & Marsh, 1994; Harris & Booth, 1987). It has been argued that experience with salty tastes probably does not play a major role in the shift from indifference or rejection of salt at birth to acceptance in later infancy (Beauchamp & Cowart, 1990). Rather, this change in response may reflect postnatal maturation of central or peripheral mechanisms, or both, underlying salt taste perception. The salt preference that emerges at approximately 4 months of age may be largely unlearned. Finally, a recent study of the infant's sensitivity to bitter taste revealed that relatively low concentrations of urea were not rejected in newborn infants, but rejection was evident among infants who were 14–180 days of age (Kajuira, Cowart, & Beauchamp, 1992). These data are consistent with the idea that there is an early developmental change in bitter perception or the ability to regulate the intake of bitter solutions.

In summary, the sensory world of the young infant is different from that of the adult; sensitivity to several different taste stimuli appears to develop at different times postnatally. Specifically, responses to sweet tastes are evident prenatally, and major changes are not known to occur postnatally. The rejection of sour taste is evidenced from birth onward. In contrast, salt and bitter sensitivities change postnatally, with salt taste providing the clearest example. The developmental changes in salt preference may reflect changes in sensitivity that are independent of experience, or may be a consequence of specific experiences, or both.

Role of Early Taste Experiences in Modifying Later Behaviors

There are suggestions that variations in sodium status during postnatal development can affect later responsiveness to salt taste. Studies with rats have demonstrated that an episode of sodium depletion produces a permanent elevation in salt appetite, and this effect has been reported to be especially robust if the depletion occurs during early development (Frankmann, Dorsa, Sakai, & Simpson, 1986; Sakai, Fine, Epstein, &

Frankmann, 1987). In humans, a variety of clinical studies suggest that early sodium depletion may predispose the individual to excessive salt consumption later in life (see the review by Beauchamp & Cowart, 1993). Moreover, analysis of salt avidity in children who were exposed to chloride-deficient diets as infants (which, in turn, resulted in sodium deficiency) indicated that the children had heightened preferences for salty foods, relative to unexposed siblings (Beauchamp & Cowart, 1993).

These data, along with those on the effects of salt balance during pregnancy as described previously, lead one to suggest that the preference for salt (and perhaps sensitivity to it as well) can be influenced by experiential events to a substantial degree. For the other taste qualities, evidence for major effects of experience is less extensive. Infants fed sweetened water during the first several months of life exhibited a greater preference for sweetened water at 2 years of age than did infants who had little or no experience with sweetened water (Beauchamp & Moran, 1985). This effect of experience was specific to the particular beverage and did not generalize to other sweetened foods, however. Finally, it has been reported anecdotally that young infants fed protein hydrolysate formulas, which because of the presence of some free amino acids are more bitter and less palatable than normal formula (Mennella & Beauchamp, 1996), were much more willing to accept such formula later in infancy and even in childhood than were infants who did not have this early experience. Whether this anecdote is true and, if it is, whether this rejection is due to the taste or odor properties, which are also different in the hydrolyzed formula, is currently under investigation at the Monell Chemical Senses Center.

Olfaction

Shortly after birth, human infants can detect and discriminate among a wide variety of volatile chemicals and are capable of complex associative learning with odors (see Leon, 1992; Schaal, 1988; Wilson & Sullivan, 1994, for reviews). Perhaps the most salient of odors for the newborn infant are those originating from the mother (MacFarlane, 1975). Within hours after birth, mothers and infants can recognize each other through the sense of smell alone (see Schaal, 1988, for a review). Breast-fed infants spent more time orienting toward a breast pad previously worn by their lactating mothers than one worn by an unfamiliar lactating woman (Schaal, 1986, 1988).

They moved their head and arms less and sucked more when they were exposed to their mothers' odors (Schaal, 1986). This ability of breast-fed infants to discriminate the odors of their mothers from those of other lactating women is not limited to odors emanating from the breast region; they can also discriminate odors originating from their mothers' underarms (Cernoch & Porter, 1985) and neck (Schaal, 1986). Moreover, newborns preferred their mothers' breast unwashed compared to thoroughly washed and thereby devoid of some of its odors (Varendi, Porter, & Winberg, 1994). As in other mammalian young, therefore, the orthonasal perception of maternal odors may play a role in guiding the human infant to the nipple area and in facilitating early nipple attachment and suckling.

Researchers failed to demonstrate that newborn bottle-fed infants can identify their mothers on the basis of odor alone (Cernoch & Porter, 1985; Schaal, 1986). It has been suggested that breast-fed infants are able to discriminate these odors because they, unlike bottle-fed infants, have prolonged periods of skin contact with their mothers, and their nostrils are in close proximity to their mothers' breasts and underarms during breast feeding (Cernoch & Porter, 1985). Recent evidence suggests that bottle-fed infants also prefer the breast odors of an unfamiliar lactating woman to the breast odors of a nonparturient woman, however (Makin & Porter, 1989). Thus, breast odors, or perhaps the volatile components of breast milk, may be particularly attractive to all human newborns. It has been suggested that the newborn's preference for such odors is due to similarities in the aromatic profile of breast milk and amniotic fluid (Stafford, Horning, & Zlatkis, 1976; Schaal, 1988).

TRANSFER OF VOLATILES TO MOTHER'S MILK AND THE ROLE OF EARLY EXPERIENCE

The retronasal route of olfaction also may be particularly salient for infants, allowing them to experience the many odors present in their mothers' milk. Studies of other mammals have revealed that a wide variety of flavors can be transmitted from the mother's diet to her milk, which, in turn, alters the milk flavor and later preferences of her young. Recent research in our laboratory has focused on human milk as a medium for early sensory experiences for the infant. In the following section, this literature is reviewed and the more recent findings on the human mother–infant dyad are discussed.

Animal Model Studies

In 1757, a treatise was published that described how cows that were fed beets and turnips produced a bitter-flavored milk (Bradley, 1757). Whether this observation represented an actual change in the taste or odor of the milk remains unknown. Since that time, there have been numerous reports that a variety of odors from various feeds (e.g., silage, rye) and weeds (e.g., garlic, onion) eaten by the cow or from the air it breathes can be transmitted to the milk while it is in the udder (Babcock, 1938; Bassette, Fung, & Mantha, 1986). Some of the volatile components associated with these flavors, such as dimethyl sulfide, have been identified (Shipe et al., 1978). Perhaps the most common and readily recognized transmitted off-flavor is produced when the cow eats and grazes on wild garlic or onions.

Research on other mammals suggests that the young develop preferences for the flavors of the foods eaten by the mother during nursing. The growth rate of weanling pigs improved when a flavor that had been incorporated into the sow's feed during lactation was added to the weanling's feed (Campbell, 1976). Moreover, weanling animals actively seek and prefer the flavor of the diet eaten by the mother during nursing (e.g., Bilkó, Altbacker, & Hudson, 1994; Capretta & Rawls, 1974; Galef & Sherry, 1973; Hunt, Kraebel, Rabine, Spear, & Spear, 1993) and are more likely to accept unfamiliar flavors if they experience a variety of different flavors during the nursing period (Capretta, Petersik, & Steward, 1975). Although the milk was not evaluated before and after the lactating females consumed the flavor or flavors, the research does suggest that the young animals were learning through flavor cues in the mother's milk rather than from other sensory cues present in the mother's breath or body odor or from food particles clinging to the mother's fur or vibrissae (Galef & Henderson, 1972; Nolte & Provenza, 1991; Wuensch, 1978). Most of the aforementioned studies evaluated the young animal's preference for a short period of time during weaning. Although some of these preferences were short-lived (Galef & Henderson, 1972), stronger and more persistent preferences were evidenced when the young animal was exposed to the flavors during both nursing and the postweaning period (Capretta & Rawls, 1974). Whether there are sensitive periods for exposure to flavors in mother's milk remain unknown (see Provenza & Balph, 1987).

At weaning, the young animal is faced with learning what to eat and how to forage. An important factor influencing the weanling's dietary choices appears to be exposure to the diet of adult conspecifics (Galef, 1971). Although pups are attracted to the feeding site of adult conspecifics (Galef & Clark, 1971, 1972), the mother appears to be more important than other conspecifics in influencing the dietary habits of her offspring. Lambs that ate mountain mahogany with their mothers formed more persistent prefer-ences for mountain mahogany than did lambs exposed to the shrub in the absence of their mother (Nolte, Provenza, & Balph, 1990). Similarly, lambs that ate novel foods with their mothers consumed approximately twice as much of these foods after weaning than did lambs that ate the foods with a dry ewe (Thorhalldottir, Provenza, & Balph, 1990). In summary, exposure to flavors in mother's milk may be one of several ways in which the mother teaches her young what foods are "safe" (Rozin, 1976). Consequently, young animals may tend to choose a diet similar to that of their mothers when faced with their first solid meal.

Human Studies

In a study of the flavor properties of human milk (Barker, 1980; McDaniel, 1980), milk samples were collected from 24 lactating women during the morning hours on three consecutive days. Within 3 hours of expression, a trained sensory panel evaluated the milk samples for the taste quality of sweetness and for textural properties such as viscosity and mouth-coating. Each of these sensory attributes varied from mother to mother, with the primary taste quality of the milk being its sweetness. The sensory panelists also reported that off-flavors were present in some of the samples. Of particular interest was the finding that panelists used the verbal descriptors hot, spicy, and peppery to describe the milk of one woman who had consumed a "spicy" meal during the test period. Thus, the types and intensity of flavors experienced by infants in their mothers' milk may be unique.

Flavor of Garlic

More recent studies have systematically explored whether flavors from wom-en's diets are transmitted to their milk and what effects, if any, this has on the behavior of their breast-fed infants (Mennella & Beauchamp, 1991a). Mothers and their exclusively breast-fed infants were tested on 2 days separated by 1 week. On one testing day, the mother ingested garlic capsules, whereas on the other testing day, she ingested placebo capsules. Each infant fed on demand, was weighed immediately before and after each feeding to determine the amount of milk consumed, and was videotaped to determine total time attached to its mother's nipples. Milk samples, obtained from each woman at fixed intervals before and after the ingestion of the capsules, were evaluated by a sensory panel of adults within hours of expression.

As in other mammals, volatiles from women's diets are transmitted to their milk. Maternal garlic ingestion significantly and consistently increased the perceived intensity of the milk odor; this increase in odor intensity peaked in strength 2 hours after ingestion and decreased thereafter (see Figure 4). There was no perceived change in the odor of the milk on the days the mothers ingested the placebo capsules. The infants breast-fed longer and sucked more when the milk smelled like garlic compared to when this flavor was absent, suggesting that they detected the sensory change in their mothers' milk. There was a tendency for the infants to ingest more milk when it was garlic-flavored as well.

Another study revealed that repeated consumption of garlic by nursing mothers modified their infants' response to garlic-flavored milk (Mennella & Beauchamp, 1993b). The infants of mothers who had repeatedly consumed garlic capsules breast-fed for similar periods of time during the 4-hour test session in which their mothers consumed garlic compared with the session in which their mothers ingested the placebo. In contrast, infants who had no or minimal exposure to garlic volatiles in their mothers' milk spent more time breast feeding when their mothers ingested garlic than when their mothers ingested the placebo (see Figure 5), thus corroborating previous findings (Mennella & Beauchamp, 1991a).

Perhaps the garlic flavor became monotonous to these infants who were repeatedly exposed to it in their mothers' milk. Over the short term, children (Birch & Deysher, 1986) and adults (Rolls, Rowe, & Rolls, 1982) report that the palatability of a food and the amount of it consumed decline following repeated consumption of that food, whereas less recently consumed foods are considered more palatable and stimulate food intake. Moreover, the garlic-flavored milk may have aroused the infants who were exposed to a

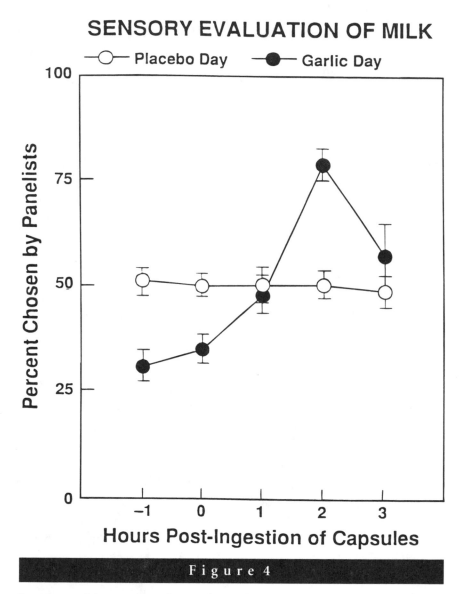

SENSORY EVALUATION OF MILK

—○— Placebo Day   —●— Garlic Day

Percent Chosen by Panelists

Hours Post-Ingestion of Capsules

Figure 4

Percentage of time panelists chose milk samples obtained before and at fixed interval after the ingestion of garlic (closed circles) and placebo (open circles) capsules. According to a forced-choice paradigm, panelists were presented individually with pairs of milk samples and asked to indicate which of the pair smelled "more like garlic" or "stronger." A value of 50% would be expected if there were no difference in the odor of the samples and hence the panelists responded at random. (Data represent mean ±SEM.) (Reprinted with permission from *Pediatrics*, 1991, *88*: 747–744.)

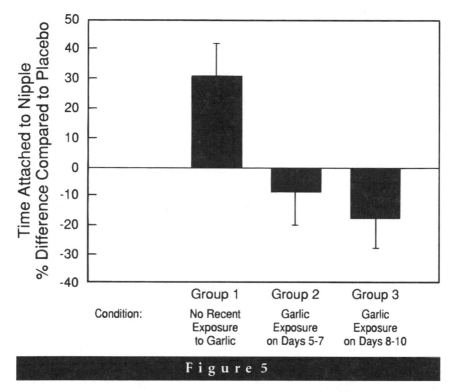

Figure 5

Percent difference in the amount of time infants were attached to nipple during 4-hour testing session in which mothers consumed garlic capsules (Day 11) versus placebo capsules (Day 4). Group 1 infants had no exposure to garlic capsules during Test Days 1–10. Group 2 infants had exposure to garlic capsules on Days 5–7 of the experimental period, and Group 3 infants had exposure to garlic capsules during Days 8–10. Each mother–infant dyad participated in the study for 11 days. The infants' behaviors were monitored on 2 separate days: on Day 4 when their mothers ingested placebo capsules and on Day 11 when she ingested garlic capsules. From J. Mennella and G. K. Beauchamp, "The Effects of Repeated Exposure to Garlic-Flavored Milk on Nursing Behavior," *Pediatric Research 34*, 805–808. Reprinted with permission.

diet of mother's milk relatively low in flavor, garliclike compounds, or both. When aroused, mammalian infants suck more (Bridger, 1962) and exhibit a variety of other oral behaviors (Korner, Chuck, & Dontchos, 1968; Terry & Johanson, 1987). This enhanced suckling time did not result in an increase in milk intake, however. The absence of an effect on the infant's milk intake may reflect milk availability, infant capacity, or both. Nonetheless, these findings suggest that the sensory attributes of mother's milk contribute to the patterning and duration of suckling at the breast.

Flavor of Vanilla

Some authorities have recently recommended that vanilla be added to follow-on formulas intended for infants who are beginning the weaning process, reportedly for both its flavoring properties and its ability to provide variety to the bottle-fed infant's otherwise "bland" diet (Food Advisory Committee, 1992). Additionally, vanilla-flavored pacifiers are currently being distributed in some hospitals. Consequently, two experiments were designed to investigate the breast- and formula-fed infants' responses to vanilla flavors in either mother's milk or formula, respectively (Mennella & Beauchamp, 1996). Consistent with what was reported previously with garlic, after nursing mothers' consumed vanilla flavor, their infants breast-fed longer and consumed more milk. An adult panel verified that the vanilla odor was apparent in the milk 1–2 hours after the mothers' consumption of the vanilla (Mennella & Beauchamp, 1994).

When studying how a change in the flavor of mother's milk affects the behavior of the infant at the breast, it is difficult to separate the direct effects on the infant from other possible influences the consumed flavors could have on the mother (e.g., changes in the odor of the mother's breath or sweat; see Mennella & Beauchamp, 1991a, for further discussion). Consequently, one cannot unequivocally conclude that the flavor change in the mother's milk was responsible for the alteration of the infant's suckling behavior. To examine this issue directly, one could study breast-fed infants' suckling response when feeding on mother's milk (unaltered or flavored) from a bottle. However, there are several methodological constraints with this approach, and many breast-fed infants do not have experience consuming mother's milk from a bottle (Auerbach & Danner, 1988).

The second experiment was designed to investigate only the effects of vanilla flavoring on exclusively formula-fed infants' feeding behaviors by adding the flavor directly into the infants' formula. Consistent with what was found for breast-fed infants, the bottle-fed infants' response to the flavored formula was altered relative to their response to the unflavored formula. In the first, short-term preference test, the infants sucked more vigorously when feeding on the vanilla-flavored formula, and in the second test, which encompassed an entire feeding, they spent more time feeding on the first bottle when it contained the vanilla flavor (Mennella & Beau-champ, 1996).

Why did the infants respond to the vanilla-flavored milk by enhanced suckling? As mentioned previously, the nursing mothers were asked to eat bland diets devoid of vanilla flavor during the 3 days preceding each testing day. Formula-feeding mothers clearly were providing a monotonous diet because formula is virtually unchanging. Perhaps the novelty was sufficient to induce increased suckling. Alternatively, the flavor of vanilla may be inherently positive as a result of either prior exposure (an unlikely explana-tion for the formula-fed infants although in utero experience is possible) or, like preference for sweet taste, a hard-wired (innate) response.

These data, along with those reported previously (Mennella & Beau-champ, 1991a, 1991b, 1993a, 1993b), demonstrate that infants can detect flavors either added to formula or transmitted to human milk from their mothers' diet and that experience with a flavor in either medium can alter how they respond to that flavor in subsequent feedings. Whether experience with vanilla-flavored pacifiers affects the infant's acceptance of similarly flavored mother's milk or formula needs to be examined experimentally.

Flavor of Alcohol

The complexities of flavor transfer from the mother to her infant, and the possible effects on the infant's suckling behaviors, are further exemplified in studies of maternal alcohol consumption. For centuries, lactating women have been given advice about drinking alcohol. Although some advisors claimed that the most frequent source of acquired alcoholism was exposure to alcohol in mother's milk, others recommended that the mother or wet nurse drink alcoholic beverages, especially beer, to increase her milk supply and strengthen her breast-feeding infant (Robinovitch, 1903; Routh, 1879). In response to the latter folklore, beer companies marketed low-alcoholic beers, or "tonics," during the early 1900s as a means for women to stimulate their appetite, increase their strength, and enhance their milk yield (Krebs, 1953).

Using methods similar to that described previously for garlic and vanilla, it was found that the odor of human milk is altered when nursing women drink a small dose of alcohol in orange juice (Mennella & Beauchamp,

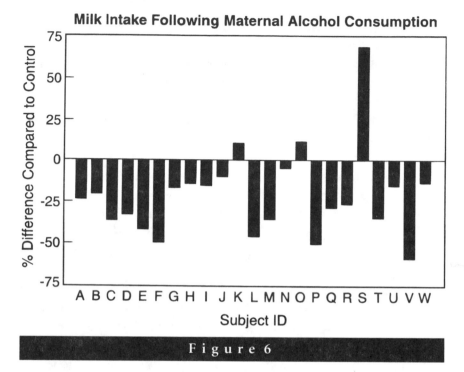

Figure 6

Percent difference in amount of milk consumed by infants during the testing session in which their mother ingested an alcoholic beverage versus a nonalcoholic beverage. Twenty of 23 infants consumed less milk when the milk was flavored with alcohol. (Data from Mennella & Beauchamp, 1991b and 1993a, combined.)

1991b) or in the form of beer (Mennella & Beauchamp, 1993a). The sensory change in the milk parallels the changing concentrations of ethanol in the milk. It was also found that, contrary to the folklore, breast-fed infants consumed less milk during the 3–4 hours after their nursing mothers drank a small dose of alcohol (see Figure 6; Mennella & Beauchamp, 1991b; 1993a).

Several factors could account for this decrease in milk intake. First, the infants may be responding to the change in the flavoring of their mothers' milk; that is, for reasons as yet unknown, the flavor of alcohol may be relatively unpalatable. This explanation seems unlikely, however, because low levels of alcohol as evidenced in the milk are often described as sweet and pleasant (Mennella & Beauchamp, 1991b).

A second explanation, that the depression in milk intake was due to a pharmacological effect of alcohol on the infant, is also unlikely because the infants tended to consume less milk during the first feeding that followed their mothers' consumption of an alcoholic beverage (Mennella & Beauchamp, 1993a). Whether short-term exposure to small amounts of alcohol affects the infants in other ways requires further study.

A third explanation is that the decrease in the infants' milk intake may represent a pharmacological effect of alcohol on the nursing mothers; that is, ethanol consumption may affect the milk-ejection reflex (but see Cobo, 1973). Moreover, ethanol consumption may alter the composition of milk such that infants consume less milk but take in the same number of calories. Chronic ethanol consumption by lactating rats during both pregnancy and lactation resulted in milk that was higher in lipid and lower in lactose content compared to the milk of control rat mothers (Vilaró, Viñas, Remesar, & Herrera, 1987). Because no alteration in protein or water content was observed, the milk of ethanol-exposed rats had a higher energy content owing to the greater energetic value of lipids compared to proteins and lactose. Whether this altered milk composition was a direct consequence of ethanol intake or caused by malnutrition is not known. Nor is it known whether ethanol intake, in the short term, has similar effects on milk composition and yield in humans or whether, by relaxing the mother, it facilitates the ejection of milk from the breast. Future research is needed to address these issues.

CLINICAL IMPLICATIONS AND CONCLUSION

The sensory world of an infant is different from that of a child or an adult. Moreover, the sensory world of a newborn infant is different from that of a 6-month-old infant. In adults, the senses of taste, retronasal olfaction, and oral irritation appear to fuse into one sensory gestalt, that of flavor. It is not known whether the same is true for the infant. Certainly, the balance of these three systems may be different for infants, with relative insensitivity to some taste components (e.g., salt, some bitter compounds) combined with adultlike or perhaps even heightened sensitivity to others (e.g., odors, perhaps irritants).

Food habits and preferences are said to be among the last characteristics of a culture to be lost during the immigration of an individual or group into a new culture (Rozin, 1980). Although this seems to imply that the kinds of foods chosen are firmly established early in life, there is little evidence to support this contention (see reviews by Ray & Klesges, 1993; Rozin, 1984). For example, similarities between the food preferences of children and their parents are often small (Birch, 1980; Burt and Hertzler, 1978; Pliner & Pelchat, 1986), and there is some evidence in primates, including humans, that younger individuals are more willing to sample novel foods (see review by Beauchamp & Maller, 1977).

How can these seemingly contradictory tendencies be reconciled? Low levels of positive correlation between the food preferences of parents, especially the mother, and their children may not mean that early experience has no effect on later flavor choice and preferences. As noted, the sensory systems of infants, children, and adults are different, so that one might not expect similar choices even if there were experiential effects of exposure. Second, there is no standardized method of measuring what constitutes a food preference agreement (Birch, 1980; also see review by Ray & Klesges, 1993). Moreover, no studies to our knowledge have evaluated the preferences for flavors, rather than foods, within and between families. Family studies need to be done to evaluate both the kinds of flavors preferred, chosen, or avoided and the intensity of the flavors most preferred, and such research should assess the child's preferences directly, because mothers' accounts of their children's preferences are often inaccurate and biased (see Birch, 1980). Finally, experimental studies, even with animal models, have often neglected the very early exposure to flavors that occurs *in utero* and through mother's milk.

Our research demonstrates that human milk is not a food of invariant flavor but one that provides the potential for a rich source of varying chemosensory experiences to the infant (Mennella & Beauchamp, 1991a, 1991b, 1993a, 1994). Moreover, the prior flavor experiences of mothers and, consequently, of their infants may modify the infants' responses to these flavors. These findings might imply that the sensory world of breast-fed infants is rich, varied, and quite different from that of bottle-fed infants, who experience a constant set of flavors from standard formulas and thus may be missing significant sensory experiences that, until recent times in human history, were common to all infants. As we have suggested (Mennella, 1995; Mennella & Beauchamp, 1991a, 1993b, 1996), early sensory experiences may be particularly important in human development, and the advent of formula feeding may not only deprive infants of important immunological and perhaps psychological benefits (see review by Goldman, Atkinson, & Hanson, 1987), but also limit their exposure to an important source of information and education about the flavor world of their mother, family, and culture.

We have also discovered that amniotic fluid is a potential flavor carrier (Mennella, Johnson, & Beauchamp 1995). Because amniotic fluid and mother's milk are under the common priming of maternal diets, their aromatic profiles may overlap and serve as a "thread of chemical continuity between the pre- and postnatal niches" (Schaal & Orgeur, 1992). Whether the apparent redundancy in exposure to flavors in amniotic fluid and mother's milk ensures that the human infant can acquire preferences for a variety of foods eaten by the mother during different stages of development (see Bilkó, Altbacker, & Hudson, 1994; Capretta, Petersik, & Steward, 1975) is clearly an area in which further research is needed. These questions not only have ramifications for understanding the development of food habits, but are also relevant for understanding such nutritional concerns as excessive salt and fat consumption, which may lead to hypertension and obesity, respectively, and the effects of early exposure to drugs such as alcohol and tobacco on later preferences.

REFERENCES

Arey, L. B. (1930). *Developmental anatomy: A textbook and laboratory manual of embryology.* Philadelphia: Saunders.

Auerbach, K. G., & Danner S. C. (1988). Measuring sucking patterns [Letter]. *Journal of Pediatrics, 112,* 159.

Babcock, C. J. (1938). Feed flavors in milk and milk products. *Journal of Dairy Science, 21,* 661–667.

Barker, E. (1980). *Sensory evaluation of human milk.* Unpublished masters thesis, University of Manitoba, Winnipeg, Canada.

Bassette, R., Fung, D. Y. C., & Mantha, V. R. (1986). Off-flavors in milk. *CRC Critical Reviews in Food Science and Nutrition, 24,* 1–52.

Beauchamp, G. K., & Cowart, B. J. (1990). Preferences for high salt concentrations among children. *Developmental Psychology, 26,* 539–545.

Beauchamp, G. K., & Cowart, B. J. (1993). Development of salt taste responses in human newborns, infants and children. In *Development, Growth and Senescence in the Chemical Senses* (NIH Publication No. 93-3483, 3, pp. 61–68). Washington DC: U.S. Department of Health and Human Services.

Beauchamp, G. K., Cowart, B. J., Mennella, J. A., & Marsh, R. R. (1994). Infant salt taste: Developmental, methodological and contextual factors. *Developmental Psychobiology, 27*, 353–365.

Beauchamp, G. K., Cowart, B. J., & Moran M. (1986). Developmental changes in salt acceptability in human infants. *Developmental Psychobiology, 19*, 17–25.

Beauchamp, G. K., & Maller O. (1977). The development of flavor preferences in humans: a review. In M. R. Kare & O. Maller, (Eds.), *The chemical senses and nutrition.* (pp. 291–311). San Diego, CA: Academic Press.

Beauchamp, G. K., & Moran M. (1985). Acceptance of sweet and salty taste in 2-year-old children. *Appetite, 5*, 291–305.

Bilkó, A., Altbacker, V., & Hudson, R. (1994). Transmission of food preference in the rabbit: the means of information transfer. *Physiology and Behavior, 56*, 907–912.

Birch, L. L. (1980). The relationship between children's food preferences and those of their parents. *Journal of Nutrition Education, 12*, 14–18.

Birch, L. L., & Deysher, M. (1986). Caloric compensation and sensory specific satiety: Evidence for self-regulation of food intake by young children. *Appetite, 7*, 323–331.

Birnholtz, J. C. (1988). On observing the human fetus. In W. P. Smotherman & S. R. Robinson (Eds.), *Behavior of the fetus* (pp. 47–60). Caldwell, NJ: Telford Press.

Bossey, J. (1980). Development of olfactory and related structures in staged human embryos. *Anatomy and Embryology (Berlin), 161*, 225–236.

Bradley, R. A. (1757). *A general treatise of agriculture.* London: W. Johnston.

Bradley, R. M. (1972). Development of the taste bud and gustatory papillae in human fetuses. In J. F. Bosma (Ed.), *The third symposium on oral sensation and perception: The mouth of the infant.* Springfield, IL: Charles C. Thomas.

Bridger, W. H. (1962). Ethological concepts and human development. *Recent Advances in Biological Psychiatry, 4*, 95–107.

Buck, L., & Axel, R. (1991). A novel multigene family may encode for odorant receptors: A molecular basis for odor recognition. *Cell, 65*, 175–187.

Burt, J. V., & Hertzler, A. A. (1978). Parental influence on the child's food preference. *Journal of Nutrition Education, 10*, 127–130.

Campbell, R. G. (1976). A note on the use of feed flavour to stimulate the feed intake of weaner pigs. *Animal Production, 23*, 417–419.

Capretta, P. J., Petersik, J. T., & Stewart, D. J. (1975). Acceptance of novel flavours is increased after early experience of diverse taste. *Nature, 254*, 689–691.

Capretta, P. J., & Rawls, L. H. (1974). Establishment of a flavor preference in rats: Importance of nursing and weaning experience. *Journal of Comparative and Physiological Psychology, 86*, 670–673.

Cernoch, J. M., & Porter, R. H. (1985). Recognition of maternal axillary odors by infants. *Child Development, 56*, 1593–1598.

Cobo, E. (1973). Effect of different doses of ethanol on the milk-ejecting reflex in lactating women. *American Journal of Obstetrics and Gynecology, 115*, 817–821.

Conel, J. L. (1939). *The post-natal development of the human cerebral cortex: I. Cortex of the newborn*. Cambridge, MA: Harvard University Press.

Crook, C. K. (1978). Taste perception in the newborn infant. *Infant Behavior and Development, 1*, 52–69.

Crystal, S., & Bernstein, I. (1994, August). Morning sickness: Impact on offspring salt preference. Abstract presented at the meeting of the Society for the Study of Ingestive Behavior, McMaster University, Canada.

De Casper, A. J., & Fifer, W. (1980). Of human bonding: Newborns prefer their mothers' voices. *Science, 208*, 1174–1176.

De Casper, A. J., & Prescott, P. A. (1984). Human newborn's perception of male voices: Preference, discrimination and reinforcing value. *Developmental Psychobiology, 17*, 481–491.

De Casper, A. J., & Spence, M. J. (1986). Newborns prefer a familiar song over an unfamiliar one. *Infant Behavior and Development, 9*, 133–150.

DeSnoo, K. (1937). Das trinkende kind in uterus. *Monatssch fur Gebürtshilfe Gynaekol, 105*, 88–97.

Desor, J. A., Maller, O., & Andrews, K. (1975). Ingestive responses of human newborns to salty, sour and bitter stimuli. *Journal of Comparative and Physiological Psychology, 89*, 966–970.

Desor, J. A., Maller, O., & Turner, R. E. (1977). Preference for sweet in humans: Infants, children and adults. In J. M. Weiffenbach (Ed.), *Taste and development: The genesis of sweet preference*. Washington, DC: U.S. Government Printing Office.

Duenholter, J. H., & Pritchard, J. A. (1976). Fetal respiration: Quantitative measurements of amniotic fluid inspired near term by human and rhesus fetuses. *American Journal of Obstetrics and Gynecology, 125,* 306–309.

Fifer, W. P., & Moon, C. (1988). Auditory experience in the fetus. In W. P. Smotherman & S. R. Robinson (Eds.), *Behavior of the fetus* (pp. 175–188). Caldwell, NJ: Telford Press.

Food Advisory Committee. (1992). *Report on the review of additives in foods specially prepared for infants and children.* (FdAC/REP/12. MAFF, HMSO) London.

Frankmann, S. P., Dorsa, D. M., Sakai, R. R., & Simpson, J. B. (1986). A single experience with hyperoncotic colloid dialysis persistently alters water and sodium intake. In J. M. Weiffenbach (Ed.), *The physiology of thirst and sodium appetite* (pp. 161–172). Washington, DC: U.S. Government Printing Office.

Galef, B. G. (1971). Social effects in the weaning of domestic rat pups. *Journal of Comparative and Physiological Psychology, 75,* 358–362.

Galef, B. G., & Clark, M. M. (1971). Social factors in the poison avoidance and feeding behavior of wild and domesticated rat pups. *Journal of Comparative and Physiological Psychology, 75,* 341–357.

Galef, B. G., & Clark, M. M. (1972). Mother's milk and adult presence: Two factors determining initial dietary selection by weanling rats. *Journal of Comparative and Physiological Psychology, 78,* 220–225.

Galef, B. G., & Henderson, P. W. (1972). Mother's milk: A determinant of the feeding preferences of weaning rat pups. *Journal of Comparative and Physiological Psychology, 78,* 213–219.

Galef, B. G., & Sherry, D. F. (1973). Mother's milk: A medium for transmission of cues reflecting the flavor of mother's diet. *Journal of Comparative and Physiological Psychology, 83,* 374–378.

Ganchrow, J. R., Steiner, J. E., & Munif, D. (1983). Neonatal facial expressions in response to different qualities and intensities of gustatory stimuli. *Infant Behavior and Development, 6,* 473–484.

Goldman, A. S., Atkinson, S. A., & Hanson, L. Å. (Eds.). (1987). *Human lactation: 3. The effects of human milk on the recipient infant.* New York: Plenum Press.

Harris, G., & Booth, D. A. (1987). Infants' preference for salt in food: Its dependence upon recent dietary experience. *Journal of Reproductive and Infant Psychology, 5,* 97–104.

Hauser, G. J., Chitayat, D., Berbs, L., Braver, D., & Mulbauer B. (1985). Peculiar odors in newborns and maternal pre-natal ingestion of spicy foods. *European Journal of Pediatrics, 44,* 403.

Hepper, P. G. (1987). The amniotic fluid: An important priming role in kin recognition. *Animal Behavior, 35,* 1343–1346.

Hepper, P. G. (1988). Adaptive fetal learning: Prenatal exposure to garlic affects postnatal preferences. *Animal Behavior, 36,* 935–936.

Hill, D. L., & Mistretta, C. M. (1990). Developmental neurobiology of salt taste sensations. *Trends in Neuroscience, 13,* 188–195.

Hill, D. L., & Prezekop, O. R. (1988). Influences of dietary sodium on functional taste receptor development: A sensitive period. *Science, 241,* 1826–1828.

Hunt, P. S., Kraebel, K. S., Rabine, H., Spear, L. P., & Spear, N. E. (1993). Enhanced ethanol intake in preweanling rats following exposure to ethanol in a nursing context. *Developmental Psychobiology, 26,* 133–153.

Kajuira, H., Cowart, J., & Beauchamp, G. K. (1992). Early developmental changes in bitter taste responses in human infants. *Developmental Psychobiology, 25,* 375–386.

Korner, A. F., Chuck, B., & Dontchos, S. (1968). Organismic determinants of spontaneous oral behavior in neonates. *Child Development, 39,* 1145–1157.

Krebs, R. (1953). *Making friends is our business: 100 years of Anheuser-Busch.* St. Louis, MO: A-B Inc.

Leon, M. (1992). The neurobiology of filial learning. *Annual Review of Psychology, 43,* 77–98.

Liley, A. W. (1972). Disorders of amniotic fluid. In N. S. Assali (Ed.), *Pathophysiology of gestation: Fetal placental disorders (Vol. 2).* San Diego, CA: Academic Press.

Mace, J. W., Goodman, S. I., Centerwall, W. R., & Chinnock, R. F. (1976). The child with an unusual odor: A clinical resumé. *Clinical Pediatrics, 15,* 57–62.

MacFarlane, A. J. (1975). Olfaction in the development of social preferences in the human neonate. *Ciba Foundation Symposium, 33,* 103–117.

Makin, J. W., & Porter, R. H. (1989). Attractiveness of lactating females' breast odors to neonates. *Child Development, 60,* 803–810.

Maone, T. R., Mattes, R. D., Bernbaum, J. C., & Beauchamp, G. K. (1990). A new method for delivering a taste without fluids to preterm and term infants. *Developmental Psychobiology, 23,* 179–191.

McDaniel, M. R. (1980). Off-flavors in human milk. In G. Charalambous (Ed.), *The analysis and control of less desirable flavors in foods and beverages* (pp. 267–291). San Diego, CA: Academic Press.

Mennella, J. A. (1995). Mother's milk: A medium for early flavor experiences. *Journal of Human Lactation, 11,* 39–45.

Mennella, J. A., & Beauchamp, G. K. (1991a). Maternal diet alters the sensory qualities of human milk and the nursling's behavior. *Pediatrics, 88,* 737–744.

Mennella, J. A., & Beauchamp, G. K. (1991b). The transfer of alcohol to human milk: Effects on flavor and the infant's behavior. *New England Journal of Medicine, 325,* 981–985.

Mennella, J. A., & Beauchamp, G. K. (1993a). Beer, breast feeding and folklore. *Developmental Psychobiology, 26,* 459–466.

Mennella J. A., & Beauchamp, G. K. (1993b). The effects of repeated exposure to garlic-flavored milk on the nursling's behavior. *Pediatric Research, 34,* 805–808.

Mennella, J. A., & Beauchamp, G. K. (1994). The infant's responses to flavored milk. *Infant Behavior and Development, 17,* 819.

Mennella, J. A., & Beauchamp, G. K. (1996). The contribution of taste and olfaction to the flavor properties of milk-based, soy-based, and protein hydrolysate formulas. Unpublished raw data.

Mennella, J. A., & Beauchamp, G. K. (1996). The infant's responses to vanilla flavors in mother's milk and formula. *Infant Behavior and Development,* 13–19.

Mennella, J. A., Johnson, A., & Beauchamp, G. K. (1995). Garlic ingestion by pregnant women alters the odor of amniotic fluid. *Chemical Senses, 20,* 207–209.

Nakashima, T., Kimmelman, C. P., & Snow, J. B. (1985). Immunohistopathology of human olfactory epithelium, nerve and bulb. *Laryngoscope, 95,* 391–396.

Nicholaides, S., Galaverna, O., & Meltzer, C. H. (1990). Extracellular dehydration during pregnancy increases salt appetite of offspring. *American Journal of Physiology, 258,* R281–R283.

Nolte, D. L., & Provenza, F. D. (1991). Food preferences in lambs after exposure to flavors in milk. *Applied Animal Behavior Science, 32,* 381–389.

Nolte, D. L., Provenza, F. D., & Balph, D. F. (1990). The establishment and persistence of food preferences in lambs exposed to selected foods. *Journal of Animal Science, 68,* 998–1002.

Pliner, P., & Pelchat, M. L. (1986). Similarities in food preferences between children and their siblings and parents. *Appetite, 7,* 333–342.

Pritchard, J. A. (1965). Deglutition by normal and anencephalic fetuses. *Obstetrics and Gynecology, 25,* 289–297.

Provenza, F. D., & Balph, D. F. (1987). Diet learning by domestic ruminants: Theory, evidence and practical implications. *Applied Animal Behaviour Science, 18,* 211–232.

Ray, J. W., & Klesges, R. C. (1993). Influences on the eating behavior of children. *Annals of the New York Academy of Sciences, 699*, 57–69.

Robinovitch, L. G. (1903). Infantile alcoholism. *Quarterly Journal of Inebriety, 25*, 231–236.

Rolls, B. J., Rowe, E. S., & Rolls, E. T. (1982). How sensory properties of foods affect human feeding behavior. *Physiology and Behavior, 29*, 407–417.

Rosenstein, D., & Oster, H. (1990). Differential facial responses to four basic tastes in newborns. *Child Development, 59*, 1555–1568.

Routh, C. H. F. (1879). *Infant feeding and its influence on life.* New York: William Wood.

Rozin, P. (1976). The selection of food by rats, humans and other animals. In J. Rosenblatt, R. A. Hinde, C. Beer, & E. Shaw (Eds.), *Advances in the study of behaviors* (Vol. 6, pp. 21–76). San Diego, CA: Academic Press.

Rozin, P. (1980). Human food selection: Why do we know so little and what can we do about it? *International Journal of Obesity, 4*, 333–337.

Rozin, P. (1982). "Taste-smell confusions" and the duality of the olfactory sense. *Perception and Psychophysics, 31*, 397–401.

Rozin, P. (1984). The acquisition of food habits and preferences. In J. D. Mattarazzo, S. M. Weiss, J. A. Herd, N. E. Miller, & S. M. Weiss (Eds.), *Behavioral health: A handbook of health enhancement and disease prevention* (pp. 590–607). New York: Wiley.

Sakai, R. R., Fine, W. B., Epstein, A., & Frankmann, S. P. (1987). Salt appetite is enhanced by one prior episode of sodium depletion in the rat. *Behavioral Neuroscience, 101*, 724–731.

Schaal, B. (1986). Presumed olfactory exchanges between mother and neonate in humans. In J. Le Camus, & J. Conier (Eds.), *Ethology and psychology* (pp. 101–110). Toulouse: Privat IEC.

Schaal, B. (1988). Olfaction in infants and children: Development and functional perspectives. *Chemical Senses, 13*, 145–90.

Schaal, B., & Orgeur, P. (1992). Olfaction in utero: Can the rodent model be generalized? *Quarterly Journal of Experimental Psychology, 44*, 245–278.

Schaal, B., Orgeur, P., & Rognon, C. (1995). Odor sensing in the human fetus: Anatomical, functional and chemo-ecological bases. In: J. P. Lecanuet, N. A. Krasnegor, W. Fifer, & W. P. Smotherman (Eds.), *Prenatal development: Psychobiological perspectives* (pp. 205–237). Hillsdale, NJ: Lawrence Erlbaum Associates.

Schaffer, J. P. (1910). The lateral wall of the cavum nasi in man with special reference to the various developmental stages. *Journal of Morphology, 21,* 613–617.

Shipe, W. F., Bassette, R., Deane, D. D., Dunkley, W. L., Hammond, E. G., Harper, W. J., Kleyn, D. H., Morgan, M. E., Nelson, J. H., & Scanlan, R. A. (1978). Off-flavors of milk: Nomenclature, standards and bibliography. *Journal of Dairy Science, 61,* 855–868.

Smotherman, W., & Robinson, S. R. (Eds.), (1988). *Behavior of the fetus.* Caldwell, NJ: Telford Press.

Spielman, A. I., Huque, T., Nagai, H., Whitney, G., & Brand, J. G. (1994). Generation of inositol phosphates in bitter taste transduction. *Physiology and Behavior, 56,* 1149–1155.

Stafford, M., Horning, M. C., & Zlatkis, A. (1976). Profiles of volatile metabolites in bodily fluids. *Journal of Chromatography, 126,* 495–502.

Steiner, J. E. (1977). Facial expressions of the neonate infant indicating the hedonics of food-related chemical stimuli. In JM Weiffenbach (Ed.), *Taste and development: The genesis of sweet preference.* Washington, DC: U.S. Government Printing Office.

Tatzer, E., Schubert, M. T., Timischl, W., & Simbruner, G. (1985). Discrimination of taste and preference for sweet in premature babies. *Early Human Development, 12,* 23–30.

Terry, L. M., & Johanson, I. B. (1987). Olfactory influences on the ingestive behavior of infant rats. *Developmental Psychobiology, 20,* 313–332.

Thorhallsdottir, A. G., Provenza, F. D., & Balph, D. F. (1990). Ability of lambs to learn about novel foods while observing or participating with social models. *Applied Animal Behaviour Science, 25,* 25–33.

Varendi, H., Porter, R. H., & Winberg, J. (1994). Does the newborn baby find the nipple by smell? *Lancet, 334,* 989–990.

Vasquez, M., Pearson, P. B., & Beauchamp, G. K. (1982). Flavor preferences in malnourished Mexican infants. *Physiology and Behavior, 28,* 513–519.

Vilaró, S., Viñas, O., Remesar, X., & Herrera, E. (1987). Effects of chronic ethanol consumption on lactational performance in the rat: Mammary gland and milk composition and pups' growth and metabolism. *Pharmacology Biochemistry and Behavior, 27,* 333–339.

Wilson, D. A., & Sullivan, R. M. (1994). Neurobiology of associative learning in the neonate: Early olfactory learning. *Behavioral and Neural Biology, 61,* 1–18.

Wuensch, K. L. (1978). Exposure to onion taste in mother's milk leads to enhanced preference for onion diet among weanling rats. *Journal of General Psychology, 99,* 163–167.

5

The Role of Experience in the Development of Children's Eating Behavior

Leann L. Birch and Jennifer A. Fisher

I n this chapter, we present a developmental perspective in delineating the ways in which early experience shapes the controls of food intake in children. In so doing, we draw on both normative and individual-difference perspectives to describe (a) how experience supports the normal development of feeding in infants and children and (b) ways in which early experience contributes to the development of individual differences in food preferences, food-acceptance patterns, and styles of intake control that have emerged by adulthood, such as dietary restraint, chronic dieting, and eating disorders.

The recurring theme throughout this chapter is that learning is central to the development of the controls of food intake. Associative learning, which is particularly important in shaping our emotional responses to things and events, also plays a central role in the child's developing controls of food intake. For example, eating can produce positive or negative physiological consequences, and children's eating usually occurs in a social context, which can be either pleasant or unpleasant. These contexts and consequences can produce either positive or negative emotions in the child. When these responses are associated with sensory cues from foods, they shape the child's affective reaction to the food itself. In addition, there are many opportunities for children to learn that particular social and physical settings predict the presence or absence of food and eating and, in turn, that eating particular foods predicts pleasant feelings of satiety or unpleasant physiological consequences. This learning affects the timing of meals and can influence meal size.

Although energy expenditure and the demand for nutrients is continuous, eating behavior is periodic. Eating is a discrete behavioral event, and the quantity and quality of the diet depends on (a) how frequently meals are taken, or the intervals between meals, (b) how much is consumed at each meal, and (c) what foods the individual selects for consumption. Varying one or a combination of these three behavioral parameters can dramatically alter food intake and dietary quality. We have organized this review around what is known regarding the developing control of the timing of meals, meal size, and food selection.

Initially, infants are totally dependent on the caregiver for food, but they are already capable of assuming a degree of control over meal timing and meal size; however, young infants consume an exclusive milk diet, so that food selection is not an issue. During the early years of life, the controls of food intake are shared between parent and child, and developmental change entails shifts in the "balance of power" in the feeding relationship. In general, these developmental changes reflect children's increasing control and autonomy. We propose that individual differences among children in the controls of food intake can also be viewed in terms of differences in this balance of power in feeding. Finally, we argue that the individual differences in styles of intake control that emerge by adolescence and adulthood, including chronic dieting, eating disorders, and "out-of-control," disinhibited eating, have their beginnings in the early balance of control in the feeding context. As is described in more detail subsequently, the limited evidence suggests that the course of development of shared control differs for intermeal interval, food selection, and meal size.

In the three sections that follow, we examine how experience shapes the child's developing capacity for self-control in feeding, including control over the intervals between meals, meal size, and food selection. The review reveals that descriptive information is lacking in many areas concerning the normal development of the controls of food intake. With respect to individual differences, we present some data indicating that differences in parental control in child-feeding practices can produce individual differences in children's developing ability to control meal timing and meal size and can also have an impact on food selection.

EARLY EXPERIENCE AND THE CONTROL OF INTERMEAL INTERVAL

When food availability is not limited, free-feeding animals adjust the intervals between meals, thus taking more or fewer meals as the primary means of adjusting food intake (Le Magnen, 1985). For many human adults, however, adjusting the timing of meals is not a particularly useful strategy because cultural rules and other demands constrain the number and timing of meals. To the extent that there are restrictions on when meals can be taken, food selection and meal size become more important determinants of total food intake.

Although the adult's opportunities for adjusting meal timing may be limited, for the infant, varying intermeal intervals to take more or fewer meals is the major mechanism for controlling intake. Food selection is not an issue during early infancy; the infant consumes an exclusive milk diet. In addition, the size of feedings is somewhat limited by the infant's gastric capacity. Across cultures and throughout history, the prevailing approach to infant feeding has been to allow the infant to determine the timing of meals and to feed "on demand" when distress cues seem to indicate hunger. Only in recent history in the United States has experts' advice departed from this view: During the 1920s and 1930s, the prevailing advice was to feed infants on a strict schedule, typically with 4 hours between feedings. Over time, there has been a return to the idea that the infant should be fed "on demand." Whether parents have chosen breast or formula feeding, they are encouraged to be sensitive to the infant's cues to allow the infant to take the lead in determining when feedings will occur as well as how much is consumed at a feeding (Satter, 1990). An implicit assumption underlying demand feeding is that the infant "knows" when she is hungry and when she is full and that, given the opportunity to control meal timing and meal size, the infant will consume the quantities of milk needed to maintain growth and health.

Parents are encouraged to allow their infants control over the timing of meals as well as meal size. For formula-feeding parents, however, it is easy to monitor the infant's intake, which makes it easy for motivated parents to control how much the infant consumes at a feeding. In contrast, during breast feeding, the mother cannot readily determine how much the infant has consumed, and in the absence of such information, the mother may allow the infant greater control over the size and timing of feedings. Fomon (1993) pointed out that allowing the infant control of the size and timing of feedings creates a circumstance that is "conducive to establishing habits of eating in moderation" (p. 114). Put in other terms, demand feeding allows the infant to learn to associate meal initiation with feelings of hunger, and meal termination with normal satiety. We hypothesize that such learning is critical in shaping individual differences in styles of intake control in infancy and early childhood, although research to support this view is limited. It should be emphasized that little attention has been given to whether parents who profess to demand-feed actually allow the child to control the timing and size of feedings. Fomon (1993) argued persuasively that few infants are truly fed on demand. Failure to feed on demand may occur because the parent is not sufficiently motivated to do so owing to scheduling conflicts or because the parent has difficulty accurately differentiating whether the infants' distress cues signal hunger or other discomfort. We have been unable to locate systematic studies of the effects of demand versus schedule feeding on infants' physical growth and health.

Meal size influences the timing of meals: Large meals are associated with long intervals between meals, and small meals with shorter intermeal intervals. However, the sequential nature of the meal size and meal interval relationship changes with development (Le Magnen, 1985). In mature, free-feeding animals and in adult humans living in environments without the usual social constraints (Bernstein, 1981), the size of a meal is positively related to the time that elapses until the next meal. In this case, there is a *postprandial* relationship between meal size and intermeal interval: The size of the meal determines the period of satiation that follows the meal. However, in young animals, there are strong *preprandial* relationships between meal size and meal intervals. In this case, the size of a meal is strongly related to the duration of the previous interval; the time since the last feeding seems to dictate the volume consumed at a feeding.

When researchers examined the patterning of meals of breast-fed infants, they found that intermeal intervals were related to meal size, and these findings were consistent with developmental data from animal models. In exclusively breast-fed infants (whose parents reported feeding on demand), positive relationships between meal size and meal interval were noted. Strong preprandial relationships were seen, at least in the first 3 months of life (Matheny, Birch, & Picciano, 1990; Pinilla & Birch, 1993). In a recent study, Pinilla and Birch (1993) explored behavioral procedures to teach breast-fed infants to self-soothe and to sleep through the night (Pinilla & Birch, 1993). As periods of sleep between midnight and 5 a.m. lengthened in response to the procedures, the volume of the first morning feeding increased, so that as they began to sleep through the night, 8-week-old infants took the largest meal of the day at their early morning feeding, following the overnight fast, consistent with a preprandial relationship between meal interval and meal size.

Peter Wright and colleagues (Wright, Fawcett, & Crow, 1980) reported similar relationships between meal interval and meal size for breast-fed infants. At about 8 weeks, Wright's breast-fed infants' diurnal meal patterns revealed that their largest feeding was taken early in the morning, following the overnight fast. However, by the time the infants were 6 months old, they showed the more adultlike postprandial pattern: The size of a meal predicts the size of the subsequent intermeal interval. These older infants were taking a large feeding late at night, just before the long, overnight fast. Wright and colleagues (Wright et al., 1980) proposed that through early learning, the relationships between feeding interval and feeding size change during the first year of life from a predominantly preprandial pattern to the more mature adultlike postprandial pattern. At about 6 months of age, infants learn that certain environmental cues predict a long, overnight fast, and they begin taking a large meal before that long period without food; the size of a meal anticipates the size of the subsequent intermeal interval. In summary, in at least among breast-fed infants who are fed on demand, meal size is positively related to meal interval during infancy, but the sequential patterning of the relationship may change during early development. In early infancy, large meals are taken in response to long, overnight fasts, but by about 6 months, there is some evidence that large meals are eaten in anticipation of a long period without food, so that large meals begin to precede long, overnight fasts. These findings suggest that whereas meal size is initially a reaction to a prior period of deprivation, with development, infants may learn to adjust intake at a meal in anticipation of how long it will be until the next meal.

The relationships between meal size and meal interval that were observed in breast-fed infants were not obtained for formula-fed infants (Wright et al., 1980). Formula-fed infants' meal sizes were not related to intermeal intervals, and they did not show the diurnal patterns in meal size seen in breast-fed infants. Wright and colleagues pointed out that the formula-fed infants were not fed on demand; their scheduled feedings caused meal intervals and feeding volumes to be relatively fixed, not free to vary, because they were determined by the parent. Therefore, although there is some evidence that infants adjust meal intervals and meal size to regulate intake, in the presence of parental controls, evidence for such regulation disappears.

As infants become young children, they must begin to forgo demand feeding as they are socialized into the temporal patterns of meals for their culture, and their control over the timing of meals becomes more limited. With intermeal intervals fixed, the child's options are limited to adjustments in meal size and food selection. However, in our culture and others, children are allowed some flexibility in this regard: Although children partake of scheduled meals, snacking on demand is relatively common. Unfortunately, there is little information on how the timing of meals and snacks might impact on children's food intake and growth patterns. Even Clara Davis's (Davis, 1928, 1939) classic research on self selection of diets by young children (see next section) provided no evidence concerning this issue, because children were fed three or four meals at regularly scheduled times. Fortunately, recent research by Dewey and colleagues explored relationships between the timing and number of meals and snacks taken by children and their total daily energy intake, using a sample of malnourished children (Garcia, Kaiser, & Dewey, 1990a, 1990b).

Dewey and colleagues' (Garcia et al., 1990a, 1990b) findings revealed that young children's caloric intake was directly related to feeding frequency. In addition to the two regularly scheduled meals each day, the 3- to 5-year-old Mexican children in their sample requested food frequently and were usually given snacks when they requested them, so that the children had a mean of 13.5 eating occasions each day. Children who ate more than the average number of meals had significantly higher energy intakes than those who ate less frequent meals and snacks. The authors also reported that far more food was available to the children than they ate, so that intake was not limited by availability. Because many of the foods offered to the children were of relatively low energy density, the bulkiness of the food may have been a factor limiting intake within an eating occasion. The results indicated that when children were given the opportunity to have frequent snacks, the low energy density of the foods did not limit children's total daily energy intake. However, the data did not answer the question of whether variations in meal frequency can produce differences in growth even when diets are of equivalent total energy content. Because the sample was drawn from chronically malnourished children, extrapolation to well-nourished populations must be made with caution.

The timing of meals taken "on demand" is not exclusively controlled by hunger cues; environmental and social cues begin to play a role in initiating eating (Birch, McPhee, Sullivan, & Johnson, 1989). In research to investigate the extent to which social and environmental cues play a role in initiating meals during childhood, preschool children in day care were given repeated opportunities to play in two different playrooms. In one playroom, snack foods were always available, whereas in the other playroom, food was never present. The researchers tested whether children would be more likely to initiate a meal in the playroom previously associated with food, *even when they were not hungry.* They made sure the children were not hungry by feeding them just before the test session. Right after eating, the children went into the playrooms, and during this session, food was readily available in both rooms. It was found that when the children were in the room previously associated with food and eating, they initiated a meal more quickly and took a larger meal than when they were in the room that had never been associated with food and eating. These findings indicate that the "depletion driven" (Weingarten, 1985) eating of infancy was altered through learning and experience by the preschool period.

LEARNING, EXPERIENCE, AND THE CONTROL OF MEAL SIZE

Satter (1986, 1987, 1990) advocates a division of responsibility in feeding and argues persuasively that although parents need to take responsibility for providing children with an array of healthful foods, children must assume responsibility for how much they eat (or whether they eat at all). This advice is based on the assumption that, left to their own devices, children can regulate how much they ingest to maintain positive energy balance and sustain growth and health. What is the evidence that children can regulate energy intake? Clara Davis's classic study of the self selection of diets by newly weaned infants is certainly relevant (Davis, 1928, 1939). The infants and toddlers who participated in Davis's studies had no control over the timing of meals, which were served at fixed times, but they were free to select whatever foods they liked and to consume as much as they liked of the foods served to them. Children's participation typically started at weaning, so that all the solid foods served were initially novel to them. Most continued in the study for a minimum of several months; some participants were followed for several years. In addition to looking at the infants' food selections, meal patterns, and dietary intake, Davis obtained data on growth and morbidity. Davis's reports of infants' and children's energy and macronutrient intakes were consistent with current guidelines (Fomon, 1993). The children obtained about 35% of energy from fat and 17% from protein, and they grew well and had few childhood illnesses. The size and composition of individual meals varied dramatically, with children rarely consuming more than 2 or 3 of the 10–12 foods presented at any meal. The children also went on "food jags," eating only one or a few foods for several meals and then abandoning that food in favor of others. There were large individual differences in what was consumed and in the patterning of meal size, but all children developed well during the course of the study. She concluded that her findings, showing the children's success at self selecting a healthy diet, suggested "the existence of some innate, automatic mechanism for its accomplishment, of which appetite is a part" (Davis, 1939, p. 260).

The "food jags" of Davis's children were quite different from typical meal patterns of adults. Work by Barbara Rolls and colleagues (Rolls, 1986) has revealed that for adults, the variety of foods available influences meal size, with greater variety stimulating greater intake. When a variety of palatable foods is present, meals are larger than when only one or a few palatable foods are present; increased variety leads to increased intake (Rolls, 1986). This increased meal size is a result of the specificity of satiety; that is, preference for a food eaten declines during eating, but preference for uneaten foods remains relatively high, so that if a variety of foods is available, and satiety increases for the foods being eaten, the individual can simply switch to eating another food. Despite their propensity to consume meals consisting of one or only a few foods, 3- to 5-year-olds also show sensory-specific satiety (Birch & Deysher, 1986), although it is not known whether sensory-specific satiety increases meal size in children as it does in adults.

The energy density of the diet is an important determinant of meal size during infancy and early childhood. Perhaps because maintaining positive energy balance is so critical during the rapid growth of the early years of life, infants and young children adjust meal size on the basis of the energy density of food available, eating relatively large amounts of energy-dilute meals and much smaller amounts of energy-dense ones. Research conducted by Fomon (1993) with human infants revealed evidence for such adjustments in the volume of formula taken by infants as young as 6 weeks. Infants compensated for energy differences and adjusted the volume of intake of formula, consuming more energy-dilute (54 kcal/dl) than energy-dense formula (100 kcal/dl), so that total energy intake was similar to that of infants fed standard formula of 67 kcal/dl energy density.

Recently, researchers conducted a study to determine the extent to which the energy density of foods influences children's food intake, particularly their energy intake. They monitored children's energy intake within two-course meals and across 24-hour periods. In the experiments investigating children's ability to regulate energy intake within meals, children consumed a fixed amount of a first-course "preload," which was either high or low in energy density. The experimenters varied energy density by varying carbohydrate or fat content, keeping protein content constant. These preloads were consumed on different days, followed in each case by the same array of palatable foods as a second course. The child self-selected an ad lib meal from among these foods, and the data of interest were derived from intake in the second course, including the energy and macronutrient content of the foods selected as well as which foods were selected. In all cases, the food consumption data were derived from pre- and postweighing of all foods, which were analyzed using nutrient composition data. The children were responsive to these changes in the energy content of the first course; they adjusted their food intake in the ad lib second course, eating more following the energy-dilute than following the energy-dense first course (Birch & Deysher, 1985, 1986; Birch, McPhee, Shoba, Steinberg, & Krehbiel, 1987; Birch, McPhee, Steinberg, & Sullivan, 1990; Birch, McPhee, & Sullivan, 1989).

Additional evidence that the size of children's meals is influenced by the energy content of the foods eaten comes from research investigating whether children can learn to associate the sensory cues of food with the consequences of eating those foods. In this research, children had repeated opportunities to consume fixed volumes of high- and low-energy-density versions of a single type of food, such as yogurts or puddings. The high- and low-energy versions of the food typically contained about 170 kcal and 50 kcal per 4-oz serving, respectively, and were distinctively flavored, with a flavor cue consistently paired with each energy density. For example, a child had repeated opportunities to consume low-energy vanilla yogurt on some days and high-energy almond yogurt on others. After the children had several opportunities to consume each one, the researchers tested whether they had learned to associate the flavor cue with the postingestive consequences of the differences in energy content. In the test situation, children again consumed fixed volumes of the two flavors of yogurt, this time prepared so that both flavors were of the same energy density. The yogurts were consumed as first-course preloads on two different days, followed in each case by the same self-selected, ad lib lunch. Results confirmed that children were learning associations between foods' flavor cues and the postingestive consequences of eating those foods. Children ate less ad lib after they were given the flavor previously paired with high energy density, indicating that they had learned to associate the high-energy-paired flavor with the postingestive consequences of high energy density and adjusted subsequent food intake accordingly (Johnson, McPhee, & Birch, 1991; Kern, McPhee, Fisher, Johnson, & Birch, 1993). These findings, consistent with those obtained with animal models (Sclafani, 1990), indicate that satiety is influenced by learning and can be conditioned (Booth, 1985). The ability to learn about the satiety value of familiar foods may explain how meals can be terminated before postingestive cues signaling satiety have a chance to develop. As a result of repeatedly consuming familiar foods, people learn about the "fillingness and fatteningness" of familiar foods and make anticipatory adjustments in intake (Stunkard, 1975).

The research employing single-meal protocols has provided evidence that meal size is strongly influenced by energy density and has revealed that infants and children can be responsive to cues resulting from the energy density of the diet in determining the size of individual meals. Is there evidence that energy intake is regulated over 24-hour periods? Is the size of a meal influenced by energy intake at previous meals as well as by the energy content of the current meal? To investigate these questions, researchers measured the 24-hour food intake of 15 2- to 5-year-old children for 6 days (Birch, Johnson, Andresen, Petersen, & Schulte, 1991). The same menus were offered to the children on all 6 days, and food intake was not limited by availability. Energy intake was derived from pre- and postweighing of all foods consumed by each child.

One of the central issues addressed was the variability of individual children's intake (a) at individual meals and (b) over 24-hour periods. For example, Davis reported an apparently paradoxical finding—children self selecting their diets grew well, were healthy, and had normal energy intake (Davis, 1928, 1939)—but she also indicated that their intake at individual meals was highly unconventional, erratic, and unpredictable. To examine the variability of children's food intake at individual meals and for 24-hour periods, our group used coefficients of variation as an index of variability. These coefficients were calculated for each child for each of the six meals per day and for 24-hour total energy intake. Results revealed that although intake at individual meals was highly variable, total daily energy intake was relatively constant for each child. The mean coefficient of variation for each child's energy intake at individual meals was 33.6%, whereas the mean coefficient of variation for each child's 24-hour energy intake was 10.4%. In most cases, there was evidence for adjustments in energy intake *across* successive meals; high-energy intake at one meal was followed by low-energy intake at the next, or vice versa. Therefore, although intake at individual meals was highly variable and seemingly erratic, the adjustments in meal size across successive meals produced relatively tight regulation of energy intake for 24-hour periods.

Subsequently, the experimenters covertly altered the energy content of several foods in the diet by substituting olestra for about 14 g of dietary fat in several foods served during the first three meals of the day (Birch, Johnson, Jones, & Peters, 1993). Olestra (Procter & Gamble, Cincinnati, OH) is a nonenergy fat substitute that has the sensory characteristics of fat but is not absorbed and hence has no energy value. Participants were 29 2- to 5-year-olds, whose food intake at all eating occasions was monitored for 8 days by pre- and postweighing of all foods. Again, intake was not limited by availability, and the same menus were used throughout the study. Results revealed adjustments in meal size in response to the manipulation of energy density, so that total energy intake across 2-day blocks was nearly identical across conditions (13,673 vs. 13,573 kJ in the full-fat vs. fat-substitute conditions). As an index of variability, coefficients of variation showed the same pattern as in the previous work: For individual meals, the coefficients of variation were large, but for 24-hour energy intake, they were much smaller. Consistent with the previous findings and confirming parents' informal observations, children's individual meals were highly variable; however, we again noted evidence for adjustments in intake across successive meals, with large meals followed by small ones, and vice versa. This pattern, in conjunction with the evidence for adjustments in meal size across successive meals, suggests that children regulate energy intake and that regulation of meal size in response to the energy density of foods constitutes one mechanism controlling children's food intake.

These findings indicate that children are responsive to the energy density of foods and regulate meal size in response to energy density of foods consumed. However, the child's early experience with feeding can shape the extent to which the child is responsive to the energy content of the diet. Specifically, child-feeding practices can profoundly influence the child's responsiveness to energy density and the size of meals taken. A study was done to investigate the impact of contrasting child-feeding practices on children's responsiveness to energy density as a control of meal size. Children participated in single-meal protocols similar to those previously described, in which the energy content of a first course was either high or low and the second course was ad lib; the child-feeding strategies used by the adults who were present at mealtimes were varied (Birch, McPhee, Shoba, Steinberg, & Krehbiel, 1987). In one condition, adults focused the children on their internal hunger and satiety cues and discussed how those feelings help people know how much to eat. In the contrasting condition, children were focused on cues other than hunger and satiety that can control eating: The children ate at specific times, they were focused on how much food remained on the plate, and they were rewarded for finishing their portions. The children who were focused on internal cues of hunger and satiety showed clear evidence of adjusting energy intake in response to the energy content of foods, consistent with our previous findings. In contrast, when children were focused on external factors, no evidence of responsiveness to energy density was noted. These findings emphasize that child-feeding practices can shape the extent to which children are responsive to the energy content of foods in regulating meal size and that individual differences in the controls of food intake emerge from differences in the "balance of power" in child feeding. We believe that differences in responsiveness to energy density are the basis for individual differences in styles of intake control.

Johnson and Birch (1994) subsequently investigated how young children's responsiveness to energy density is influenced by parental control of child feeding. A laboratory measure was developed to test children's responsiveness to energy density; it was based on the single-meal protocol described previously. On two different occasions, children consumed two-course meals, consisting of a first-course preload and an ad-lib self-selected meal. From the child's energy intake on these two eating occasions, we calculated a compensation index for each child. This compensation index (COMPX) is the difference in ad-lib energy intake on the two occasions divided by the difference in the energy content of the preloads, transformed to a percentage. A value of 100% would indicate "calorie-for-calorie" adjustments in intake; smaller values reflect partial, incomplete compensation, and larger values, overcompensation. Results indicated that the best predictor of the child's responsiveness to energy density was parenting style in the feeding context; in particular, children's regulation of energy intake was negatively related to the imposition of authoritarian parental controls on their eating. Children's regulation of energy intake was also negatively related to their adiposity.

When the data were analyzed separately for boys and girls, relationships between the child's adiposity, child-feeding practices, and the child's responsiveness differed by sex of child. The extent to which girls showed regulation of energy intake was negatively related to their adiposity; fatter girls showed less evidence of regulating energy intake. In boys, this relationship was not obtained. In addition, parental reports of difficulties in controlling their own food intake, especially as measured by the dietary disinhibition scale of the Eating Inventory (Stunkard & Messick, 1985), were strongly related to their children's ability to regulate intake. Parents who reported difficulty in controlling their own eating, as indicated by high disinhibition scores on the Eating Inventory, had children who showed evidence of difficulty in regulating their energy intake in response to changes in energy density. These results reveal that differences in how young children regulate energy intake are related to parents' own eating styles as well as their child-feeding practices. We believe that these early differences in the regulation of energy intake are precursors of later individual differences as well as sex differences in styles of intake control. We have hypothesized that the chronic dieting and dietary restraint that have become normative in young women and adolescent girls may have their beginnings in the early regulation of energy intake and in the differences in how boys and girls are parented in the feeding context, particularly the extent to which parental controls are imposed on eating.

EARLY EXPERIENCE AND FOOD SELECTION: CHILDREN'S FOOD PREFERENCES

Children are responsive to the energy density of foods, and that energy density can serve as a control of meal size. Through early learning and experience, energy density also influences food *selection* in two ways. First, the energy density of foods consumed at a first course in a meal can influence which foods are selected in subsequent courses (Birch, McPhee, & Sullivan, 1989). Second, associative conditioning shapes preferences for energy-dense foods. With respect to subsequent food selection, we have indicated that energy density of foods consumed at one meal can influence the size of the next meal: The consumption of a high-energy meal leads to reduced consumption at the next eating occasion. How do children adjust their food intake in the second meal to accomplish this? The reduced intake following energy-dense meals occurs because children reduce the variety of foods eaten following eating of energy-dense foods: *Which* foods children consume in the next meal are affected by the energy density of foods consumed in the previous meal. After consuming a high-energy first course, the children consumed fewer foods ad lib. Data on the children's food preferences revealed that, relative to intake following the low-energy first course, the children simply eliminated the less preferred foods from meals that followed the more energy-dense first course, but they continued to consume their preferred foods. In fact, their preferred foods tended to be relatively energy-dense ones with high levels of sugar and fat, and those not eaten tended to be good sources of micronutrients, generally lower in energy density (Birch, McPhee, Bryant, & Johnson, 1993; Birch, McPhee, & Sullivan, 1989). Because foods eliminated tended to be nonpreferred foods such as vegetables, which are lower in sugar and fat content but high in micronutrients, the resulting reduced variety, over a period of time, may have negative effects on dietary quality.

Children's food preferences are the major determinants of their food intake; children do not eat what they do not like, and the correlations between preferences and intake are strong, ranging from about .60 to .80 (Birch, 1979a, 1979b). Given the powerful role of food preferences in children's food selection and intake patterns, much of this section is focused on what is known about factors shaping children's food preferences. Children's preferences for foods are learned through repeated experiences with food and eating, and associative conditioning to the social contexts and physiological consequences of eating is particularly important. Only the preference for sweet and the rejection of sour and bitter substances appear to be unlearned and are present in the newborn (Cowart, 1981); a preference for salt emerges by about 4 months. For very young children who are just being introduced to the adult diet, all foods are initially unfamiliar. A brief review of research on factors influencing acceptance of novel food reveals that children, like other omnivores, tend to reject unfamiliar foods, and this initial rejection can be modified by repeated opportunities to eat the new food. Recent findings reveal that the energy density of foods also shapes children's food preferences and their food selection through associative learning.

Although previous work has indicated that children's food preferences are predictors of their consumption patterns, discussions of pediatric nutrition typically focus on the role that parents and caregivers play in providing children with nutritionally adequate diets. The impact of children's food selections on their dietary intake is frequently overlooked. Recent research (Fisher & Birch, 1995) indicated that children's food preferences influence not only the types of foods they choose to consume, but also the overall quality of their diets. Preschool children's ($N = 18$) food intake, including their consumption of high-fat foods and total dietary fat intake, were measured during six 30-hour periods of observation. In addition to assessing children's fat preferences and intake, the researchers obtained measurements of children's and parents' adiposity. Although the same menus were offered to all children, children's food-selection patterns produced variability in the quality of their diets. The percentage of energy from fat in the menus offered was 33%, but across individual children the percentage of energy from dietary fat ranged from 25% to 41%. Children's preferences for high-fat foods were significantly related to their selection and consumption of high-fat foods, their total dietary fat intake, and parental adiposity. Children indicating strong preferences for high-fat foods had the greatest triceps skinfolds, a measurement of relative adiposity. Children who preferred high-fat foods had higher fat intakes, obtaining a large percentage of their energy intake from high-fat foods, and had the heaviest parents. This research indicates that although the nutritional adequacy of young children's diets is constrained by the foods provided to them, the children's choices from among those foods exert a considerable influence on the overall quality of their diets. Providing children with a variety of healthful foods from which to select their diets is necessary but not sufficient to ensure nutritional adequacy. Finally, the fact that children's fat preferences, consumption of high-fat foods, and total dietary fat intake were related to parental adiposity highlights the central role of familial factors on food selection and the controls of food intake.

Children consume foods they like, and many of these preferred foods are energy-dense foods, high in fat or carbohydrate content. Why do children and adults like these energy-dense foods? There are a variety of reasons, ranging from cultural habits to sensory aspects: "Rich" foods are high-fat foods, often foods reserved for feasts, holidays, and special occasions. From a sensory perspective, many of the volatile substances that impart flavor to food are fat-soluble, so that high-fat foods are often flavorful ones (Birch, 1992; Mela, 1992). In addition, to the extent that the energy content of a food comes from simple sugars, the foods are also sweet, and the preference for sweetness is strong, unlearned, and well established at birth. Other high-energy foods are high in salt content. An apparently unlearned preference for salt emerges at about 4 months after birth (Beauchamp, Cowart, & Moran, 1986), and infants and children tend to prefer higher levels of salt in food than do adults. High-energy, high-fat, and high-carbohydrate foods also have specific physiological effects (Smith & Greenberg, 1992) that can produce pleasurable feelings of satiety.

Associative learning contributes to the acquisition of food preferences through the formation of associations between sensory cues of foods and the contexts and consequences of eating. The gastrointestinal consequences of ingestion can serve as powerful unconditioned stimuli in associative conditioning of food preferences and food aversions. In particular, this associative conditioning contributes to preferences for high-fat, high-energy foods (Birch, 1992). In this form of learning, the postingestive gastrointestinal consequences of eating a food are associated with the food's sensory cues. For example, when consumption of a food is followed by the negative gastrointestinal consequences of nausea and vomiting, and the sensory cues of the food are associated with these negative consequences, a food aversion results. In a similar fashion, associations between foods and positive postingestive consequences, such as the pleasant feelings of satiety that can follow eating energy-dense foods, can produce learned food preferences. Research with animal models first confirmed the existence of these learned preferences: Given repeated opportunities to consume foods, rats learned to associate sensory cues of foods with positive postingestive consequences of ingested nutrients, and they subsequently learned to prefer high-energy-density foods over low-energy-density versions of the same foods. These learned preferences that are based on high-energy density result whether the high-energy content is due to carbohydrate or fat (Sclafani, 1990).

Inspired by the animal research on these learned food preferences, our research group conducted a number of experiments that have confirmed that such learned associations between sensory cues of foods and the postingestive consequences of high-energy content contribute to children's preferences for high-energy foods (Birch, McPhee, Steinberg, & Sullivan, 1990; Johnson, McPhee, & Birch, 1991; Kern et al., 1993). These protocols are similar to those described earlier that were used to explore children's responsiveness to energy density. Children are given repeated opportunities to consume high- and low-energy versions of foods, such as yogurts, drinks, and puddings, that vary in energy density. The high- and low-energy versions of the foods are distinctively flavored, whereas sensory characteristics of the two versions, such as texture and mouthfeel, are similar. After the child's initial preferences for the foods were assessed, each child consumed equivalent, fixed amounts of a high-energy, almond-flavored yogurt on some days and a low-energy peppermint yogurt on other days (other children had the reverse energy density–flavor pairing). Following several opportunities to eat the high- and low-energy versions, the child's preferences for both flavors were assessed. Preferences were assessed by having the experimenter how well they liked a food on the basis of tasting small food samples, a procedure that has been shown to yield reliable, valid preferences that are good predictors of children's consumption in a self-selection setting (Birch, 1979a, 1979b, 1980). Using this preference measure, the results confirmed that through association of flavor cues with the postingestive consequences of high-energy density, children learned to prefer flavors repeatedly associated with high-energy density. Like learned aversions, in which children learn to avoid flavors previously associated with gastrointestinal illness, learned preferences could serve an adaptive function, allowing children to learn that particular flavor cues predict pleasurable feelings of satiety that result from high-energy-dense foods.

As indicated earlier, eating is usually a social occasion for children, often involving siblings, peers, and adults who can serve as models, as well as adults who may attempt to control children's eating. Associative conditioning contributes to the formation of children's food likes and dislikes through associations of food cues with the social contexts in which ingestion occurs. Evidence suggests that children learn to prefer foods associated with positive contexts and dislike foods presented in negative ones. Unfortunately, a confounding exists in our culture between affective tone of these social contexts and the palatability of foods: Foods that are not highly palatable initially (e.g., foods without sugar, fat, and salt) tend to be presented in coercive, negative contexts ("eat your vegetables"), whereas palatable foods (those high in sugar, fat, and salt) tend to be presented in positive contexts. These confoundings tend to potentiate both children's liking of palatable high-energy, high-fat, sweet foods and their dislike of less palatable foods that parents believe are healthy for children. These palatable foods are often served in positive contexts: as rewards, as desserts at the ends of meals, and as a part of holidays and celebrations. Foods presented to children in the context of a positive interaction with a friendly adult or served as rewards become preferred (Birch, Zimmerman, & Hind, 1980).

On the other hand, the social contexts in which children eat can also be negative. For example, children are sometimes coerced to eat foods in greater quantities than they would like, especially when those foods are "good for them." To the extent that one applies pressure, coercing and forcing children to eat these foods, associative conditioning can produce dislikes for the very foods we want children to consume. When researchers rewarded children for consuming foods, their preference for those foods declined significantly. In fact, the children who were rewarded for consuming a novel drink liked it less after they were rewarded for consuming it than they did when it was novel (Birch, Birch, Marlin, & Kramer, 1982; Birch, Marlin, & Rotter, 1984). This was particularly impressive evidence for the role of social context in shaping food preferences, because children tend to dislike and reject novel foods. In contrast, children who simply sampled the drink on the same number of occasions but were not rewarded for drinking it came to prefer the drink as it became more familiar.

Children do not readily accept new foods, with the notable exception of foods high in sugar, which they do not have to learn to like. This *neophobia,* or fear of the new, is normal in children and is found among other omnivorous species; it arises from what Rozin (1977) called the "omnivore's dilemma": As omnivores, we need a variety of foods, and we must compose the diet from available edible substances. However, ingesting new substances is a risky business; the substance may prove to be toxic. This view suggests an evolutionary basis for neophobia, which can protect against the ingestion of potentially dangerous items. Typically, neophobia is reduced by repeated consumption of a new food that is not followed by any negative gastrointestinal consequences. For the child who is just being introduced to the adult diet, all foods are initially novel, and young children's neophobic responses can have particularly powerful effects on their food selection and eating behavior.

In her research on dietary self selection, Davis (1939) described the dramatic changes that occurred in food acceptance as children were introduced to new foods and had repeated opportunities to sample them. When the weanling infants first began to self-select their diets, they initially tasted many of the foods, sampling widely from among the new foods. Davis described how with repeated opportunities for the infants to eat the foods, they developed food preferences. They began avidly to seek out some foods and reject others; food preferences emerged before her eyes. Davis was careful to emphasize that the "trick" of her experiment was the array of foods that were offered to the children: a set of healthy foods, simply prepared, without additional salt or sugar. These foods bear little resemblance to many of the foods available today, especially many foods that are marketed for children. Davis stated that one should "leave the selection of the foods to be made available to young children in the hands of their elders where everyone has always known it belongs" (Davis, 1939, p. 260). When the children self-selected their diets from a limited array of healthful foods, the children did well. Davis's work is often misquoted and used to support the theory of the "wisdom of the body": Children "know" what nutrients they need and will seek out the foods containing those nutrients. In fact, there are no human data to support this view. Except for a few substances (e.g., sodium), the evidence for such wisdom of the body and for "specific hungers" is weak, even in experimental animals who are severely deprived of an essential nutrient (Galef, 1991).

Our group investigated the effects of repeated exposure to new foods on children's preferences for those foods and found that with repeated exposure, many new foods that children initially rejected were accepted (Birch & Marlin, 1982). However, acceptance does not come immediately but may take 8–10 exposures and must involve tasting the food; looking at and smelling it are not sufficient to induce increased acceptance (Birch, McPhee, Shoba, Pirok, & Steinberg, 1987). Unfortunately, parents do not often appreciate that the child's initial rejection of a new food (a) is normal, (b) reflects an adaptive process, and (c) may be followed by increased acceptance of the food after the child has repeated opportunities to eat it. The commonly held view is that the child's initial rejection of a food reflects a fixed, immutable dislike for the food. As a result, the child may be viewed as finicky, and the new food may not be offered to the child again, eliminating any opportunity for the child to learn to like the food. The child's neophobia plays a central role in early food acceptance. The fact that early and repeated opportunities to eat new foods can change initial rejection to acceptance underscores the critical role of parents in selecting the array of foods offered to their children.

Our group recently investigated infants' responses to their first solid foods and whether their acceptance of new foods was enhanced with repeated exposure (Sullivan & Birch, 1994). Infants 4–6 months old were fed a novel vegetable on 10 occasions, several times each week by their mothers, and intake of the vegetable was measured before, during, and after their opportunities to eat the food. Infants were videotaped while eating, and adults rated the videotapes for the infants' acceptance of the foods. Over the exposure series, infants showed dramatic increases in intake of the vegetables, doubling their intake from about 30 g to about 60 g. An unanticipated result was that the results differed for formula-fed and breast-fed infants; increases in intake were most dramatic for the breast-fed infants. We hypothesize that this greater acceptance of a novel food by the breast-fed infants is due to their greater experience with a variety of flavors, which pass from the maternal diet into breast milk. Recent research reveals that flavors ingested by mothers are present in breast milk and that infants respond systematically to these flavors (Mennella & Beauchamp, 1991a, 1991b). Research with animal models has shown that young animals who experience dietary variety show much more ready acceptance of novel diets than do animals whose dietary experience is limited to a single diet (Capretta, Petersik, & Stewart, 1975). Additional research is needed to determine ways in which human infants' early experience during the suckling period influences subsequent preferences and food-acceptance patterns.

IMPLICATIONS FOR CHILD-FEEDING PRACTICES AND CONCLUSION

In infancy there are relationships between meal size and meal interval that reflect an emerging regulatory process. Children are sensitive to the energy content of food and regulate meal size and food selection. These early regulatory processes are modified by learning and experience. With respect to the timing of meals, demand feeding initially is desirable, allowing the infant a high degree of control over meal timing. When infants are fed on demand, there is evidence that through experience and learning, the meal size, meal timing, and relationships between size and timing of meals change with experience and learning. In addition, over time, the infant relinquishes a degree of control over meal timing as a gradual transition to scheduled meals at culturally specified times occurs. Finally, with respect to food selection, children come into the world predisposed to learn about food: to learn what to eat and what to like and to prefer some foods and reject others. This learning is based on repeated experience with food and eating and on associations formed between the sensory cues of foods and the affect generated by the social contexts and physiological consequences of eating.

We have presented evidence that infants and young children are capable of assuming a high degree of self-control over meal timing and meal size and, within constraints on what foods are offered, over food selection. Children differ in their responsiveness to internal cues of hunger and satiety in regulating meal size and total daily energy intake and in the extent to which they have learned to use other cues to control the timing and size of meals. These other cues include the presence of food, time of day, and social or environmental contexts previously associated with food and eating. Research has begun to reveal that individual differences in the control of food intake emerge during childhood and that differences among children are related to parenting style in child feeding, especially differences in the balance of parent–child control in child feeding. By adulthood, after years of learning and experience, the controls of food intake become complex. A variety of learned controls of food intake may operate either in addition to or instead of internally generated cues signaling hunger and satiety. The increasingly high incidence of obesity and eating disorders suggests that for many in our society, hunger and satiety signals are not functioning as controls of food intake to maintain energy balance: Chronic dieters consistently ignore hunger cues, and binge eaters continue eating well beyond normal satiety.

What does research on the developing controls of food intake in children imply regarding child-feeding practices? What practices should parents follow to facilitate the development of styles of intake control that maintain energy balance and result in healthy diets? We encourage parents to focus on the long-term goal of developing healthy self-control of feeding in children and to look beyond their immediate concerns regarding composition and quantity of foods children consume. Research supports the view that children should be given substantial control over food intake, especially meal size. While allowing children control over how much is eaten, parents should work toward shaping the timing of the child's meals to the adult pattern of the culture by imposing some control over meal intervals. Because children's food preferences and food selection are tightly linked to the familiarity of foods, parents can have a powerful positive influence on the nutritional adequacy of children's diets through the array of foods that they offer the child (Satter, 1986, 1987, 1990). Research on associative conditioning of food preferences suggests that parents should forgo the temptation to control children's eating by imposing contingencies and coercive practices. Although rewarding children for eating, coercing them to eat, or using foods as rewards can give parents control over children's eating in the short run, the learned food preferences that result tend to be antithetical to the selection of healthy diets. Such child-feeding practices can be harmful because, in addition to limiting opportunities for self-control, children learn to dislike the foods that are "good for them" and to love the "junk" foods that should be consumed only in moderation.

To facilitate healthy self-control of eating, one should give children repeated opportunities to sample healthful foods in noncoercive, positive contexts, so that through associative learning processes, some of the foods offered will become preferred and accepted. Although evidence is limited, we also caution that parents should not severely restrict access to highly palatable "junk" foods—foods high in sugar, salt, and fat—because we suspect that such restricted access may make these forbidden foods even more attractive. Parental influence should not be focused on controlling intake at individual meals, but it should operate to allow children to develop preferences and food-selection patterns consistent with a healthy diet.

We do not imply that children should be given total control over food selection, as advocated in one recent book on child feeding (Hirschmann & Zaphiropoulos, 1985). This position is not consistent with the literature on the development of children's food preferences and the controls of food intake. First, research does not support the view that specific hungers and the "wisdom of the body" will lead the child to select an adequate diet when the choices are unlimited. In addition, children have an unlearned preference for sweet and salty tastes (Cowart & Beauchamp, 1986). Children are neophobic and reject new foods (especially those that are not sweet or salty). Finally, children have a propensity to learn to prefer energy-dense foods. Given these propensities and the array of foods available in supermarkets today, consider the likely outcome of the following hypothetical experiment. Using Clara Davis's dietary self-selection protocol, we give weaning infants and toddlers complete freedom to select their diets by allowing them to select from among all the foods available in U.S. supermarkets today. Similar to Davis's infants, our participants begin the study at weaning, so that all foods are initially novel to them. However, in striking contrast to Davis's findings, we predict that children's "supermarket" diets would not be nutritionally adequate; from among the foods available, they would select foods high in sugar, salt, and fat, and it is unlikely that the children would ever learn to like and consume other novel, less inherently palatable foods. As Davis pointed out, the "trick" of her successful dietary self-selection studies was in what the children were offered.

To increase the likelihood that children will select foods that constitute an adequate diet, parents must be provided with information about how children learn to accept new foods. Armed with such information, parents would not expect that new foods (especially those low in sugar, salt, and fat) would be accepted the first time they were offered, and would be prepared to offer new foods repeatedly, with the expectation that acceptance would emerge gradually. In addition, once parents appreciate the role of social context in shaping children's food likes and dislikes, they may be motivated to provide opportunities for children to eat foods in positive social contexts, in the absence of coercion. Many healthful foods, such as vegetables, that we want children to consume are not inherently palatable. Especially for foods that are not sweet or salty, associative learning can be pivotal in determining whether these foods will be accepted or rejected.

Finally, providing accurate information regarding appropriate portion sizes for young children can reduce parental anxiety about the adequacy of their children's diets. In our informal discussions with parents of young children, we find that many parents frequently overestimate the amounts of food that young children need to eat. The discrepancy between what parents think children should eat and the child's actual intake can make parents anxious and may underscore parental convictions that the child is not capable of controlling his or her own food intake. This can lead parents to attempt to assume greater control over feeding, particularly over how much the child eats. Certainly, parents with misconceptions about portion sizes are not well prepared to assume responsibility for controlling children's meal size. We have found that providing parents with information about more appropriate portion sizes for their young children can help to reduce their anxiety about whether their child is getting enough to eat, allowing parents to relinquish some control over meal size.

Let us return to Clara Davis's advice, given more than 60 years ago: During children's transition to the adult diet, parents should restrict themselves to assuming responsibility for what foods are made available to children. The current research findings support the view that given experience with an adequate variety of healthful foods in a noncoercive feeding environment, the normally developing child will learn to accept the consume a variety of foods in sufficient quantities to constitute a nutritionally adequate diet and to sustain growth and health. These same views are reflected in Satter's more contemporary advice to parents (1986, 1987, 1990). With respect to meal size, all the evidence suggests that children have some capacity to regulate energy intake by adjusting meal size. If presented with a healthy array of foods, the child will obtain adequate nutrients; parents should not assume control of meal size or resort to coercing or controlling tactics to induce the child to eat. Preliminary findings suggest that parental control can have adverse effects on children's responsiveness to the energy content of food, which can serve as an effective control of food intake. In summary, parents should provide children with a variety of healthful foods, set limits to shape the child toward adult meal patterns, but allow the child control of whether and how much to eat.

REFERENCES

Beauchamp, G. K., Cowart, B. J., & Moran, M. (1986). Developmental changes in salt acceptability in human infants. *Developmental Psychobiology, 19*, 17–25.

Bernstein, I. (1981). Meal patterns in "free running humans." *Physiology & Behavior, 27*, 621–624.

Birch, L. L. (1979a). Dimensions of preschool children's food preferences. *Journal of Nutrition Education, 11*, 189–192.

Birch, L. L. (1979b). Preschool children's food preferences and consumption patterns. *Journal of Nutrition Education, 11*, 77–80.

Birch, L. L. (1980). Effects of peer models' food choices and eating behaviors on preschooler's food preferences. *Child Development, 51,* 489–496.

Birch, L. L. (1992). Children's preferences for high-fat foods. *Nutrition Reviews, 50,* 249–255.

Birch, L. L., Birch, D., Marlin, D., & Kramer, L. (1982). Effects of instrumental eating on children's food preferences. *Appetite, 3,* 125–134.

Birch, L. L., & Deysher, M. (1985). Conditioned and unconditioned caloric compensation: Evidence for self-regulation of food intake by young children. *Learning and Motivation, 16,* 341–355.

Birch, L. L., & Deysher, M. (1986). Caloric compensation and sensory specific satiety: Evidence for self-regulation of food intake by young children. *Appetite, 7,* 323–331.

Birch, L. L., Johnson, S. L., Andresen, G., Petersen, J. C., & Schulte, M. C. (1991). The variability of young children's energy intake. *New England Journal of Medicine, 324,* 232–235.

Birch, L. L., Johnson, S. L., Jones, M. B., & Peters, J. C. (1993). Effects of a non-energy fat substitute on children's energy and macronutrient intake. *American Journal of Clinical Nutrition, 58,* 326–333.

Birch, L. L., & Marlin, D. W. (1982). I don't like it; I never tried it: Effects of exposure to food on two-year-old children's food preferences. *Appetite, 4,* 353–360.

Birch, L. L., Marlin, D. W., & Rotter, J. (1984). Eating as the "means" activity in a contingency: Effects on young children's food preference. *Child Development, 55,* 432–439.

Birch, L. L., McPhee, L. S., Bryant, J. L., & Johnson. S. L. (1993). Children's lunch intake: Effects of midmorning snacks varying in energy density and fat content. *Appetite, 20,* 83–94.

Birch, L. L., McPhee, L., Shoba, B. C., Pirok, E., & Steinberg, L. (1987). What kind of exposure reduces children's food neophobia? *Appetite, 9,* 171–178.

Birch, L. L., McPhee, L., Shoba, B. C., Steinberg, L., & Krehbiel, R. (1987). Clean up your plate: Effects of child feeding practices on the conditioning of meal size. *Learning and Motivation, 18,* 301–317.

Birch, L. L., McPhee, L., Steinberg, L., & Sullivan, S. (1990). Conditioned flavor preferences in young children. *Physiology and Behavior, 47,* 501–505.

Birch, L. L., McPhee, L., & Sullivan, S. (1989). Children's food intake following drinks sweetened with sucrose or aspartame: Time course effects. *Physiology and Behavior, 45,* 387–396.

Birch, L. L., McPhee, L., Sullivan, S., & Johnson, S. (1989). Conditioned meal initiation in young children. *Appetite, 13,* 105–113.

Birch, L. L., Zimmerman, S., & Hind, H. (1980). The influence of social–affective context on preschool children's food preferences. *Child Development, 51,* 856–861.

Booth, D. A. (1985). Food conditioned eating preferences and aversions with interoceptive elements: Conditioned appetites and satieties. *Annals of the New York Academy of Sciences, 443,* 22–41.

Capretta, P. J., Petersik, J. T., & Stewart, D. J. (1975). Acceptance of novel flavours is increased after early experience of diverse tastes, *Nature, 254,* 689–691.

Cowart, B. (1981). Development of taste perception in humans: Sensitivity and preference throughout the life span. *Psychological Bulletin, 90,* 43–73.

Cowart, B. J., & Beauchamp, G. K. (1986). Factors affecting acceptance of salt by human infants and children. In M. R. Kare & J. G. Brand (Eds.), *Interaction of the chemical senses with nutrition* (pp. 25–44). San Diego, CA: Academic Press.

Davis, C. M. (1928). Self-selection of diet by newly weaned infants. *American Journal of Diseases of Children, 36,* 651–679.

Davis, C. M. (1939). Results of the self-selection of diets by young children. *Canadian Medical Association Journal, 41,* 257–261.

Fisher, J. A., & Birch, L. L. (1995). Fat preferences and fat consumption of 3– to 5–year–old children are related to parental adiposity. *Journal of The American Dietetic Association, 95,* 759–764.

Fomon, S. J. (1993). *Nutrition of normal infants.* St. Louis, MO: Mosby–Year Book.

Galef, B. G., Jr. (1991). A contrarian view of the wisdom of the body as it relates to dietary self-selection. *Psychology Review, 98,* 218–223.

Garcia, S. E., Kaiser, L. L., & Dewey, K. G. (1990a). The relationship of eating frequency and caloric density to energy intake among rural Mexican preschool children. *European Journal of Clinical Nutrition, 44,* 381–387.

Garcia, S. E., Kaiser, L. L., & Dewey, K. G. (1990b). Self-regulation of food intake among rural Mexican preschool children. *European Journal of Clinical Nutrition, 44,* 371–380.

Hirschmann, J. R., & Zaphiropoulos, L. (1985). *Solving your child's eating problems.* New York: Ballantine Books.

Johnson, S. L., & Birch, L. L. (1994). Parent's and children's adiposity and eating style. *Pediatrics, 94,* 653–661.

Johnson, S. L., & McPhee, L., & Birch, L. L. (1991). Conditioned preferences: Young children prefer flavors associated with high dietary fat. *Physiology & Behavior, 50,* 1245–1251.

Kern, D. L., McPhee, L., Fisher, J., Johnson, S., & Birch, L. L. (1993). The postingestive consequences of fat condition preferences for flavors associated with high dietary fat. *Physiology & Behavior, 54,* 71–76.

Le Magnen, J. (1985). *Hunger.* New York: Cambridge University Press.

Matheny, R., Birch, L. L., & Picciano, M. F. (1990). Control of intake by human milk fed infants: Relationships between feeding size and interval. *Developmental Psychobiology, 23,* 511–518.

Mela, D. J. (Ed.). (1992). *Dietary fats.* Essex, England: Elsevier Science.

Mennella, D. J. A., & Beauchamp, G. K. (1991a). Maternal diet alters the sensory qualities of human milk and the nursling's behavior. *Pediatrics, 88* 737–744.

Mennella, J. A., & Beauchamp, G. K. (1991b). The transfer of alcohol to human milk: Effects on flavor and the infant's behavior. *New England Journal of Medicine, 325,* 981–985.

Pinilla, T., & Birch, L. L. (1993). Help me make it through the night: Behavioral entrainment of breast-fed infants' sleep patterns. *Pediatrics, 91,* 436–444.

Rolls, B. J. (1986). Sensory-specific satiety. *Nutrition Reviews, 44,* 93–101.

Rozin, P. (1977). The use of characteristic flavorings in human culinary practice. In C. M. Apt (Ed.), *Flavor: Its chemical, behavioral, and commercial aspects.* Boulder, CO: Westview Press.

Satter, E. (1986). *Child of mine.* Palo Alto, CA: Bull Publishing.

Satter, E. (1987). *How to get your kid to eat . . . but not too much.* Palo Alto, CA: Bull Publishing.

Satter, E. (1990). The feeding relationship: Problems and interventions. *The Journal of Pediatrics, 117,* S181–S189.

Sclafani, A. (1990). Nutritionally based learned flavor preferences in rats. In E. Capaldi & T. Powley (Eds.), *Taste, experience, and feeding* (pp. 139–156). Washington, DC: American Psychological Association.

Smith, G. P., & Greenberg, D. (1992). The investigation of orosensory stimuli in the intake and preference of oils in the rat. In D. Mela (Ed.), *Dietary fats* (pp. 167–178). Essex, England: Elsevier Science.

Stunkard, A. (1975). Satiety is a conditioned reflex. *Psychosomatic Medicine, 37,* 383–389.

Stunkard, A. J., & Messick, S. (1985). The three-factor eating questionnaire to measure dietary restraint, disinhibition, and hunger. *Journal of Psychosomatic Research, 29,* 71–83.

Sullivan, S. A., & Birch, L. L. (1994). Infant dietary experience and acceptance of solid foods. *Pediatrics, 93,* 271–277.

Weingarten, H. P. (1985). Stimulus control of eating: Implications for a two-factor theory of hunger. *Appetite, 6,* 387–401.

Wright, P., Fawcett, J., & Crow, R. (1980). The development of differences in the feeding behaviour of bottle and breast fed human infants from birth to two months. *Behavior Processes, 5,* 1–20.

PART FOUR

How Biology Affects Eating Patterns

6

Sensory Factors in Feeding

Valerie B. Duffy and Linda M. Bartoshuk

Foods and beverages excite all of the sensory modalities present in the oral and nasal cavities (i.e., taste, olfaction, touch, temperature, pain). Surprisingly, the language used to describe these sensations is often confusing. The specialist's narrow definition of *true taste* refers only to sensations arising from receptors on the tongue and palate. However, in ordinary conversation the term *taste* is used to refer to the perception of flavor, a combination of true taste and smell. There is no verb in the English language (we are not sure about other languages) to express the perception of flavor; thus, the word *taste* must serve both the specialist and the consumer. Rozin (personal communication) suggested a new term, "mouthsense," to refer to the integration of oral sensations. Following his lead, we begin this chapter with a discussion of the contributions of taste and smell to mouthsense. Because individuals can experience alteration of mouthsense through clinical pathologies of taste and smell, we discuss some of these alterations and their potential influence on the sensory experience of food. Next, we provide an overview of the history of genetic variation in true taste and the recent developments suggesting that this genetic variation may be even more important to the sensory processing of food than its discoverers realized. Finally, we discuss the nutritional functions of taste and smell.

TASTE AND OLFACTORY QUALITIES

Taste

There is general agreement that taste sensations can be classified as sweet, salty, sour, or bitter. A few other terms have been suggested as potential

145

taste qualities (e.g., metallic, alkaline, and *umami*, the savory taste of gluta-mate), but these are not universally accepted. Sweet, salty, sour, and bitter share an important characteristic. Their hedonic attributes serve as meta-phors to express value in nontaste situations. For example, one can express clear meaning in the phrase "Shirley Temple is sweet" or "Scrooge is bitter." The universal affect of taste is established from birth; humans are born liking sweet and disliking bitter.

Olfaction

Names for olfactory qualities also share an important characteristic. The name of the odor is often derived from the object that produced the odor (e.g., minty, smoky, vanilla, lemon, chocolate). It is important to note that the common substances that one smells (e.g., bacon, evergreen, pizza) are mixtures of odorants. Cain (1987) suggested that people form templates to recognize these mixtures; that is, one recognizes odor mixtures holistically. This permits recognition of a variety of objects by their unique smells even if those objects have some odors in common. In sum, the olfactory system is able to sense many odor molecules. An individual's experience with specific combinations of those molecules results in that individual's learned ability to recognize and name the combinations that are important in his or her life. Although the number of molecules that can be sensed by the olfactory system may be quite large (this has never been determined experimentally despite the frequent citation of the number 10,000), the number that can be recognized and named is relatively small (Engen, 1982).

Liking or disliking the odor combinations that one learns to recognize involves conditioning. Nausea paired with an odor makes the odor disliked (Pelchat, Grill, Rozin, & Jacobs, 1983; Pelchat & Rozin, 1982). Positive experiences (e.g., calories, sweet taste, mood elevation, social reward) paired with an odor make the odor liked (Birch, McPhee, Steinberg, & Sullivan, 1990; Zellner, Rozin, Aron, & Kulish, 1983). These findings have implications for the human predilection to build cuisines. When we create a new food dish (i.e., a complex mixture of food constituents), the olfactory signature of this dish is learned holistically. Positive conditioning then makes the dish liked. The ability of the olfactory system to provide distinct sensory labels for new combinations of foods can lead to a continually expanding set of food items that can become pleasurable.

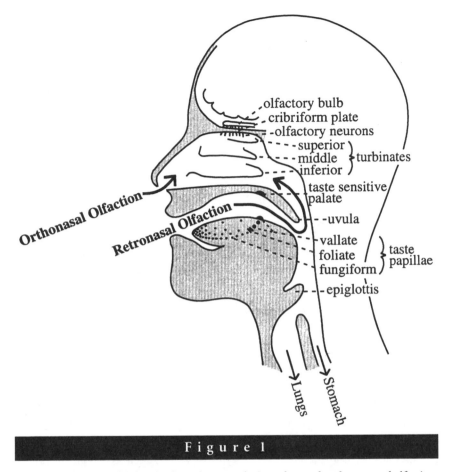

olfactory bulb
cribriform plate
olfactory neurons
superior ⎫
middle ⎬ turbinates
inferior ⎭
taste sensitive palate
uvula
vallate ⎫
foliate ⎬ taste papillae
fungiform ⎭
epiglottis

Orthonasal Olfaction

Retronasal Olfaction

Lungs

Stomach

Figure 1

Schematic diagram of the paths that odorants take in orthonasal and retronasal olfaction. The locations of taste papillae and the taste-sensitive portion of the palate are also shown. (Adapted from Amoore, Johnston, and Rubin, 1964; Mozell, Smith, Smith, Sullivan, and Swender 1969).

MOUTHSENSE

Taste and olfactory qualities perceptually blend to produce the flavor sensations attributed to the mouth. Figure 1 shows the relation between orthonasal and retronasal olfaction, the location of taste papillae on the tongue, and the taste-sensitive area at the margin of the hard and soft palates. In addition to being found on taste papillae, taste buds are found on the uvula and in the throat. Sniffing pulls odorants into the nasal cavity through the nostrils (orthonasal olfaction). The air carrying the odorants is made turbulent by passing over the turbinate bones. This permits a small sample of the air to reach the olfactory mucosa located at the top of the nasal cavity between the septum (the tissue separating the two halves of the nose) and the superior turbinate. (The space the odor molecules must pass through to reach the receptors is called the *olfactory cleft*.) Olfactory neurons carrying signals from the mucosa form small bundles that pass through holes in the cribriform plate and enter the olfactory bulb.

Odorants can also reach the mucosa from the mouth (retronasal olfaction). The mouth movements during chewing and swallowing pump odorants up into the nasal cavity behind the palate. During eating, taste sensations are added to retronasal sensations, producing flavor. In spite of the importance of retronasal olfaction, people commonly speak only of "tasting" food. This is not simply an error but rather reflects the fact that perceptual localization is provided by touch. Odorants sniffed through the nostrils are localized to the nose, whereas those pumped into the nasal cavity by chewing and swallowing are localized to the mouth.

Orthonasal Versus Retronasal Olfaction

Do orthonasal and retronasal olfaction produce the same qualitative experiences? The same odor molecules reach the olfactory mucosa whether an individual sniffs or consumes a food. However, retronasal olfaction requires the efficient transport of odorants from the mouth through normal oral movements during chewing and swallowing (Burdach & Doty, 1987). A number of factors could diminish the intensity of odorants perceived retronasally by impairing the release or transport of volatiles to the olfactory receptors (e.g., dry mouth, poorly fitting dentures, limited time that food is in the mouth). Active diaphragmatic exhalation can enhance transport of volatiles and thus enhance retronasal olfaction (Pierce & Halpern, 1995).

Even if the concentration of volatiles from orthonasal and retronasal olfaction were identical at the olfactory mucosa, the simultaneous presence of true taste sensations can affect flavor experience (see Hornung & Enns, 1987, for a review). For example, an orally sampled solution is often reported to have a "taste" sensation even if it contains primarily odorant and little or no true taste (Murphy & Cain, 1980; Murphy, Cain, & Bartoshuk, 1977). On the other hand, the presence of a true taste may suppress a retronasal olfactory sensation. When sucrose was added to coffee flavor, the intensity of coffee flavor was reduced (Calvino, Garcia-Medina, & Cometto-Muniz, 1990). This latter observation is of particular interest in light of the genetic variation in sweet taste discussed later in this chapter. For example, individuals who perceive more intense sweet tastes from sugar might be expected to show greater suppression of the coffee flavor. This possibility deserves examination.

Rozin (1982) raised the possibility that some odors that are disliked when perceived orthonasally are liked when perceived retronasally. He queried undergraduates and found that they often disliked the smell but liked the taste of strong cheese, fish, and eggs. Because the "taste" of these foods is largely produced by retronasal olfaction, this suggests that the odors may vary qualitatively between orthonasal and retronasal perception. In a second experiment, Rozin asked participants to smell four juices and four soups (selected to be unfamiliar odors) and to learn to identify the smells by assigned numbers. Once the odors were learned orthonasally (i.e., correct identification on two successive trials), the juices and soups were introduced into the mouth with a syringe (to bypass orthonasal olfaction), and the participants were asked to identify them retronasally. Participants scored above chance but were less skilled at retronasal than orthonasal identification (Rozin, 1982). This finding could reflect weaker perceived intensities if the retronasal stimulation resulted in lower concentrations of odorants at the mucosa. However, these observations support the possibility that the qualitative experiences during orthonasal and retronasal olfaction are not identical.

Dissociation Between Orthonasal and Retronasal Olfaction

Any damage to the olfactory mucosa, neurons, or central structures causes losses in the ability to perceive volatiles no matter what path they take to the receptors (i.e., orthonasal or retronasal paths). However, clinical conditions that change the way volatiles are released and pumped into the nasal cavity during eating may impair retronasal olfaction but leave orthonasal olfaction intact. A comparison of orthonasal and retronasal perception in a group of elderly women supported this dissociation. In this study (Duffy, 1992), the two measures of olfactory perception correlated significantly; however, approximately 33% of the participants had normal orthonasal perception but elevated retronasal sensitivity. Those with complete maxillary dentures were more likely to show the elevated retronasal sensitivity. Future investigations could determine whether poorly fitting dentures alter chewing and mouth movements enough to diminish retronasal olfactory perception.

Impaired orthonasal with intact retronasal olfaction is also observed clinically in patients with laryngectomies. After laryngectomy, patients usually report losses in the ability to smell, but they do not typically complain of a loss in the ability to perceive flavor (Ritter, 1964). Normally, one breathes air in through the nose or mouth, and the air travels through the trachea into the lungs. Laryngectomy interrupts this path, so that patients do not breathe through the nose or mouth but rather breathe through a stoma, an opening created in the throat that allows air to be drawn directly into the trachea, bypassing the nose and mouth. The major reason for loss of the ability to smell is that air carrying odorants does not pass through the nose during breathing (see Doty & Frye, 1989; Mozell et al., 1986, for reviews). During eating, odors can still enter the nose by the retronasal route; therefore, these patients do not lose their ability to perceive food flavors.

Chemesthesis, Touch, and Thermal Sensations

Mouthsense also includes the oral sensations of touch, irritation or burn, pain, and temperature. On the anterior, mobile tongue, these sensations are mediated by the trigeminal nerve (V), and on the posterior tongue, they are mediated by the glossopharyngeal nerve (IX). Later in this chapter, we provide support for the existence of genetic variation in the perception of oral irritation. Irritation (e.g., pungency) and thermal sensations are also produced in the nasal cavity by way of the trigeminal nerve (V). Irritation sensations interact with both taste and smell (e.g., see Cain & Murphy, 1980; Lawless & Stevens, 1984). Furthermore, touch sensations also serve to localize taste and olfactory sensations as noted previously (e.g., Todrank & Bartoshuk, 1991).

ABERRATIONS OF TASTE AND SMELL

Losses of taste and smell can be dangerous because they deprive individuals of important information (e.g., the warning provided by the odorant added to natural gas). Equally important, losses of taste and smell impair the quality of life by removing a valuable source of pleasure.

Taste

Patients with damage to the olfactory system often report taste loss as well as olfactory loss because of the confusion between true taste and retronasal olfaction. When the distinction is clarified, true taste loss appears to be much less common than olfactory loss (Deems et al., 1991; Goodspeed et al., 1986; Smith, 1991). This poses an interesting puzzle. Even when portions of the taste system are known to have been damaged, patients often fail to report any change in their taste experiences. An understanding of the answer to this puzzle requires consideration of the anatomy of the taste system. Three cranial nerves innervate the taste system: VII innervates the fungiform papillae on the anterior tongue (chorda tympani branch) and the taste buds on the palate (greater superficial petrosal branch); IX (glossopharyngeal) innervates the foliate papillae on the rear edges of the tongue (there remains controversy about whether or not VII innervates these papillae as well; Catalanotto, Lecadre, Robinson, & Bartoshuk, 1992; Tomita, Ikeda, & Okuda, 1986) and the circumvallate papillae on the back of the tongue; and X (vagus) innervates receptors in the throat. Incidentally, the tongue map so commonly found in taste chapters in physiology books that depicts sweet on the tip of the tongue, bitter on the back, and so on, is wrong. All four taste qualities are perceived by all cranial nerves mediating taste (Bartoshuk, 1993a, 1993b; Collings, 1974).

Almost 175 years ago, Brillat-Savarin wrote about a man whose tongue had been cut out (the anterior, mobile part of the tongue that is innervated by VII) but who could still taste (Brillat-Savarin, 1825). More recently, Pfaffmann documented his own experience with damage to some of the taste nerves (Pfaffmann & Bartoshuk, 1989, 1990). In his 70s, Pfaffmann developed herpes zoster oticus, a reactivation of the virus responsible for chicken pox. Herpes zoster oticus can do extensive damage to cranial nerves; in Pfaffmann's case, it damaged both VII and IX on the left side of his mouth. The damage was so severe that no taste function remained on the left tongue and palate. In spite of this damage, Pfaffmann experienced no change in his taste world.

Halpern and Nelson (1965) first proposed interactions between VII

151

and IX that explain why taste is maintained despite extensive damage. They anesthetized the chorda tympani (VII) at the point where it crosses the eardrum on its path to the brain. This caused neural responses (in the medulla) produced by the stimulation of tongue areas innervated by IX (rear of the tongue) to increase. They hypothesized that VII normally inhibits IX. When VII is anesthetized, its inhibition of IX is released, and responses to stimulation of IX increase. This hypothesis has been supported and generalized in human studies (Bartoshuk, Kveton, Yanagisawa, & Catalanotto, 1994; Catalanotto, Bartoshuk, Östrum, Gent, & Fast, 1993; Lehman, Bartoshuk, Catalanotto, Kveton, & Lowlicht, 1995; Yanagisawa et al., 1992); that is, both VII and IX appear to inhibit one another through their projection fields in the central nervous system (CNS) such that damage to one releases inhibition on the other. The release of inhibition thus compensates for the loss caused by the damage. It is interesting that the observer does not detect this compensation because the spatial localization of taste experience is controlled by touch (L. Green, 1991; Todrank & Bartoshuk, 1991), just as the localization of olfactory and thermal sensations are controlled by touch (B.G. Green, 1977). As long as touch sensations are normal, taste sensations seem to arise from whatever area is touched in the mouth.

The most common causes of taste damage are head trauma (Bartoshuk, Catalanotto, Scott, & Solomon, 1989; Costanzo & Zasler, 1991; Schechter & Henkin, 1974; G. M. Solomon, 1991; G. M. Solomon, Catalanotto, Scott, & Bartoshuk, 1991; Sumner, 1967) and upper respiratory infection (Deems et al., 1991; Duncan, Seiden, Paik, & Smith, 1991; Goodspeed et al., 1986; Henkin, Larson, & Powell, 1975; Smith, 1991; G. M. Solomon, 1991; G. M. Solomon et al., 1991). The chorda tympani taste nerve is particularly vulnerable when upper respiratory infections are associated with otitis media (infections of the middle ear) because the nerve travels through the middle ear on its way to the brain (DiLisio, 1990; Urbantschitsch, 1876; Williams, 1995).

Damage to taste was observed in a group of otherwise healthy young adults ($N = 147$) recruited for genetic taste testing from the Yale University community. Participants were given a spatial taste test that included bilateral testing of all cranial nerves mediating taste (Kveton & Bartoshuk, 1994) and completed a questionnaire that included items about head trauma and otitis media. Participants who reported chronic otitis media had elevated taste intensities on the anterior tongue, whereas those with a significant history of head trauma had depressed taste intensities on the anterior tongue. These taste-related pathologies may influence the classification of genetic taste status. This relation was demonstrated in 366 participants in a screening for genetic taste status (rated bitterness of filter paper impregnated with 6-n-propylthiouracil; PROP). Those who reported a history of otitis media were more likely to rate the PROP as very intense (i.e., be classified as supertasters), and those who reported a history of head trauma were more likely to rate the PROP as tasteless (i.e., be classified as nontasters; Bartoshuk, Duffy, Reed, & Williams, 1995).

The elderly tend to have higher taste thresholds than young people (Grzegorczyk, Jones, & Mistretta, 1979; Moore, Nielsen, & Mistretta, 1982; Murphy, 1986; Schiffman, Hornack, & Reilly, 1979; Weiffenbach, 1989; Weiffenbach, Baum, & Burghauser, 1982). The suprathreshold data are more difficult to interpret because of the many different methods, some inappropriate, used to assess perceived intensity (Bartoshuk & Duffy, 1995). Conservative interpretation of the literature suggests that there is little loss of taste with age and that when it does occur, it is most likely to be for sour and bitter substances. However, sensory losses in aging must be the combination of age-related loss (if any) with losses associated with pathology. Scientists do not have the means for totally distinguishing age-related loss from pathology-related loss, but careful evaluation of pathology demonstrates the distinction.

Another explanation for loss of taste with aging may relate to sex differences in perception of bitterness. If the perception of bitter is enhanced for women during childbearing years, what appears to be a taste loss in elderly women may reflect, at least in part, a loss of the extra taste ability conferred at menarche.

Olfaction

The most common sources of olfactory loss are head trauma, viral infection, and nasal disease (Deems et al., 1991; Goodspeed et al., 1986; Smith, 1991). Head trauma may produce central damage, but there is a peripheral explanation for the loss as well. As noted previously, olfactory neurons pass through the cribriform plate on their way to the olfactory bulb. A blow to the head can fracture that bone, severing the olfactory neurons. Viral infections are believed to damage olfaction by invading and destroying olfactory neurons.

Nasal disease causes olfactory loss by simple obstruction. Swelling of tissue near the olfactory cleft causes the cleft to close, preventing access of odors to the olfactory receptors.

Olfactory perception declines with the normal process of aging, but this change may reflect disease and environmental insults (e.g., head trauma, upper respiratory tract viruses, nasal sinus disease; (Ship & Weiffenbach, 1993). Older individuals show a range of function in olfaction from that equal to younger cohorts to total loss. A precipitous loss suggests pathology.

Older individuals generally show blunted perception of orthonasal perception from very weak to very strong. Their thresholds are elevated, therefore, and the perceived intensities of suprathreshold odorants are reduced (D. A. Stevens & Lawless, 1981; J. C. Stevens & Cain, 1985, 1987; J. C. Stevens, Plantinga, & Cain, 1982). One area of debate concerns whether or not all odors show equal losses. The National Geographic Smell Survey, a six-item scratch and sniff test given to 1.2 million individuals, suggested that losses with age are not equivalent for all odorants (Gilbert & Wysocki, 1987). As noted previously, even in individuals who do not suffer severe damage to the olfactory system, retronasal olfaction can be impaired if volatiles are not released normally during chewing and swallowing. Not surprisingly, elderly individuals show impaired ability to rely on olfactory cues to identify food flavors (Cain, Reid, & Stevens, 1990; Schiffman, 1977).

GENETIC VARIATION IN TASTE

Humans live in different taste worlds because of genetic variation (e.g., see Bartoshuk, Duffy, & Miller, 1994). The accidental discovery of genetic taste blindness to phenylthiocarbamide (PTC; Fox, 1931) led to family studies (Blakesleeand Fox, 1932; Snyder, 1931) that confirmed that PTC tasting resulted from a dominant allele (T). Nontasters have two recessive alleles (tt), and tasters have only one (Tt or tT) or two dominant alleles (TT). Although the early studies often involved tasting PTC crystals or concentrated solutions (e.g., see Fernberger, 1932), Harris and Kalmus (1949) developed a threshold procedure that became the "gold standard" evaluation technique. Plotting the distribution of Harris–Kalmus thresholds as a function of PTC concentration resulted in a bimodal curve that looked like two normal distributions overlapping slightly with the nontaster distribution

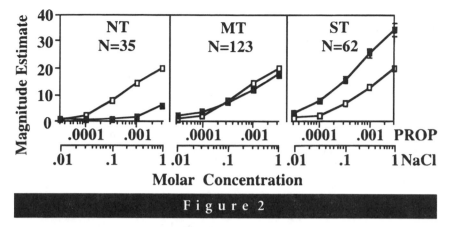

Figure 2

Magnitude estimates (± *SE*) of taste intensities of NaCl (open squares) and PROP (filled squares) for nontasters (NT), medium tasters (MT), and supertasters (ST). NaCl and PROP functions are superimposed to permit comparisons. ST: PROP ratio ≥ 1.2. MT: 0.4 ≤ PROP ratio < 1.2. NT: PROP ratio < 0.4.

making up about 25% of the total. Studies on a variety of bitter compounds revealed that only those containing the N − C = S group produced this bimodal distribution. One of those compounds, 6-n-propylthiouracil (PROP), lacked the sulfurous odor associated with PTC and so came to be used in its place in later research (Fischer & Griffin, 1964). Safety concerns also favor use of PROP (Lawless, 1980). Because PROP is a medication used to treat hyperthyroidism, safety limits on exposure can be set with reference to pharmaceutical doses. Taste testing uses quantities far smaller than those ingested by patients using PROP under physician guidance.

The exclusive use of thresholds to establish PROP status seems, in retrospect, unfortunate. It is now known that thresholds do not reflect suprathreshold taste perception (Bartoshuk, 1978; Pangborn, 1980); that is, an individual can have a very low threshold, but as concentration rises, the perceived intensity can grow so slowly that even the highest concentrations produce only weak taste sensations. On the other hand, an individual can have a high threshold, but the perceived intensity can increase with concentration so rapidly that the highest concentrations produce extremely strong taste sensations. Evaluation of PROP tasting of suprathreshold concentrations seemed warranted, therefore, to assess an individual's genetic status properly. Figure 2 shows the results from an experiment in which participants were asked to estimate the magnitudes of the tastes of NaCl and PROP. Earlier work suggested that NaCl tastes approximately the same to all people (Marks et al., 1988); therefore, NaCl was used as the standard. As Figure 2 shows, nontasters were easy to classify because they reported the bitterness of PROP to taste very weak compared to the saltiness of NaCl. However, the tasters showed a considerable amount of variation; some tasters found the most concentrated PROP to be only moderately bitter, whereas others found it to be intensely bitter. To quantify this difference, we formed a PROP ratio:

$$PROP\ ratio = [(.001\ M\ PROP/.32\ M\ NaCl)$$
$$+ (.0032\ M\ PROP/1\ M\ NaCl)]/2$$

where .001 M PROP refers to the magnitude estimate for PROP, and so on. We used the PROP ratio to separate tasters into medium tasters and supertasters (see Figure 2). We suspect, but have yet to prove, that medium tasters have one dominant allele (tT or Tt) and supertasters have two (TT). For many years, PTC–PROP taste blindness was considered to be simply a curiosity in taste. Those who were taste-blind were believed to lack a particular receptor mechanism for PTC, PROP, and their chemical relatives but to be normal for all other tastes. However, the advent of suprathreshold scaling techniques and their application to this phenomenon has changed that view dramatically. The earliest of these studies (done before supertasters were recognized) showed that tasters perceived greater bitterness from caffeine (Hall, Bartoshuk, Cain, & Stevens, 1975) and KCl (Bartoshuk, Rifkin, Marks, & Hooper, 1988), bitter compounds that do not contain the N − C = S group. Furthermore, the taster–nontaster difference extended even to sweet compounds; tasters perceived greater sweetness from saccharin (Bartoshuk, 1979) and sucrose (Gent & Bartoshuk, 1983). Subdivision of PROP tasters into medium tasters and supertasters showed that PROP supertasters perceived the greatest taste intensities (Bartoshuk, 1993a, 1993b).

Miller and Reedy (1990) found evidence for an anatomical explanation of the variation in PROP tasting with a technique using dyes (methylene blue or ordinary blue food coloring) that stain some structures on the tongue but not others. The dyes stain filiform papillae (which do not contain

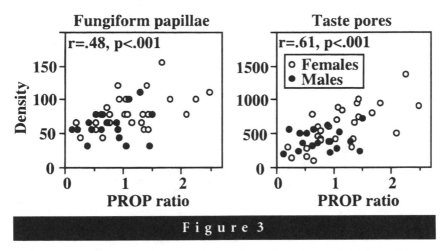

Figure 3

PROP ratio versus densities of fungiform papillae and taste pores. Participants have no histories of otitis media or head trauma. If the nontasters are removed, the correlations remain significant (fungiform papillae: $r = .38$, $p < .05$; taste pores: $r = .57$, $p < .001$).

taste buds) but do not stain fungiform papillae (which do contain taste buds); thus, the fungiform papillae can be seen as pink circles against a blue background. Examination of the fungiform papillae with a microscope reveals small blue dots on the papillae. These are taste pores, the conduits that lead to the taste buds. Miller and Reedy found that PROP tasted more intense to individuals who had more taste buds. In collaboration with these researchers, we extended their observations to supertasters (Reedy et al., 1993). Supertasters had the most taste buds, and nontasters, the least (see Figure 2). Note that the densities of both fungiform papillae and the taste buds on these papillae increase with increasing ability to taste PROP as measured by the PROP ratio (Figure 3).

Sex and PROP Tasting

The data shown in Figure 3 are separated by sex. The PROP ratios and the densities of fungiform papillae and taste pores reached higher values for women (Bartoshuk, Duffy, & Miller, 1994). The distribution of perceived bitterness of the PROP paper also showed the sex difference (see Figure 4). PROP papers were constructed by soaking Whatman #1 filter paper in a saturated solution of PROP (near-boiling temperature), allowing the paper to dry, and cutting it into 1-inch squares. As the paper dries, the saturated

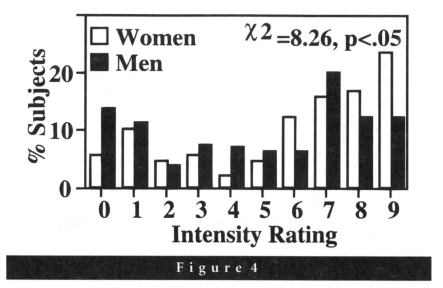

Figure 4

Distributions of intensity ratings of PROP papers for women ($n = 90$) and men ($n = 81$). Frequencies are expressed as a percentage for each sex. Participants have no histories of otitis media or head trauma. The distributions were tested with a chi-square analysis of the frequencies in the following rating groups (0–5, 6, 7, 8–9).

PROP crystallizes into the paper. The PROP paper is a convenient way to provide a measured quantity of crystals to the participant (each PROP paper contains about 1.2 mg of PROP). Marketed tablets of PROP sold for the treatment of hyperthyroidism contain 50 mg each, and the maintenance dosage for this medication varies from 50 to 200 mg/day (D. H. Solomon, 1986); thus, the PROP paper contains a small fraction of a pharmacologically active dose. Participants were instructed to place the paper in the mouth, moisten it with saliva, and report the maximum taste intensity on a 9-point scale on which 1 = *very weak,* 5 = *medium,* and 9 = *very strong.* This sex effect was also uncovered by reanalyzing earlier published PTC–PROP threshold and suprathreshold data with modern statistical procedures (Bartoshuk, Duffy, & Miller, 1994).

The reason for the sex difference is as yet unknown. Superior bitter detection in women would help to ensure a healthy pregnancy, because in nature, bitters are often poisonous. Sex hormones may modify the phenotypic display of the taste genotype. Bitter sensitivity increases during the first trimester of pregnancy (unpublished data collected in the laboratory of J. Rodin) and varies across menstruation (Aaron, 1975; Bhatia, Sharma, & Mehta, 1981; Glanville & Kaplan, 1965a, 1965b; Parlee, 1983; Than, Delay, & Maier, 1994). The female superiority in bitter tasting may disappear with age, possibly owing to diminished production of sex hormones. There are many anecdotal accounts of cravings for sweets associated with the menstrual cycle. The association between PROP tasting and sex hormones suggests that PROP tasting should be studied in conjunction with changes in preferences for sweets.

Other Oral Sensations and PROP Tasting

Capsaicin (found in chili peppers) produces burning sensations when applied to the tongue. Before the development of the distinction between medium tasters and supertasters, it was found that capsaicin (applied to the anterior tongue) produced greater burn to tasters than to nontasters (Karrer & Bartoshuk, 1991). In a more recent study (Karrer et al., 1992), that finding was extended to supertasters and other irritants were added. Participants were divided into PROP nontasters, medium tasters, and supertasters using the threshold and suprathreshold criteria (see Figure 2). Supertasters gave the highest ratings of intensity to the burn of capsaicin (chili pepper), piperine (black pepper), ginger, and ethanol. Whitehead and colleagues (Whitehead, Beeman, & Kinsella, 1985; Whitehead & Kachele, 1994) showed that the taste buds in fungiform papillae are surrounded by trigeminal neurons. Because supertasters have more taste buds, they may also have more trigeminal neurons and thus a greater capacity to feel pain. This hypothesis was tested by applying 100 ppm capsaicin to tongue loci with and without taste buds. Supertasters rated burn as more intense on areas with more taste buds, supporting the hypothesis (Karrer et al., 1992). Because women are more likely than men to be supertasters and have, on average, more taste buds, women also experience, on average, more intense oral burn from capsaicin (Bartoshuk et al., 1995).

Supertasters may be particularly aware of fat in food. Fat has no taste or smell but does produce tactile sensations that may be more salient to supertasters, because tactile sensations, like oral irritation, are mediated by the trigeminal nerve. Recent data show highest creaminess ratings of high-fat milk products in PROP supertasters (Duffy, Bartoshuk, Lucchina, Snyder, Tym, in press). The question is, does perception of fat correlate with preference for fat? Preference for high-fat foods varies with both PROP tasting and sex; that is, in women, preference for high-fat foods fell as PROP tasting increased, whereas in men, preference for high-fat foods tended to rise as PROP tasting increased. In elderly women, PROP tasting was associated with measures of body fat and serum lipids: Women who were more responsive to PROP were thinner and had serum lipid values that were reflective of lower cardiovascular disease risk (Lucchina, Bartoshuk, Duffy, Marks, & Ferris, 1995).

RELATIONSHIP OF TASTE AND OLFACTION TO NUTRIENTS

Taste and olfaction play very different roles in nutrition, a fact that becomes clear if one examines the tastes and smells of nutrients. The macronutrients consist of proteins, carbohydrates (starch and sugar), and fats. Contrary to popular belief, the only one of these detectable by taste or smell is sugar (which tastes sweet). Protein, starch, and fat molecules are too large to stimulate taste or smell receptors. Some proteins (e.g., bacon, chicken) and fats (e.g., olive oil, sesame oil) seem to have distinct flavors, but these are due to volatiles mixed with the protein or fat. Micronutrients consist of vitamins (too dilute in food to be detected by taste or smell) and minerals. Minerals in the form of salts taste salty (e.g., NaCl) or salty plus bitter when the cation is larger than sodium (e.g., KCl, $CaCl_2$). Many poisons— important nutrients in the sense that they must be avoided—are bitter.

No nutrients can be identified by smell; however, certain nutrients can be identified by taste. These are sodium (salty), sugar (sweet), and poison (bitter). For sodium and sugar, there is evidence that the palatability of the taste is altered by the need for the nutrient, for example, salt deprivation increases preference for NaCl (e.g., Richter, 1942–43), and injection of insulin lowers blood glucose and increases preference for sweet (e.g., Mayer-Gross & Walker, 1946).

Taste

In the older literature on PTC–PROP, the ability of tasters to perceive greater bitterness was associated with a greater number of food dislikes (see Drewnowski, 1990, for a review). Because PTC-related compounds occur in some bitter vegetables, there was early interest in the evaluation of vegetable preferences in nontasters and tasters. Although marginal effects were observed, studies failed to support a clear association between PROP–PTC thresholds and bitter vegetable preference (Jacobs, 1958; Jerzsa-Latta, Krondl, & Coleman, 1990). A reevaluation seems warranted now that supertasters can be identified. In addition, predictions of food liking must take into account the totality of sensations evoked by the food; that is, supertasters and nontasters might experience sensations from vegetables that differ more than in simple bitterness.

Bitterness is an important taste quality in dairy products. In one study, PROP–PTC tasters perceived more bitterness in some dairy products, including cheddar cheese (Marino et al., 1991), and in another study, these tasters showed less preference for strong cheese, cottage cheese, buttermilk, and whipped cream (Forrai & Bankovi, 1984). A study with children (Anliker, Bartoshuk, Ferris, & Hooks, 1991) used Birch's (1979) technique to provide a ranking of foods and beverages by preference. With this technique, children were asked to sample the foods of interest and then select their favorite. The favorite item was removed, and the children were asked to select the favorite of those remaining, and so on. One of the foods was cheddar cheese. The average position of the cheddar cheese in the ranking of eight foods and beverages was 1.4 for nontasters, 3.2 for medium tasters, and 5.4 for supertasters.

PROP supertasters were found to perceive more bitterness and more oral irritation from ethanol than medium tasters and nontasters (Bartoshuk et al., 1993). This finding is interesting in light of the data suggesting that alcoholics tend to be nontasters (Pelchat & Danowski, 1992). The possibility exists that supertasters might be protected from alcoholism to some extent because the sensory properties of alcohol are more aversive to them.

Although the early studies on PTC–PROP tasting focused on bitterness, later psychophysical studies showed that tasters also perceived greater sweetness (Bartoshuk, 1979; Gent & Bartoshuk, 1983). Recent work suggests that there is a PROP–sweet preference connection that was previously unsuspected. Looy and Weingarten (1992) studied a sample of young adults (primarily females) who were classified as PROP tasters or nontasters by their PROP thresholds. Nontasters were sucrose likers, whereas tasters were more likely to be sucrose dislikers. Working with Weingarten, we extended

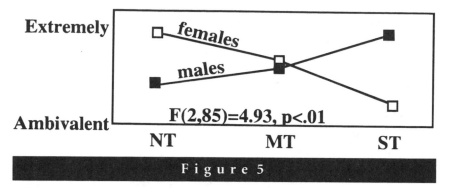

Figure 5

PROP × Sex interaction on preference for sweet foods and beverages in women ($n = 52$) and men ($n = 40$), aged 18–35 years, who are nontasters (NT), medium tasters (MT), and supertasters (ST) of PROP. Pairwise comparisons were significant for female NT and ST ($p < .01$) and for female ST and male ST ($p < .05$).

those observations by examining the association between sweet preference and PROP tasting in nontasters, medium tasters, and supertasters with both male and female participants. The results showed an interaction between sex and PROP tasting. Figure 5 shows that a composite preference score for 12 sweet foods or beverages (including candy, sweet dairy products, baked goods, sweeteners, and sugar-sweetened soda) fell as ability to taste PROP increased in women (confirming Looy & Weingarten, 1992). The opposite was seen in men (Duffy, Weingarten, & Bartoshuk, 1995). The sex difference could result because female supertasters perceive sweets as too intense and thus less pleasant. It could also result, however, because female supertasters show more concern with weight and thus may reject sweet because of its association with calories.

Olfaction

As we have shown, olfaction is not tuned to nutrients; rather, it labels foods and provides an important source of pleasure. Because olfactory perception is much more vulnerable to loss than is taste, the question arises concerning the consequences of olfactory loss to food behavior. In a group of health-seeking individuals, olfactory dysfunction did not cause overt malnutrition (Ferris & Duffy, 1989; Mattes & Cowart, 1994). However, these individuals experienced less pleasure from eating and may have compensated in part by increased attention to taste. In fact, those with olfactory dysfunction, especially older women, showed a dietary pattern that increased chronic disease risk (Duffy, Backstrand, & Ferris, 1995). Lower olfactory perception was associated with lower preference for fruits and vegetables, higher intakes of high-fat sweets, and higher intakes of total fat and saturated fats. This pattern could increase the difficulty of elderly persons in controlling chronic disease risk through diet. Increases in the concentration of odorants (Schiffman & Warwick, 1993), visual displays, and textural variation in food may enhance food enjoyment, especially for the institutionalized elderly.

CONCLUSION

Foods evoke several qualitatively different sensations as the result of contacting receptors in the oral and nasal cavities. Although one can attend to each of these sensations in turn, normal experience results from the integration of these sensations into perceived food objects. The nervous system constructs ice cream, pizza, or chili peppers from the stream of taste, olfactory, touch, thermal, and pain sensations that flow from the sensory receptors. The pleasure gotten from taste reflects hard-wired neural mechanisms (people are born loving sweet and hating bitter), but the pleasure obtained from smells (orthonasally or retronasally perceived) reflects experience (one learns to love chocolate and hate feces). Pathology can alter the sensations produced by foods; because taste and smell evoke pleasure, chemosensory pathology can produce devastating impairments to the quality of life. Genetic variation results in substantial differences in taste experiences across individuals that impact on the pleasure of eating and affect food choices and, ultimately, nutrition.

REFERENCES

Aaron, M. (1975). Effect of the menstrual cycle on subjective ratings of sweetness. *Perceptual and Motor Skills, 40,* 974.

Amoore, J. E., Johnston, J. W., & Rubin, M. (1964). The stereochemical theory of odor. *Scientific American, 210,* 42–49.

Anliker, J. A., Bartoshuk, L. M., Ferris, A. M., & Hooks, L. D. (1991). Children's food preferences and genetic sensitivity to the bitter taste of PROP. *Americal Journal of Clinical Nutrition, 54,* 316–320.

Bartoshuk, L. M. (1978). The psychophysics of taste. *American Journal of Clinical Nutrition, 31,* 1068–1077.

Bartoshuk, L. M. (1979). Bitter taste of saccharin: Related to the genetic ability to taste the bitter substance 6-n-propylthiouracil (PROP). *Science, 205,* 934–935.

Bartoshuk, L. M. (1993a). The biological basis of food perception and acceptance. *Food Quality and Preference, 4,* 21–32.

Bartoshuk, L. M. (Ed.). (1993b). *Genetic and pathological taste variation: What can we learn from animal models and human disease?* New York: Wiley.

Bartoshuk, L. M., Catalanotto, F. C., Scott, A. E., & Solomon, G. M. (1989). Spatial taste losses associated with head trauma, upper respiratory infection and nasal symptoms [abstract]. *Chemical Senses, 14,* 684.

Bartoshuk, L. M., Conner, E., Karrer, T., Kochenbach, K., Palcso, M., Snow, D., Pelchat, M., & Danowski, S. (1993). PROP supertasters and the perception of ethyl alcohol [abstract]. *Chemical Senses, 18,* 526–527.

Bartoshuk, L. M., & Duffy, V. B. (1995). Taste and smell in aging. In E. J. Masoro (Eds.), *Handbook of Physiology: Section II: Aging* (pp. 363–375). New York: Oxford University Press.

Bartoshuk, L. M., Duffy, V. B., Berger, A., Karrer, T., Snyder, D. & Sasaki, C. (1995). Women perceive greater oral burn from capsaicin: Clinical implications for oral pain. [abstract]. *Chemical Senses, 20,* 663–664.

Bartoshuk, L. M., Duffy, V. B., & Miller, I. J. (1994). PTC/PROP tasting: Anatomy, psychophysics, and sex effects. *Physiology and Behavior, 56,* 1165–1171.

Bartoshuk, L. M., Duffy, V. B., Reed, D., & Williams, A. (1995). Supertasting, earaches, and head injury: Genetics and pathology alter our taste worlds. *Neuroscience and Biobehavioral Reviews. 20,* 79–87.

Bartoshuk, L. M., Kveton, J., Yanagisawa, K., & Catalanotto, F. (1994). Taste loss and taste phantoms: A role of inhibition in taste. In K. Kurihara, N. Suzuki, & H. Ogawa (Eds.), *Annals of the New York Academy of Sciences, 510,* (pp. 557–560). New York: Springer-Verlag.

Bartoshuk, L. M., Rifkin, B., Marks, L. E., & Hooper, J. E. (1988). Bitterness of KCl and benzoate: Related to PTC/PROP [abstract]. *Chemical Senses, 13,* 517–528.

Bhatia, S., Sharma, K. N., & Mehta, V. (1981). Taste responsiveness to phenylthiocarbamide and glucose during menstrual cycle. *Current Science, 50,* 980–983.

Birch, L. (1979). Dimensions of preschool children's food preferences. *Journal of Nutrition Education, 11,* 77–80.

Birch, L. L., McPhee, L., Steinberg, L., & Sullivan, S. (1990). Conditioned flavor preferences in young children. *Physiology and Behavior, 47*, 501–505.

Blakeslee, A. F., & Fox, A. L. (1932). Our different taste worlds. *Journal of Heredity, 23*, 97–107.

Brillat-Savarin, J. A. (1825). *The physiology of taste* (M. F. K. Fisher, Trans.). New York: Knopf.

Burdach, K., & Doty, R. (1987). The effects of mouth movements, swallowing and spitting on retronasal odor perception. *Physiology and Behavior, 41*, 353–356.

Cain, W. S. (1987). Taste vs. smell in the organization of perceptual experience. In J. Solms, D. A. Booth, R. M. Pangborn, & O. Raunhardt (Eds.), *Food acceptance and nutrition* (pp. 63–77). San Diego, CA: Academic Press.

Cain, W. S., & Murphy, C. L. (1980). Interaction between chemoreceptive modalities of odour and irritation. *Nature, 284*, 255–257.

Cain, W., Reid, F., & Stevens, J. (1990). Missing ingredients: Aging and the discrimination of flavor. *Journal of Nutrition for the Elderly, 9*, 3–15.

Calvino, A., Garcia-Medina, M., & Cometto-Muniz, J. (1990). Interactions in caffeine-sucrose and coffee-sucrose mixtures: Evidence of taste and flavor suppression. *Chemical Senses, 15*, 505–519.

Catalanotto, F. A., Bartoshuk, L. M., Östrum, K. M., Gent, J. F., & Fast, K. (1993). Effects of anesthesia of the facial nerve on taste. *Chemical Senses, 18*, 461–470.

Catalanotto, F., Lecadre, Y., Robinson, M., & Bartoshuk, L. (1992). Effects of 7th cranial nerve anesthesia on taste [abstract] *Chemical Senses, 17*, 602.

Collings, V. B. (1974). Human taste response as a function of locus of stimulation on the tongue and soft palate. *Perception and Psychophysics, 16*, 169–174.

Costanzo, R. M., & Zasler, N. D. (1991). Head trauma. In T. Getchell, R. L. Doty, L. M. Bartoshuk, & J. B. Snow (Eds.), *Smell and taste in health and disease* (pp. 711–730). New York: Raven Press.

Deems, D. A., Doty, R. L., Settle, R. G., Moore-Gillon, V., Shaman, P., Mester, A. F., Kimmelman, C. P., Brightman, V. J., & Snow, J. B. (1991). Smell and taste disorders: A study of 750 patients from the University of Pennsylvania Smell and Taste Center. *Archives of Otolaryngology-Head and Neck Surgery, 117*, 519–528.

DiLisio, G. J. (1990). *Taste alteration in subjects with acute otitis media or middle ear fluid/taste preservation in otolaryngologic patients.* Unpublished medical school thesis, Yale University School of Medicine, New Haven, CT.

Doty, R. L., & Frye, R. (1989). Influence of nasal obstruction on smell function. *Otolaryngologic Clinics of North America, 22*, 397–411.

Drewnowski, A. (1990). Genetics of taste and smell. *World Review of Nutrition and Dietetics, 63*, 194–208.

Duffy, V. B. (1992). *Olfactory dysfunction, food behaviors, dietary intake, and anthropometric measures in single-living, elderly women.* Unpublished doctoral dissertation, University of Connecticut, Storrs.

Duffy, V. B., Backstrand, J., & Ferris, A. (1995). Olfactory dysfunction and related nutritional risk in free-living, elderly women. *Journal of the American Dietetic Association, 95*, 879–884.

Duffy, V. B., Bartoshuk, L. M., Lucchina, L. A., Snyder, D. J., Tym, A. (in press). Supertasters of PROP (6-n-propylthiouracil) rate the highest creaminess to high-fat milk products [abstract]. *Chemical senses.*

Duffy, V. B., Weingarten, H. P., & Bartoshuk, L. M. (1995). Preference for sweet in young adults associated with PROP (6-n-propylthiouracil) genetic taster status and sex. *Chemical Senses, 20*, 688.

Duncan, H. J., Seiden, A. M., Paik, S. I., & Smith, D. V. (1991). Differences among patients with smell impairment resulting from head trauma, nasal disease, or prior upper respiratory infection [abstract]. *Chemical Senses, 16*, 517.

Engen, T. (1982). *The perception of odors.* San Diego, CA: Academic Press.

Fernberger, S. W. (1932). A preliminary study of taste deficiency. *American Journal of Psychology, 44*, 322–326.

Ferris, A. M., & Duffy, V. B. (1989). The effect of olfactory deficits on nutritional status: Does age predict individuals at risk? In C. Murphy, W. S. Cain, & D. Hegsted (Ed.), *Annals of The New York Academy of Sciences, 561*, (pp. 113–123). New York: New York Academy of Sciences.

Fischer, R., & Griffin, F. (1964). Pharmacogenetic aspects of gustation. *Drug Research, 14*, 673–686.

Forrai, G., & Bankovi, G. (1984). Taste perception for phenylthiocarbamide and food choice: A Hungarian twin study. *Acta Physiologica Hungarica, 64*, 33–40.

Fox, A. L. (1931). Six in ten "tasteblind" to bitter chemical. *Science News Letter, 9*, 249.

Gent, J. F., & Bartoshuk, L. M. (1983). Sweetness of sucrose, neohesperidin dihydrochalcone, and saccharin is related to genetic ability to taste the bitter substance 6-n-propylthiouracil. *Chemical Senses, 7*, 265–272.

Gilbert, A. N., & Wysocki, C. J. (1987). The smell survey results. *National Geographic, 172*, 515–525.

Glanville, E. V., & Kaplan, A. R. (1965a). The menstrual cycle and sensitivity of taste perception. *American Journal of Obstetrics and Gynecology, 92*, 189–194.

Glanville, E. V., & Kaplan, A. R. (1965b). Taste perception and the menstrual cycle. *Nature, 206,* 930–931.

Goodspeed, R. B., Catalanotto, F. A., Gent, J. F., Cain, W. S., Bartoshuk, L. M., Leonard, G., & Donaldson, J. O. (1986). Clinical characteristics of patients with taste and smell disorders. In H. L. Meiselman & R. S. Rivlin (Eds.), *Clinical measurement of taste and smell* (pp. 451–466). New York: Macmillan.

Green, B. G. (1977). Localization of thermal sensation: An illusion and synthetic heat. *Perception and Psychophysics, 22,* 331–337.

Green, L. (1991) *Taste illusion: A partial explanation of unperceived taste loss.* Unpublished medical school thesis, Yale University School of Medicine, New Haven, CT.

Grzegorczyk, P. B., Jones, S. W., & Mistretta, C. M. (1979). Age-related differences in salt acuity. *Journal of Gerontology, 34,* 834–840.

Hall, M. J., Bartoshuk, L. M., Cain, W. S., & Stevens, J. C. (1975). PTC taste blindness and the taste of caffeine. *Nature, 253,* 442–443.

Halpern, B. P., & Nelson, L. M. (1965). Bulbar gustatory responses to anterior and to posterior tongue stimulation in the rat. *American Journal of Physiology, 209,* 105–110.

Harris, H., & Kalmus, H. (1949). The measurement of taste sensitivity to phenylthiourea (P.T.C.). *Annals of Eugenics, 15,* 24–31.

Henkin, R. I., Larson, A. L., & Powell, R. D. (1975). Hypogeusia, dysgeusia, hyposmia, and dysosmia following influenza-like infection. *Annals of Otology, Rhinology and Laryngology, 84,* 672–682.

Hornung, D. E., & Enns, M. P. (1987). Odor-taste mixtures. *Annals of the New York Academy of Sciences, 510,* 86–90.

Jacobs, H. L. (1958). Studies on sugar preference: I. The preference for glucose solutions and its modification by injections of insulin. *Journal of Comparative and Physiological Psychology, 51,* 304–310.

Jerzsa-Latta, M., Krondl, M., & Coleman, P. (1990). Use and perceived attributes of cruciferous vegetables in terms of genetically-mediated taste sensitivity. *Appetite, 15,* 127–134.

Karrer, T., & Bartoshuk, L. (1991). Capsaicin desensitization and recovery on the human tongue. *Physiology and Behavior, 49,* 757–764.

Karrer, T., Bartoshuk, L. M., Conner, E., Fehrenbaker, S., Grubin, D., & Snow, D. (1992). PROP status and its relationship to the perceived burn intensity of capsaicin at different tongue loci [abstract]. *Chemical Senses, 17,* 649.

167

Kveton, J. F., & Bartoshuk, L. M. (1994). The effect of unilateral chorda tympani damage on taste. *Laryngoscope, 104,* 25–29.

Lawless, H. T. (1980). A comparison of different methods used to assess sensitivity to the taste of phenylthiocarbamide (PTC). *Chemical Senses, 5,* 247–256.

Lawless, H., & Stevens, D. A. (1984). Effect of oral chemical irritation on taste. *Physiology and Behavior, 32,* 995–998.

Lehman, C. D., Bartoshuk, L. M., Catalanotto, F. C., Kveton, J. F., & Lowlicht, R. A. (1995). The effect of anesthesia of the chorda tympani nerve on taste perception in humans. *Physiology and Behavior, 57,* 943–951.

Looy, H., & Weingarten, H. P. (1992). Facial expressions and genetic sensitivity to 6-n-propylthiouracil predict hedonic response to sweet. *Physiology and Behavior, 52,* 75–82.

Lucchina, L., Bartoshuk, L. M., Duffy, V. B., Marks, L. E., & Ferris, A. M. (1995). 6-n-propylthiouracil perception affects nutritional status of independent-living older females [abstract]. *Chemical Senses, 20,* 735.

Marino, S., Bartoshuk, L. M., Monaco, J., Anliker, J. A., Reed, D., & Desnoyers, S. (1991). PTC/PROP and the tastes of milk products. *Chemical Senses, 16,* 551.

Marks, L. E., Stevens, J. C., Bartoshuk, L. M., Gent, J. G., Rifkin, B., & Stone, V. K. (1988). Magnitude matching: The measurement of taste and smell. *Chemical Senses, 13,* 63–87.

Mattes, R., & Cowart, B. (1994). Dietary assessment of patients with chemosensory disorders. *Journal of the American Dietetic Association, 94*(1), 50–56.

Mayer-Gross, W., & Walker, J. W. (1946). Taste and selection of food in hypoglycaemia. *British Journal of Experimental Pathology, 27,* 297–305.

Miller, I. J., & Reedy, F. E. (1990). Variations in human taste bud density and taste intensity perception. *Physiology and Behavior, 47,* 1213–1219.

Moore, L. M., Nielsen, C. R., & Mistretta, C. M. (1982). Sucrose taste thresholds: Age-related differences. *Journal of Gerontology, 37,* 64–69.

Mozell, M. M., Schwartz, D. N., Youngentob, S. L., Leopold, D. A., Hornung, D. E., & Sheehe, P. R. (1986). Reversal of hyposmia in laryngectomized patients. *Chemical Senses, 11,* 397–410.

Mozell, M. M., Smith, B., Smith, P., Sullivan, L., & Swender, P. (1969). Nasal chemoreception in flavor identification. *Archives of Otolaryngology, 90,* 367–373.

Murphy, C. (1986). Taste and smell in the elderly. In H. L. Meiselman & R. S. Rivlin (Eds.), *Clinical measurement of taste and smell* (pp. 343–371). New York: Macmillan.

Murphy, C., & Cain, W. S. (1980). Taste and olfaction: Independence vs interaction. *Physiology and Behavior, 24,* 601–605.

Murphy, C. L., Cain, W. S., & Bartoshuk, L. M. (1977). Mutual action of taste and olfaction. *Sensory Processes, 1,* 204–211.

Pangborn, R. M. (1980). *A critical analysis of sensory responses to sweetness.* San Diego, CA: Academic Press.

Parlee, M. B. (1983). Menstrual rhythms in sensory processes: A review of fluctuations in vision, olfaction, audition, taste, and touch. *Psychological Bulletin, 93,* 539–548.

Pelchat, M. L., & Danowski, S. (1992). A possible genetic association between PROP-tasting and alcoholism. *Physiology & Behavior, 51,* 1261–1266.

Pelchat, M. L., Grill, H. J., Rozin, P., & Jacobs, J. (1983). Quality of acquired responses to tastes by *Rattus norvegicus* depends on type of associated discomfort. *Journal of Comparative Psychology, 97,* 140–153.

Pelchat, M. L., & Rozin, P. (1982). The special role of nausea in the acquisition of food dislikes by humans. *Journal of Comparative Psychology, 3,* 341–351.

Pfaffmann, C., & Bartoshuk, L. M. (1989). Psychophysical mapping of a human case of left unilateral ageusia [abstract]. *Appetite, 14,* 738.

Pfaffmann, C., & Bartoshuk, L. M. (1990). Taste loss due to herpes zoster oticus: An update after 19 months. *Chemical Senses,* [abstract] *15,* 657–658.

Pierce, J., & Halpern, B. P. (1995). Orthonasal and retronasal identification of common substances presented as vapor phase stimuli [abstract]. *Chemical Senses, 20,* 757–758.

Reedy, F. E., Bartoshuk, L. M., Miller, I. J., Duffy, V. B., Lucchina, L., & Yanagisawa, K. (1993). Relationships among papillae, taste pores, and 6-*n*-propylthiouracil (PROP) suprathreshold taste sensitivity [abstract]. *Chemical Senses, 18,* 618–619.

Richter, C. P. (1942–43). Total self regulatory functions in animals and human beings. *Harvey Lecture Series, 38,* 63–103.

Ritter, F. N. (1964). Fate of olfaction after laryngectomy. *Archives of Otolaryngology, 79,* 169–171.

Rozin, P. (1982). "Taste-smell confusions" and the duality of the olfactory sense. *Perception and Psychophysics, 31,* 397–401.

Schechter, P. J., & Henkin, R. I. (1974). Abnormalities of taste and smell after head trauma. *Journal of Neurology, 37,* 802–810.

Schiffman, S. S. (1977). Food recognition by the elderly. *Journal of Gerontology, 32*, 586–592.

Schiffman, S. S., Hornack, K., & Reilly, D. (1979). Increased taste thresholds of amino acids with age. *American Journal of Clinical Nutrition, 32*, 1622–1627.

Schiffman, S. S., & Warwick, Z. S. (1993). Effects of flavor enhancement of foods for the elderly on nutritional status: Food intake, biochemical indices, and anthropometric measures. *Physiology and Behavior, 53*, 395–402.

Ship, J., & Weiffenbach, J. (1993). Age, gender, medical treatment and medication effects on smell identification. *Journal of Gerontology, 48*, M26–M32.

Smith, D. V. (1991). Taste and smell dysfunction. In M. M. Paparella, D. A. Shumrick, J. L. Gluckman, & W. L. Meyerhoff (Eds.), *Otolaryngology: head and neck* (pp. 1911–1934). Philadelphia: Saunders.

Snyder, L. H. (1931). Inherited taste deficiency. *Science, 74*, 151–152.

Solomon, D. H. (1986). Treatment of Graves' hyperthyroidism. In S. H. Ingbar & L. E. Braverman (Eds.), *The thyroid: A fundamental and clinical text* (pp. 987–1014). Philadelphia: Lippincott.

Solomon, G. (1991) *Patterns of taste loss in clinic patients with histories of head trauma, nasal symptoms, or upper respiratory infection.* Unpublished medical school thesis, Yale University School of Medicine, New Haven, CT.

Solomon, G. M., Catalanotto, F., Scott, A., & Bartoshuk, L. M. (1991). Patterns of taste loss in clinic patients with histories of head trauma, nasal symptoms, or upper respiratory infection. *Yale Journal of Biology and Medicine, 64*, 280.

Stevens, D. A., & Lawless, H. T. (1981). Age-related changes in flavor perception. *Appetite, 2*, 127–136.

Stevens, J. C., & Cain, W. S. (1985). Age-related deficiency in the perceived strength of six odorants. *Chemical Senses, 10*, 517–529.

Stevens, J. C., & Cain, W. S. (1987). Old-age deficits in the sense of smell as gauged by thresholds, magnitude matching, and odor identification. *Psychology and Aging, 2*, 36–42.

Stevens, J. C., Plantinga, A., & Cain, W. S. (1982). Reduction of odor and nasal pungency associated with aging. *Neurobiology of Aging, 3*, 125–132.

Sumner, D. (1967). Post-traumatic ageusia. *Brain, 90*, 187–202.

Than, T. T., Delay, E. R., & Maier, M. E. (1994). Sucrose threshold variation during the menstrual cycle. *Physiology and Behavior, 56*, 237–239.

Todrank, J., & Bartoshuk, L. M. (1991). A taste illusion: Taste sensation localized by touch. *Physiology and Behavior, 50*, 1027–1031.

Tomita, H., Ikeda, M., & Okuda, Y. (1986). Basis and practice of clinical taste examinations. *Auris Nasus Larynx (Tokyo), 13(Suppl. I)*, S1–S15.

Urbantschitsch, V. (1876). *Beobachtungen über anomalien des geschmacks der tastempfindungen und der speichelsecretion in folge von erkrankungen der paukenhöhle.* Stuttgart: Verlag von Ferdinand Enke.

Weiffenbach, J. M. (1989). Assessment of chemosensory functioning in aging. In C. Murphy, W. S. Cain, & D. M. Hegsted (Eds.), *Nutrition and the chemical senses in aging: Recent advances and current research needs* (pp. 56–64). New York: New York Academy of Sciences.

Weiffenbach, J. M., Baum, B. J., & Burghauser, R. (1982). Taste thresholds: Quality specific variation with human aging. *Journal of Gerontology, 37*, 372–377.

Whitehead, M. C., Beeman, C. S., & Kinsella, B. A. (1985). Distribution of taste and general sensory nerve endings in fungiform papillae of the hamster. *American Journal of Anatomy, 173*, 185–201.

Whitehead, M. C., & Kachele, D. L. (1994). Development of fungiform papillae, taste buds, and their innervation in the hamster. *Journal of Comparative Neurology, 340*, 515–530.

Williams, A. (1995). *Effects of otitis media on taste in children.* Unpublished senior thesis, Yale University School of Medicine, New Haven, CT.

Yanagisawa, K., Bartoshuk, L. M., Karrer, T. A., Kveton, J. F., Catalanotto, F. A., Lehman, C. D., & Weiffenbach, J. M. (1992). Anesthesia of the chorda tympani nerve: Insights into a source of dysgeusia [abstract]. *Chemical Senses, 17*, 724.

Zellner, D. A., Rozin, P., Aron, M., & Kulish, C. (1983). Conditioned enhancement of human's liking for flavor by pairing with sweetness. *Learning and Motivation, 14*, 338–350.

7

Brain Mechanisms and the Physiology of Feeding

Neil E. Rowland, Bai-Han Li, and Annie Morien

Introductory psychology texts challenge students about some fundamental philosophies concerning the nature of behavior; these include nature versus nurture and determinism versus free will. Although these issues can be illustrated and debated in almost any area of psychology, they are particularly involved in a discussion of the mechanisms of food intake and food choice. The first of these issues is fairly easy to address: The environment modifies, within limits, gene expression, which in turn endows the organism with particular structures and functions. The second issue is more difficult to evaluate, especially with regard to humans, yet is at the heart of the biological approach to brain and behavior. The philosophy of determinism states that a full knowledge of the content and structure of the brain will completely account for behavior. In the following, we implicitly assume this position with regard to eating behavior. We first review briefly some of the theoretical models of feeding behavior and relevant underlying physiology. We next describe some of the factors that inhibit food intake. Finally, we discuss the clinical implications for the biological basis of eating or body weight abnormalities.

THEORETICAL MODELS OF INGESTIVE BEHAVIOR

Homeostasis and Negative Feedback

The dominant paradigm in the biological sciences in general and in the study of the control of food intake in particular is fundamentally homeostatic

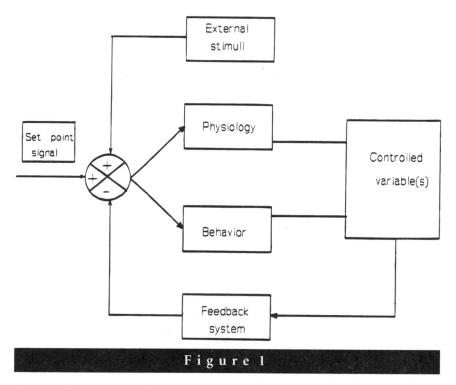

Figure 1

Diagram of a simple negative feedback control system. The present value of a variable is compared with an ideal or set point. Any difference is computed as an error signal that activates an effector mechanism or mechanisms (e.g., physiological and behavioral). The action of this mechanism is to change the present value of the variable toward the set point, thus reducing the error signal and terminating the action of the effector mechanism.

(Figure 1). The 19th-century French physiologist Claude Bernard was among the first to comment on the constancy of the *milieu interieur* of mammals. This idea was extended in the early part of this century by Walter Cannon, who coined the term *homeostasis* to refer to mechanisms that serve actively to maintain biological variables within defined limits (i.e., consistent with a high level of organismal function). It seems, however, that some internal variables are more closely regulated than others. For example, quite small excursions in blood gas concentrations are fatal, whereas large fluctuations in body mass are not immediately life threatening. In the former case, it is easy to define the variables and to locate the sensory and effector mechanisms, and so to validate the homeostatic model.

To simplify this problem as it might apply to feeding, one could liken the body to an energy reservoir or buffer between inputs and outputs. This model is appealing when the body is a single cell, but it becomes much more difficult to work with when applied to organisms that are composed of many different types of cells (e.g., neurons, muscle, fat cells). Such organisms supply most of their cells with energy by using circulating metabolic fuels whose storage and release are performed by specialized cells such as those in fat and liver. In the 1950s, Jean Mayer and Gordon Kennedy were the first to grapple with this problem. Mayer (1953) emphasized the pivotal role of blood glucose as a fuel and proposed a *glucostatic hypothesis,* according to which animals would be hungry when glucose was low and sated when it was high. Kennedy (1953) noted that body fat accounts for the overwhelming majority of the usable stored fuels in mammals and therefore ascribed a pivotal role to fat regulation in his *lipostatic hypothesis:* When fat stores declined, organisms would be hungry. These theories explicitly link a physiological deficit to activation of food intake, which then reduces the deficit.

This *negative feedback* type of model assumes that a variable has a set point (or range) against which the actual value of that variable is compared (Figure 1). Once the discrepancy between the value and the set point exceeds a threshold, corrective responses are engaged. These responses continue until either the value is restored within range or feedforward inhibitory signals "veto" the discrepancy. This paradigm has been most useful as a heuristic because it makes one ask questions about single variables; for this reason it is particularly attractive to physiologists and neurochemists. Some researchers believe that it has been overused, however, excluding other models that may be more complex but are probably more realistic (e.g., Davis, 1980; Houk, 1988; Rowland, 1995; Weingarten, 1990).

Most theorists would agree that human feeding is extremely complex and that physiological variables form at best a crude template on which the many aspects of the behavior are sculpted in an ever-changing way. Indeed, one of the outcomes of learning is that behavior can be modified in the absence of the physiological precipitator, or unconditional stimulus (Elizalde & Sclafani, 1990). It is also agreed that feeding behavior in humans is less dependent on physiological variables and more dependent on learned and cognitive aspects than in animals with less complex brains. Furthermore, even if researchers can agree on how to look for physiological variables and their transducers, it is only the first step of the journey. To draw an analogy with the much better analyzed visual system, even when one knows the physical stimulus (photons) and has identified several dominant streams of low-level signal processing, the details and concepts of concurrent processing and decision making at multiple levels still present formidable challenges (Van Essen & Deyoe, 1995).

Interacting Systems

It is generally believed that the human brain evolved to its present stage along with a hunter–gatherer style of living. It is not hard to imagine that improved procurement of food was indeed one of the adaptive advantages of our larger brain. If one accepts this general position, one should view the human brain as a complex of interacting systems involved in varying ways in feeding. To make this general model useful, it is necessary to articulate general principles of operation for the system that may transcend homeostasis of any one subsystem. Some attempts have been made to articulate this problem, although none have as yet attained the status of "paradigm." Mrosovsky (1990) advocated the use of the term *rheostasis* as an alternative to homeostasis, a term emphasizing that systems may vary across time in their apparent set points. Examples of this include programmed growth and daily or seasonal cycles. Moore-Ede (1986) advocated the use of a "predictive homeostasis" model to complement the more traditional "reactive" model of homeostasis. In the reactive mode, the organism is slavishly trying to resolve the last problem rather than to anticipate the next. In the case of food intake, cyclic changes could be programmed into a set point mechanism and so appear to anticipate future needs. Collier (1989) hypothesized that an interaction occurs between a "resident physiologist" (mechanisms that are responsible for maintaining a suitable *milieu interieur*) and a "house economist" (mechanisms that embody the pragmatics of procuring food in the real world). Weingarten (1990) discussed an "adaptive control" mechanism that could modulate the working of negative feedback mechanisms on the basis of current or anticipated events that might include learned factors. Houk (1988) previously used this term to describe interacting physiological systems: Once behavior and learning are introduced, the nature of the problem is surely amplified by several orders of magnitude.

We have introduced these theoretical positions not because we favor any one over the other—they are not in any way mutually exclusive—but because they highlight the current lack of a useful conceptual model for studying interacting systems in the physiological laboratory. The physiological models and data that we describe in the following pages were almost all driven by the single-factor negative feedback model. We ask that readers contemplate and excuse the limitations of this approach (see also chapter 1, this volume).

Macronutrients and Metabolism

As we noted previously, glucose and fats were among the earliest signal molecules considered in the metabolic control of food intake. There are three main classes of macronutrient:

1. Carbohydrates are either monosaccharides (e.g., glucose, fructose) or polysaccharides (e.g., maltodextrins, starch) composed of units of simple sugars.
2. Fats are triglycerides, which are fatty acid esters of glycerol; the nature of the aliphatic chains that form the esters determines the fat type (e.g., saturated).
3. Proteins are chains of amino acids, of which 20 occur naturally.

The stomach and intestines break down the food we eat, which varies greatly in macronutrient type and ratio, into monosaccharides, amino acids, and triglycerides. These then enter the bloodstream via the mesenteric veins that drain the intestines and join into the hepatic portal vein, which serves the liver. In the liver and in other tissues, both catabolic (breaking down the nutrients into cellular energy) and anabolic (building up nutrients into storage forms such as glycogen) processes are carefully regulated. A simplified scheme for catabolism is shown in Figure 2. This figure emphasizes that cellular energy, in particular adenosine triphosphate (ATP) and reducing agents such as NADH, is the common outcome of catabolism of each of these macronutrients. More recent metabolic theories of feeding have focused on ATP and cellular energy, rather than any single energy

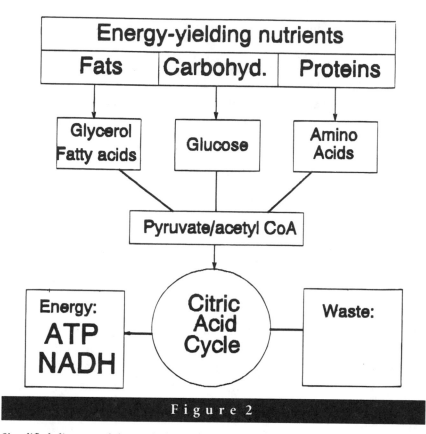

Figure 2

Simplified diagram of the catabolism of ingested macronutrients (fats, carbohydrates, and proteins). These are absorbed as small molecules that eventually are broken down to pyruvate and acetyl coenzyme A, which then enter a metabolic chain called the *citric acid cycle*. Energy-rich products from the cycle are adenosine triphosphate (ATP) and NADH, which are used to fuel numerous cellular processes. Waste (low-energy) products from the cycle are water and carbon dioxide as well as ammonia from the amino acids.

substrate (e.g., Langhans, Egli, & Scharrer, 1985; Rawson, Blum, Osbakken, & Friedman, 1994).

Neurobiology of Food Intake

One of the principal questions facing the neurobiologist is where in the brain to look for correlates of food intake. The first clues were provided by patients with tumors of the basal hypothalamus, who develop massive obesity. Hetherington and Ranson (1939) were able to reproduce this effect with experimentally produced lesions (so-called hypothalamic hyperphagia). Ranson (1939) was also the first to describe aphagia, affective and motivational changes, and postlesion recovery after damage to the lateral hypothalamic axis and subthalamic regions in monkeys. However, it was Stellar (1954) who offered the first neural model of feeding. That model was based on Sherrington's metaphor of excitation and inhibition, and it postulated that the medial hypothalamus was a "satiety center" and the lateral hypothalamus, a "feeding center." Reciprocal interaction between these systems determined net food intake and, ultimately, body weight. These and other historical findings have been treated in more detail by Woods, Taborsky, and Porte (1986) and Le Magnen (1992).

Just as the glucostatic hypothesis proved to be an oversimplification of metabolic models, the hypothalamic models turned out to be singularly deficient descriptions of the neurology of feeding. For example, by showing that ingestive and aversive responses were present in animals with transections of the brain below the level of the hypothalamus (Grill & Kaplan, 1990) and that lesions of some brain stem regions produced feeding abnormalities, it has become evident that feeding must be organized hierarchically at several levels of the nervous system. Figure 3 presents a simplified cartoon of the situation, for which we borrowed heavily from other areas of cognitive neuroscience in which hierarchically organized, parallel-distributed processing seems to be a normal type of organization for sensory systems (e.g., Van Essen & Deyoe, 1995). Our model includes only some of the areas and connecting pathways known to be involved. It is not comprehensive but is designed to challenge readers to consider the coactivation of several levels of the nervous system in food-related behaviors. In particular, the areas and roles of the cerebral cortex in human feeding are completely unknown, and only a small minority of articles on animal feeding examine cortical mechanisms.

The methods that we have available to study neural correlates of feeding in animals and humans have shown some formidable advances over the years, but they still are poorly suited to examining the type of schema shown in Figure 3. There are three principal ways in which the neural substrates of feeding behavior may be approached; these are complementary to each other:

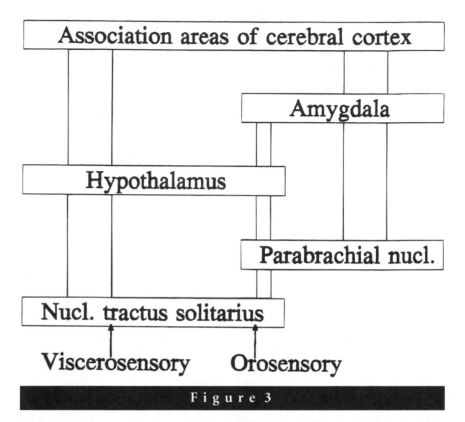

Figure 3

Schematic of some of the important brain regions involved in feeding behavior. The diagram emphasizes hierarchical and distributed parallel processing of information, primarily from visceral and oral chemosensors. The nucleus tractus solitarius is representative of hindbrain regions, the hypothalamus of the diencephalon, and the amygdala of the "primitive" cortex. (Other known regions have been omitted for clarity. These regions also have functional subdivisions that are not indicated). The regions and ways in which the cerebral cortex modifies operation of the lower systems (in humans) are completely unknown, indicating some degree of speculation in this schematic.

1. Surgery: evaluation of changes in behavior after damage to selected sites.

2. Neurochemistry: effects of specific neurotransmitters, antagonists, or agonists either systemically applied or introduced into discrete parts of the brain with a cannula.

3. Direct measurement: electrical, immediate early gene mapping, or measurement of the content or release of transmitters in defined brain areas.

Surgical and lesion methods suffer from several problems. Lesions that produce disruptions of tissue (e.g., electrocoagulation) damage both cell bodies and fibers of passage. Furthermore, even if one can accurately describe the functional deficits, it is still difficult to ascribe that function to that tissue, because disruption in one site causes dysfunctions at distal sites that may be involved in the function. Specific chemical toxins such as ibotenic acid, which damages cells but not fibers of passage, and 6-hydroxydopamine, which destroys catecholamine-containing cells, produce more selectivity than tissue-disrupting lesions, but the method suffers from the same problems of interpretation. Still more specific lesion methods (e.g., immunotargeting) are under development but will suffer from the same general problems of interpretation. As an addendum, genetic lesions ("knockout") fall into this same conceptual category. Lesions alone are not infallible indicators of functional localization; however, when complementary data on site-specific delivery of agonists or antagonists are obtained, greater confidence can be placed in the functional inferences.

Direct measurement methods are generally available only for use in animals. Early studies used whole-tissue measurements of transmitters or their metabolites as measures of synaptic release or turnover. More recently, use of microdialysis with relatively small probes inserted into discrete brain regions allows an "on-line" measurement of extracellular transmitter concentrations. This constitutes a "chemoencephalogram" (CEG), and the temporal and spatial resolution of this method is continuously improving. Nonetheless, one is usually limited to a single location and a single transmitter and so one needs a good "road map" (Figure 3) to position chemical traffic recorders strategically.

Functional mapping is a relatively new method, and advances with functional magnetic resonance imaging (FMRI) and other in vivo techniques in humans may have a bright future. In animals, the *immediate early gene (IEG) mapping* makes use of the fact that most if not all neurons are capable of expressing IEGs on adequate stimulation. Because this includes transsynaptically activated neurons, *in principle* entire neural circuits may be amenable to mapping. This method clearly provides an enormous advantage for evaluation of schematics of the type shown in Figure 3. The data relevant to feeding and the brain that have been collected to date surely represent only initial attempts and almost certainly suffer from shortcomings of sensitivity, specificity, and interpretation (see Sharp, Sagar, & Swanson, 1993, for an overview of the method and its limitations). In this chapter, we include some of the new findings using immunocytochemical mapping of the IEG protein product c-Fos, with single-cell resolution in rat brain.

Armed with a background in the nomenclature, brain systems, and methods used, we now review some of the most basic findings with regard to transmitters and feeding. As we start this overview, the reader should consider that a great many basic science findings on single transmitters (or genes) in single regions of the brain have been escalated into popular "single-factor" theories of eating disorders in humans. We discuss these clinical implications at the end of this chapter.

FACTORS THAT INCREASE FOOD INTAKE

Natural Stimuli

Hunger is the psychological sensation that leads to motivated behavior to seek and consume food. Food deprivation or restriction, viewed as a temporary abrogation of energy input, is perhaps the most powerful stimulus of hunger in humans and causes animals to exhibit food-motivated behavior. Increases in energy requirements, such as chronic exposure to cold (heat loss), gestation and lactation (the energy to grow offspring), or high levels of exercise (muscle demand), also stimulate appetite. Each of these stimuli involves changes in fuel catabolism that may either cause or be correlated with hunger (Figure 2). Many researchers have attempted to identify these metabolic signals by studying them in isolation.

Metabolic Stimuli

The lack of metabolizable glucose (glucoprivation) is a powerful stimulus of food intake in laboratory studies. Historically, the brain was considered the key site of transduction, and insulin-induced hypoglycemia and hyperphagia were used as key experimental evidence (Epstein, Nicolaidis, & Miselis, 1975; Le Magnen, 1992). The use of antimetabolites, chemicals that block the catabolism of endogenous fuels, has proved helpful in the functional analysis of these systems. These antimetabolites include 2-deoxy-D-glucose (2-DG; for glucose), 2,5-anhydro-D-mannitol (2,5-AM; for fructose), and mercaptoacetate (MA; for fatty acids). They block the production of pyruvate from the targeted fuel (Figure 2), although energy production from the other fuels remains viable.

Stricker, Rowland, Fredman, and Sahu (1977) showed that feeding induced in rats by low doses of insulin could be reversed by intravenous infusions of either glucose or fructose. Unlike glucose, fructose is a monosaccharide that does not cross the blood–brain barrier, and so it cannot directly alleviate the insulin-induced hypoglycemia to which neurons are exposed in this paradigm. Thus, insulin-stimulated adrenal catecholamine secretion was reversed by infusions of glucose, but *not* fructose. Together, these findings suggest that insulin stimulates feeding from a peripheral site to which fructose has access (see also Bellin & Ritter, 1981; Rowland, 1991; Rowland, Bellush, & Carlton, 1985). Data with 2,5-AM and inhibitors of fatty acid oxidation such as MA are even more compelling with regard to peripheral action. Rats injected with these agents show vigorous feeding, which can be prevented by cutting the hepatic branch of the vagus nerve (Ritter & Taylor, 1990; Tordoff, Rawson, & Friedman, 1991). The mechanism of action of 2,5-AM may involve reduced hepatic levels of phosphates and ATP (Rawson et al., 1994).

Treatment of rats with either insulin or 2-DG increases release–turnover of norepinephrine (NE) in the hypothalamus (Bellin & Ritter, 1981; Rowland et al., 1985). Because central administration of NE can increase feeding (see the section, Neurotransmitters and Modulators), it is possible that some antimetabolites cause feeding through release of NE. However, Rowland (1992) reported that neither 2,5-AM nor methylpalmoxirate increased NE turnover in the hypothalamus of rats. Clearly, these peripherally acting antimetabolites are not engaging, at least to the same degree, the same mechanisms as more aggressive treatments that may directly engage brain systems. (There is an analogy here with thermoregulation: There are clearly temperature sensors in the hypothalamus, but under normal conditions it is thermal-sensitive nerve endings in the skin that act as a first line of sensing and responding, such as with vasconstriction in the cold).

IEG mapping studies have added the new dimension of a systems approach to this problem. The antimetabolites MA and 2-DG each induce c-Fos in a clearly defined pathway: the nucleus of the solitary tract (NST), the lateral parabrachial nucleus (LPBN), and the central nucleus of the amygdala (CNA; cf. Figure 3). These agents may activate different cell populations within each of these areas, especially the LPBN (Ritter & Dinh, 1994). It was found that 2,5-AM induced c-Fos in NST and LPBN with a distribution similar to that seen after MA (Ritter, Dinh, & Friedman, 1994). Hepatic-branch vagotomy blocked both the food intake and the induction of Fos in brain by both MA and 2,5-AM but not by 2-DG. The NST, LPBN, and CNA are known to be involved in processing of visceral information (cf. Figure 3), in this case related to food, and so the identification of specific cells within these nuclei constitutes an important step toward understanding the ways in which diverse signals may be integrated at each of these levels.

Neurotransmitters and Modulators

Ultimately, signals relating to either actual or anticipated metabolic need, or even purely conditioned or hedonic factors, must use specific neural pathways and their associated signal molecules. Modern views of synaptic function include the concept of more than one transmitter (colocalization–release), with modulation of the action of the "primary" transmitter either by the cotransmitter or by other actions on the postsynaptic membrane; these actions include hormonal–paracrine–diffusible factors as well as other incoming transmitters that may in turn affect the efficacy of the second messenger system or systems that may be engaged by the primary transmitter. In this section, we review selectively some of the well-established signal molecules that stimulate food intake.

Norepinephrine

Norepinephrine (NE) was the first neurotransmitter linked to changes in feeding behavior. Injections of NE into the hypothalamus have both orexigenic (appetite-stimulating) effects at sites such as the paraventricular nucleus (PVN) and anorexic (appetite-reducing) effects at sites such as the perifornical area (Leibowitz, 1986). The orexigenic effects of NE are mimicked by the alpha-2-adrenergic agonist clonidine, suggesting that these are the critical receptors involved. Furthermore, exogenously applied NE is most effective when given at mealtimes, and it is more effective in the late day–early night period than at other parts of the nycthemeron. This time corresponds to peaks in levels of both circulating glucocorticoid and alpha-2-adrenergic receptors in the PVN (Leibowitz, 1988).

CEG studies have complemented these data. The extracellular concentrations of NE, detected either by push–pull cannula or microdialysis in the PVN, increase with various hunger-related treatments and also peak about the time of nightfall. Insofar as these levels reflect release from local presynaptic terminals and the alpha-2 receptors are postsynaptic, the postreceptor signal should be much greater in the evening than at other times (Stanley, Schwartz, Hernandez, Hoebel, & Leibowitz, 1989).

Leibowitz (1988) argued, on the basis of both spontaneous and NE-induced food-selection studies, that the action of NE in the PVN may not only increase caloric intake but also selectively engage an appetite for carbohydrate (CHO). There are at least two questions concerning the generality of this proposed mechanism. The first is that CHO self selection implies there is a specific appetite for postingestive CHO (and quite distinct from the tastes of CHOs). Although it is clear that the *postingestive* effects of CHOs are sufficient to produce extremely robust preferences for neutral flavors (flavor–calorie conditioning; see chapter 3, this volume), there are no data proving either an absolute nutritional requirement for or regulation of CHO intake (e.g., Ashley, 1985). Indeed, Figure 2 indicates how alternative fuels can completely substitute for CHO. The second concern is empirical: Many authors have noted that the appetite for CHO seems to be modulated by taste and texture rather than or in addition to a common postingestive effect (Blundell, 1983). Both of these concerns pose constraints on the specificity of any proposed relationship between a single transmitter and intake of CHO or other single macronutrients.

Neuropeptide Y

Neuropeptide Y (NPY) is a 33–amino acid peptide that is found in cell bodies and nerve terminals in many areas of the brain; there are prominent concentrations in the PVN and perifornical hypothalamus and in brain stem regions such as NST and LPBN (Chronwall et al., 1985; Krukoff, Vu, Harris, Aippersbach, & Jhamandas, 1992). Injection of NPY into the hypothalamus causes sated rats to eat large amounts of food (Clark, Kalra, Crowley, & Kalra, 1984). As with NE, a preference for CHO has often been identified in association with NPY injection (Jhanwar-Uniyal, Beck, Jhanwar, Burlet, & Leibowitz, 1993; Leibowitz, 1986). The PVN has received much attention as one of the regions involved, although careful studies by Stanley et al. (1993) have identified the perifornical hypothalamus as the most sensitive site for the orexigenic action of NPY. Administration of NPY into the PVN over a period of several days causes sustained hyperphagia with increase in carcass fat (Stanley, Magdalin, Salrafi, Thomas & Leibowitz, 1986). Cerebroventricular injection of NPY induces c-Fos in the medial (parvocellular) division of the PVN and perifornical hypothalamus as well as in the LPBN, bed nucleus of the stria terminalis (BNST), CNA, and other regions (Li, Xu et al., 1994).

Either the extracellular or whole-tissue concentrations of NPY or the expression of the gene encoding it (prepro-NPY mRNA) shows regionally specific increases in physiological conditions that are associated with increased food intake: these include deprivation and genetic hyperphagia–obesity (Beck, Burlet, Nicolas, & Burlet, 1990; Beck, Jhanwar-Uniyal, et al., 1990; Sahu, Kalra, & Kalra, 1988; Sahu, White, Kalra, & Kalra, 1992; Sanacora, Kershaw, Finkelstein, & White, 1990). Furthermore, neutralization of endogenous NPY with an antiserum decreased food intake (Dube, Xu, Crowley, Kalra, & Kalra, 1994; Shibasaki, Oda, Imaki, Ling, & Demura, 1993).

In summary, one or more functional systems containing NPY in the brain seem to be importantly modulated by food and energy-related stimuli. A start has been made in identifying the sites of action and interactions with other molecules. NPY is the best-characterized peptidergic stimulant of food intake. There are certainly others, only two of which are considered in the following sections.

Galanin

Galanin is a 29–amino acid peptide that, like NPY, is widespread in the brain but has particularly high concentrations in the PVN (Levin, Sawchenko, Howe, Bloom, & Polack, 1987). Injections of galanin into the PVN acutely stimulate food intake in rats, but unlike the case of NPY, there is often a preference for fat (Kyrkouli, Stanley, Seirafi, & Leibowitz, 1990; Tempel, Leibowitz, & Leibowitz, 1988). Also unlike the results with NPY, repeated administration of galanin into the ventricles does not produce sustained hyperphagia and weight gain; instead, elevated daytime intake is compensated for by reduced nocturnal intake (Smith, York, & Bray, 1994). The similarities and differences in behaviors induced by NPY and galanin may be due to interactions between NE, galanin, and NPY (Kyrkouli, Stanley, Hutchinson, Seirafi, & Leibowitz, 1990; Lambert et al., 1993). Further work is needed to clarify this issue.

Opioids

Several types of endogenous opioids seem to be involved in stimulation of food intake, but the strongest effects are observed with dynorphin, acting through kappa receptors (Morley, 1987). The PVN is perhaps the most sensitive, but not the only, site of action. In self-selection studies, fat intake is preferentially stimulated (Morley, 1987; Romsos, Gosnell, Morley, & Levine, 1987). Either peripheral or central administration of opioid receptor antagonists reduces food intake in most acute paradigms, but it becomes less effective with chronic use.

FACTORS THAT DECREASE FOOD INTAKE

We define *satiation* as the process that terminates ongoing feeding bouts and *satiety* as the process that inhibits food-seeking behavior or intake between meals (Le Magnen, 1992). These processes operate with different but overlapping time courses. Although they may be conceptually distinct, this need not imply mechanistic separation. An analogy is provided from studies of memory: Short-term and long-term memory can be separated in many ways, but their ultimate mechanisms of synaptic modification share common elements (Bailey & Kandel, 1995). As one studies the mechanisms involved in decreasing food intake, therefore, one should consider both the separation and the integration of processes relating to satiation and satiety. The relationship of satiety processes to hunger processes has been discussed by Stricker (1983) and is not addressed specifically in this chapter.

Natural Stimuli

The consumption of food is the most effective stimulus of satiation and satiety. Le Magnen (1992) reviewed his seminal work showing that the size of spontaneous meals in rats is correlated with the duration of the postmeal interval: Larger meals produce, on average, longer satiety. Nicolaidis and Rowland (1976) showed that slow intravenous infusion of metabolizable fuels such as glucose reduced food intake by increasing intermeal intervals;

that is, through augmentation of the prandial energy influx, satiety was prolonged. Meal size, hence satiation, was relatively unaffected. However, neither the efficiency of utilization nor the satiating power of intravenous calories was as great as for a comparable number of calories entering through the stomach or mouth. These and other studies demonstrate that sensory systems at several levels are involved in the production of satiety.

Humoral Factors and Satiety

Cross-circulation studies between pairs of rats demonstrated that the blood of rats following a meal contained a satiating factor (Davis, Gallagher, Ladove, & Turausky, 1969). A second putative type of satiety factor is that relating to endogenous depot stores of energy (i.e., adipose tissue). In animals, experimental overfeeding increases body fat; when overfeeding is stopped, the animals typically eat less for several days until their body weight (fat) returns to pretreatment levels. These and other data, first conceptualized in the lipostatic hypothesis (Kennedy, 1953), led to the idea that adipose cells secrete a signal molecule or molecules in proportion to their fat content (Weigle, 1994). These molecules would then constitute an integrated signal of body fat content that may be transduced by specific sensors, presumed to be in the brain.

Three possible candidates include *adipsin,* which is reduced in genetic obesity and hyperinsulinemia (Flier, Cook, Usher, & Spiegelman, 1987); *agouti,* which is a melanocyte-stimulating hormone receptor antagonist and has a human homologue (Lu et al., 1994); and the *ob/ob* gene product, which is overexpressed in obese mice and also has a human homologue (Zhang et al., 1994). The site or sites at which these molecules act and whether and how they appear in the brain to affect eating behavior remain to be determined. This section starts with a review of some potential bloodborne satiating and satiety factors for which some data are available on the brain mechanisms that they may engage. The first of these, satietin, is potentially similar in function to the proteins just mentioned. The next two, cholecystokinin and bombesin, appear to function more in satiation or meal termination. The next three, insulin, oxytocin, and corticotropin-releasing hormone (CRH), may function as integrators for systems involved in energy balance. Finally, the role of a monoamine transmitter, serotonin, is considered.

Satietin

Satietin is a large glycoprotein that has been isolated from serum and urine of various species, including humans (Knoll, 1988). Central administration of partially purified satietin causes anorexia in rats and mice, without apparent malaise or any metabolic changes (Bellinger & Mendel, 1995). There is a need for better identification of the factors that regulate the synthesis and release of satietin and of its sites of action. In a recent study (Rowland, Bellinger, Li, & Mendel, in press), Fos mapping was used in an attempt to assess the areas of the rat brain activated by cerebroventricular administration of partially purified satietin. Surprisingly few regions were so activated: These included the parvocellular part of the PVN, the dorsolateral bed nucleus of the stria terminalis (dlBNST), and the CNA. These regions contain cells that transcribe CRH mRNA; although the identity of the Fos- and CRH mRNA-containing cells has not been established, it is relevant that CRH itself has been implicated as a satiety factor or system (Bray, 1992; see the section on CRH, following).

Cholecystokinin

Cholecystokinin (CCK) is perhaps the best-known putative endogenous satiety factor. Injected at or shortly before a meal, CCK acts to reduce meal size by hastening the normal behavioral sequence associated with satiation (G. P. Smith & Gibbs, 1979). The anorectic effect of peripherally injected CCK is entirely absent in rats with cuts of either the gastric branches of the vagus nerve or the whole vagus nerve (G. P. Smith, Jerome, Cushin, Eterno, & Simansky, 1981), indicating that the exogenous compound has a peripheral site of action. Indeed, the 33–amino acid sequence of endogenous of CCK makes it too large to cross the blood–brain barrier readily. Endogenous CCK is released into the bloodstream during meals, but CCK is also widespread in the brain and has been implicated in multiple functions (Crawley & Corwin, 1994).

The CCK_A receptor subtype, of which devazepide (MK329) is a selective antagonist, seems to be involved in the satiety action of peripheral CCK, because devazepide effectively blocks the anorexia (Moran, Ameglio, Schwartz, & McHugh, 1992). Furthermore, administration of long-acting CCK_A agonists causes sustained anorexia and suppresses weight gain (Asin et al., 1992).

The satiety effect of exogenous CCK is enhanced in combination with oral, gastric, and duodenal food-related stimulation (Cox, 1990; Forsyth, Weingarten, & Collins, 1985; Schwartz, Netterville, McHugh, & Moran, 1991) or even a conditioned nutritive expectancy (Fedorchak & Bolles, 1988). The brain has CCK-containing neurons and receptors, and these also are related to food intake. It is interesting that lateral ventricular injection of the active octopeptide CCK-8 reduces real but not sham feeding, whereas peripheral CCK-8 suppresses both (Della-Fera, Coleman, & Baile, 1990), suggesting that centrally administered CCK acts at a level too high to allow any interaction with pregastric stimulation.

Fos mapping has been used to identify putative central sites of action of peripherally administered CCK. Doses of CCK as used in studies of anorexia (1–10 µg/kg) cause the appearance of Fos in the area postrema and adjacent medial nucleus of the solitary tract (AP-mNST) and in the inner layer of the external lateral parabrachial nucleus (LPBe), posterior BNST, anterior CNA, and parvocellular PVN (Li & Rowland, 1994; Olson, Hoffman, Sved, Stricker, & Verbalis, 1992; Verbalis, Stricker, Robinson, & Hoffman, 1991). At least some of the PVN cells may synthesize oxytocin as a transmitter and project caudally to the brain stem. The fact that lesions of the PVN attenuate peripheral CCK anorexia (Crawley & Kiss, 1985) is consistent with this view. The induction of Fos by peripheral CCK is prevented by either subdiaphragmatic vagotomy or injection of a CCK-A antagonist (Day, McNight, Poat, & Hughes, 1994; Li & Rowland, 1994), effects that parallel the reversal of CCK anorexia by these treatments.

Bombesin

A variety of other peptides are known to reduce food intake in rats without appearing to produce illness. The best-studied of these is bombesin (BBS), a 14–amino acid peptide. Gastrin-releasing peptide (GRP) is structurally related to BBS, and so it is probably more accurate to speak of BBS-like peptides in this section. The anorectic effect of peripherally administered BBS, unlike that of CCK, is not reduced by vagotomy, but it is reduced by total gut–brain disconnection (Stuckey, Gibbs, & Smith, 1985). BBS-like peptides and their receptors are found in high concentrations in several brain regions related to ingestion, including the AP-NST (Panula, Yang, & Costa, 1982). Injections of BBS into the fourth ventricle of rats are much more effective in reducing food intake than are equal doses into the lateral ventricles, and lesions of the AP-NST abolish both peripheral and fourth-ventricular bombesin-induced anorexia (Ladenheim & Ritter, 1993). Injection of a BBS receptor antagonist into the fourth ventricle increased food intake in rats, suggesting that caudal brain stem BBS is involved in suppression of feeding (Merali, Moody, & Coy, 1993).

Fos mapping of action of peripheral BBS has shown activation of the medial NST and parvocellular PVN (Bonaz, De Giorgio, & Tache, 1993). In a study in which more regions were surveyed (Li & Rowland, in press), BBS (10 μ/kg subcutaneously) induced moderate Fos in the BNST, CNA, external LPBN, and medial NST; weaker Fos was observed in the PVN, and none in the AP. This pattern differs from that of CCK insofar as the staining after BBS was throughout the rostrocaudal extent of the BNST and CNA, and both external and internal laminae of the external LPBN, whereas staining after CCK was much more pronounced in one half of each of these structures (posterior BNST, anterior CNA, internal LPBN).

Insulin

Insulin, like CCK, is normally released during and after meals and has major fuel-storage roles in the periphery. Injection of insulin into the cerebral ventricles decreases food intake of rats and primates. It has been suggested that the cerebrospinal fluid may act as a temporal integrator of plasma insulin, which then has access to select brain sites to produce anorexia (Schwartz, Figlewicz, Baskin, Woods, & Porte, 1992). Central insulin also inhibits transcription of NPY mRNA in arcuate nucleus, suggesting that there is a reciprocal interaction between these peptides. We previously noted that insulin may regulate the expression of adipsin. Peripheral injection of a high dose of insulin induced Fos in both the magnocellular and parvocellular PVN of rats. Many of the Fos-positive cells also contained oxytocin (Griffond et al., 1993).

Corticotropin-Releasing Hormone

Central injection of corticotropin-releasing hormone (CRH), a 41-amino acid peptide produced in the PVN and other sites (Swanson & Sawchenko, 1983), reduces food intake (Arase, York, Shimizu, Shargill, & Bray, 1988; Bray, 1992). The primary site of action is the PVN (Krahn, Gosnell, Levine, & Morley, 1988). The action of CRH has been correlated with increased peripheral sympathetic activity (Bray, 1992). CRH may normally inhibit NPY-mediated feeding systems, because putative damage to CRH-containing cells, by prior injection of an immunotargeted toxin for CRH into the PVN of rats, increased food intake elicited by NPY (Menzaghi, Heinrichs, Pich, Tilders, & Koob, 1993). Additionally, CRH may depend on oxytocin for its final action, because central administration of an oxytocin antagonist blocked CRH-induced anorexia (Olson, Drutarosky, Stricker, & Verbalis, 1991).

Oxytocin

Diverse treatments that cause satiety have been correlated with increases in circulating oxytocin. As noted previously, it has been suggested that this reflects the release of oxytocin at central locations, perhaps in particular the descending projections from the hypothalamus to the pons and medulla (Stricker & Verbalis, 1991; Verbalis, McCann, McHale, & Stricker, 1986). Furthermore, the actions of both insulin and CRH have been linked to activation of oxytocin-containing neurons (Griffond et al., 1993; Olson et al., 1991).

Several proteins and peptides, some of which are reviewed earlier in this chapter, are thought to participate in the inhibition of food intake. These almost certainly interact in complex ways. A case has been made for either common mediation by oxytocin or a correlate with altered sympathetic neural activity (Bray, 1992). These latter should be regarded as simplifying hypotheses: There is no a priori reason to suppose that there is in fact any one final common signal molecule involved in satiety. We now consider briefly one classic neurotransmitter, serotonin, and its role in feeding.

Serotonin

Peripheral administration of serotonin (5HT) and of more specific 5HT type 1 receptor agonists such as 5-carboxyamidotryptamine (5CT) decrease food intake (Eberle-Wang, Levitt, & Simansky, 1993; Pollock & Rowland, 1981). Although vagotomy does not affect 5CT anorexia, because these amines are not believed to cross the blood–brain barrier, peripheral sites of action seem to be indicated.

Brain 5HT systems have been implicated in satiety (Blundell, 1979, 1991). Drugs that function as indirect 5HT agonists, either by inhibiting

5HT reuptake into the presynaptic terminal or by promoting 5HT release from the terminals, are potent anorectic agents (Blundell, 1991). These include dexfenfluramine (DFEN), a drug that is in clinical use in many countries and has recently been approved in the United States, and fluoxetine. Injection of 5HT receptor antagonists blocks the actions of either fluoxetine or DFEN, strengthening the view that 5HT is critical for their action. However, the sites of action of these agents remain quite elusive. Thus, local injection of DFEN into the brain has only mild anorectic effects, possibly because of the rapid removal of this compound after central injection (Rowland & Carlton, 1986).

Recent work from our laboratory has used Fos mapping of brain areas activated by DFEN (Li & Rowland, 1993). The external part of the LPBN is one such region, and bilateral lesions of this area prevent the induction of Fos in some forebrain areas (notably, CNA and BNST) by peripheral DFEN, and *partly* attenuate its anorectic action (Li, Spector, & Rowland, 1994). It is possible, therefore, that DFEN targets several regions of the brain to exert its full anorectic action.

CCK and 5HT–DFEN share some interesting similarities in their behavioral effects. Both seem to act on satiation, attenuating food intake by decreasing meal size without change in the latency to eat. Cooper and Dourish (1990) proposed that these two factors interact. In unpublished studies, we have found that neurons in the external part of the LPBN that show Fos following peripheral administration of DFEN to rats are located in the region of the LPBN that has the densest CCK-immunoreactive fibers. Furthermore, the AP–NST has many neurons that show Fos after CCK, and we know there is a heavy 5HT projection from the AP to the LPBN. Collectively, these findings suggest several ways in which CCK and 5HT could interact to produce satiation.

One interesting observation from the foregoing is that many of the orexigenic and anorexigenic treatments reviewed activate (by the Fos measurement) the same general regions of the brain. In some cases, it is clear that different subdivisions of these regions are involved, whereas in other cases it is not yet clear whether the same or different populations of neurons are involved. In either case, these regions, which are organized hierarchically as well as in parallel (cf. Figure 3), and the circuits that they form are likely integrators of physiological information. The ways in which learned appetitive information impinges on these circuits require further study.

CLINICAL IMPLICATIONS

Obesity is perhaps the most widespread affliction of postindustrial societies. All kinds of obesity have but one ultimate cause: energy intake that exceeds energy expenditure over a prolonged period of time. Clearly, there could be several reasons for this imbalance. One general view ascribes this imbalance to an endogenous dysfunction, perhaps genetically programmed, that effectively produces an error signal when there is no deficit (Figure 1); that is, the physiological condition "pushes" the animal to eat excess food. Certainly, in animal models, there are several examples of obesity-related genes; extrapolating to humans, it is likely that only some of the obesities can be ascribed to a single gene. One of the biggest problems with the single-gene approach is that the body has many redundant systems, and if one is defective, its impact is minimized by compensation in other systems. Indeed, as dieters know, even if calorie intake is rigorously restricted over a period of time, weight loss tapers off with time until a new (lower) steady-state weight is attained. Increased metabolic efficiency is, in part, responsible for this phenomenon and may also underlie more rapid weight gain that often follows repeated (yo-yo) diets.

An alternative or complement to the "push" model is an altered responsiveness to foods, leading to a magnification of the "gain" in feedback loops. A discussion of reward pathways in feeding and their modification by learning is beyond the scope of this chapter. However, it is our belief that no "push" model of overeating can guarantee overeating without a concurrently increased affective component to food. Any study of "obesity genes" without an understanding of the way they operate on the food environment and of the brain systems involved is grossly inadequate.

In the same vein, single-chemical theories of eating disorders and the pharmacological treatments that they spawn are likely to fall into the same trap. Pharmacological agents that act on one system are likely to have limited effects on eating. In obesity, however, even small weight losses may significantly decrease the associated health risks of heart disease and diabetes.

The disorders of anorexia nervosa and bulimia nervosa are much harder to understand physiologically. First, it is difficult to devise an animal model of these disorders, in part because they involve complex sociocultural factors that evidently transcend the repertoire of rodents. Second, measurements of chemicals in select body fluids (CSF, urine, blood) of humans with these illnesses cannot dissociate cause from effect. Some of the chemicals whose dysregulation has been linked to anorexia or bulimia include NE, 5HT, CRH, NPY, BBS, CCK, and opioids. It is hoped that the data reviewed in previous sections will help readers to put the importance of these physiological measurements into an appropriate context.

CONCLUSION

It should be clear from this brief overview that there are many central and peripheral signal molecules involved in control of food intake. The sheer number and complexity of their potential interactions has only started to be appreciated. There seem to be three main levels at which such interactions occur: in the medulla and pons (notably NST, AP, LPBN), in the hypothalamus (notably the parvocellular PVN), and in the limbic forebrain (amygdala). The ways in which these regions and molecules may interact under less restricted paradigms than those typically used, including hedonic and learned factors, remain almost completely unexplored. Finally, what are the prospects for intervening pharmacologically to control appetite, at least in individuals with evident health risk from their eating habits? Serotonergic agents including DFEN have been in clinical use for some years. These agents seem most effective when used to help people adhere to a strict diet. However, we do not expect that any one agent will miraculously turn on or off a hunger signal. We return, therefore, to learned and hedonic factors that are undeniably played out in a neural context, including some of the elements described in this chapter, the details of which remain so elusive.

REFERENCES

Arase, K., York, D. A., Shimizu, H., Shargill, N., & Bray, G. A. (1988). Effects of corticotropin-releasing factor on food intake and brown adipose tissue thermogenesis in rats. *American Journal of Physiology, 255,* E255–E259.

Ashley, D. V. M. (1985). Factors affecting the selection of protein and carbohydrate from a dietary source. *Nutrition Research, 5,* 555–571.

Asin, K. E., Bednarz, L., Nikkel, A. L., Gore, P. A., Montana, W. E., Cullen, M. J., Shiosaki, K., Craig, R., & Nadzan, A. M. (1992). Behavioral effects of A71623, a highly selective CCK-A agonist tetrapeptide. *American Journal of Physiology, 263*, R125–R135.

Bailey, C. H., & Kandel, E. R. (1995). Molecular and structural mechanisms underlying long-term memory. In M. S. Gazzaniga (Ed.), *The cognitive neurosciences* (pp. 19–36). Cambridge, MA: MIT Press.

Beck, B., Burlet, A., Nicolas, J.-P., & Burlet, C. (1990). Hyperphagia in obesity is associated with a central peptidergic dysregulation in rats. *Journal of Nutrition, 120*, 806–811.

Beck, B., Jhanwar-Uniyal, M., Burlet, A., Chapleur-Chateau, M., Leibowitz, S. F., & Burlet, C. (1990). Rapid and localized alterations of neuropeptide Y in discrete hypothalamic nuclei with feeding status. *Brain Research, 528*, 245–249.

Bellin, S. I., & Ritter, S. (1981). Disparate effects of infused nutrients on delayed glucoprivic feeding and hypothalamic norepinephrine turnover. *Journal of Neuroscience, 1*, 1347–1353.

Bellinger, L. L., & Mendel, V. E. (1995). Blood profile and balance study of rats given the putative anorectic agent satietin. *American Journal of Physiology, 268*, R1–R7.

Blundell, J. E. (1979). Serotonin and feeding. In W. B. Essman (Ed.), *Serotonin in health and disease* (Vol. 5, pp. 403–450). New York: Spectrum.

Blundell, J. E. (1983). Problems and processes underlying the control of food selection and nutrient intake. In R. J. Wurtman & J. J. Wurtman (Eds.), *Nutrition and the brain* (Vol. 6, pp. 163–221). New York: Raven Press.

Blundell, J. E. (1991). Pharmacological approaches to appetite suppression. *Trends in Pharmacological Sciences, 12*, 149–157.

Bonaz, B., De Giorgio, R., & Tache, Y. (1993). Peripheral bombesin induces c-Fos protein in the rat brain, *Brain Research, 600*, 353–357.

Bray, G. A. (1992). Peptides affect the intake of specific nutrients and the sympathetic nervous system. *American Journal of Clinical Nutrition, 55*, 265S–271S.

Chronwall, B. M., DiMaggio, D. A., Massari, V. J., Pickel, V. M., Ruggiero, D. A., & O'Donohue, T. L. (1985). The anatomy of neuropeptide-Y-containing neurons in rat brain. *Neuroscience, 51*, 1159–1181.

Clark, J. T., Kalra, P. S., Crowley, W. R., & Kalra, S. P. (1984). Neuropeptide Y and human pancreatic polypeptide stimulate feeding behavior in rats. *Endocrinology, 115*, 427–429.

Collier, G. (1989). The economics of hunger, thirst, satiety and regulation. *Annals of the New York Academy of Sciences, 575,* 136–154

Cooper, S. J., & Dourish, C. T. (1990). Multiple cholecystokinin (CCK) receptors and CCK-monoamine interactions are instrumental in the control of feeding. *Physiology and Behavior, 48,* 849–857.

Cox, J. E. (1990). Inhibitory effects of cholecystokinin develop through interaction with duodenal signals. *Behavior Brain Research, 38,* 35–44.

Crawley, J. N., & Corwin, R. L. (1994). Biological actions of cholecystokinin. *Peptides, 15,* 731–755.

Crawley, J. N., & Kiss, J. F. (1985). Paraventricular nucleus lesions abolish the inhibition of feeding induced by systemic cholecystokinin. *Peptides, 6,* 927–935.

Davis, J. D. (1980). Homeostasis, feedback and motivation. In F. M. Toates & T. R. Halliday (Eds.), *Analysis of motivational processes* (pp. 23–37). San Diego, CA: Academic Press.

Davis, J. D., Gallagher, R. J., Ladove, R. F., & Turausky, A. J. (1969). Inhibition of food intake by a humoral factor. *Journal of Comparative and Physiological Psychology, 67,* 407–414.

Day, H. E. W., McKnight, A. T., Poat, J. A., & Hughes, J. (1994). Evidence that cholecystokinin induces immediate early gene expression in the brainstem, hypothalamus and amygdala of the rat by a CCK_A, receptor mechanism. *Neuropharmacology, 33,* 719–727.

Della-Fera, M. A., Coleman, B. D., Baile, C. A. (1990). CNS injection of CCK in rats: Effects on real and sham feeding and gastric emptying. *American Journal of Physiology, 258,* R1165–R1169.

Dube, M. G., Xu, B., Crowley, W. R., Kalra, P. S., & Kalra, S. P. (1994). Evidence that neuropeptide Y is a physiological signal for normal food intake. *Brain Research, 646,* 341–344.

Eberle-Wang, K., Levitt, P., & Simansky, K. J. (1993). Abdominal vagotomy dissociates the anorectic mechanisms for peripheral serotonin and cholecystokinin. *American Journal of Physiology, 265,* R602–R608.

Elizalde, G., & Sclafani, A. (1990). Flavor preferences conditioned by intragastric polycose infusions: A detailed analysis using an electronic esophagus preparation. *Physiology and Behavior, 47,* 63–77.

Epstein, A. N., Nicolaidis, S., & Miselis, R. R. (1975). The glucoprivic control of food intake and the glucostatic theory of feeding behaviour. In G. J. Mogenson &

F. R. Calaresu (Eds.), *Neural integration of physiological mechanisms and behaviour* (pp. 148–168). Toronto: Toronto University Press.

Fedorchak, P. M., & Bolles, R. C. (1988). Nutritive expectancies mediate cholecystokinin's suppression-of-intake effect. *Behavioral Neuroscience, 102,* 451–455.

Flier, J. S., Cook, K. S., Usher, P., & Spiegelman, B. M. (1987). Severely impaired adipsin expression in genetic and acquired obesity. *Science, 237,* 405–408.

Forsyth, P. A., Weingarten, H. P., & Collins, S. M. (1985). Role of oropharyngeal stimulation in cholecystokinin-induced satiety in the sham feeding rat. *Physiology and Behavior* 35:539–543.

Griffond, B., Deray, A., Bahjaoui-Bouhaddi, M., Colard, C., Bugnon, C., & Fellman, D. (1993). Induction of Fos-like immunoreactivity in rat oxytocin neurons following insulin injections. *Neuroscience Letters, 178,* 119–123.

Grill, H. J., & Kaplan, J. M. (1990). Caudal brainstem participates in the distributed neural control of feeding. In E. M. Stricker (Ed.), *Handbook of behavioral neurobiology: Vol. 10. Food and water intake* (pp. 125–149) New York: Plenum Press.

Hetherington, A. W., & Ranson, S. W. (1939). Experimental hypothalamicohypophyseal obesity in the rat. *Proceedings of the Society for Experimental Biology and Medicine, 41,* 465–466.

Houk, J. C. (1988). Control strategies in physiological systems. *FASEB Journal, 2,* 97–107.

Jhanwar-Uniyal, M., Beck, B., Jhanwar, Y. S., Burlet, C., & Leibowitz, S. F. (1993). Neuropeptide Y projection from arcuate nucleus to parvocellular division of the paraventricular nucleus: Specific relation to the ingestion of carbohydrate. *Brain Research, 631,* 97–106.

Kennedy, G. C. (1953). The role of depot fat in the hypothalamic control of food intake in the rat. *Proceedings of the Royal Society, Series B, 140,* 578–592.

Knoll, J. (1988). Endogenous anorectic agents: Satietin. *Annual Review of Pharmacology and Toxicology, 28,* 247–268.

Krahn, D. D., Gosnell, B. A., Levine, A. S., & Morley, J. E. (1988). Behavioral effects of corticotropin-releasing factor: Localization and characterization of effects. *Brain Research, 443,* 63–69.

Krukoff, T. L., Vu, T., Harris, K. H., Aippersbach, S., & Jhamandas, J. H. (1992). Neurons in the rat medulla oblongata containing neuropeptide Y-, angiotensin II-, or galanin-like immunoreactivity project to the parabrachial nucleus. *Neuroscience, 47,* 175–184.

Kyrkouli, S. E., Stanley, B. G., Hutchinson, R., Seirafi, R. D., & Leibowitz, S. F. (1990). Peptide-amine interactions in the hypothalamic paraventricular nucleus: Analysis of galanin and neuropeptide Y in relation to feeding. *Brain Research, 521,* 185–191.

Kyrkouli, S. E., Stanley, B. G., Seirafi, R. D., & Leibowitz, S. F. (1990). Stimulation of feeding by galanin: Anatomical localization and behavioral specificity of this peptide's effects in the brain. *Peptides, 11,* 995–1001.

Ladenheim, E. E., & Ritter, R. C. (1993). Caudal hindbrain participation in the suppression of feeding by central and peripheral bombesin. *American Journal of Physiology, 264,* R1229–R1234.

Lambert, P. D., Wilding, J. P. H., Al-Dokhayel, A. A. M., Bohuon, C., Comoy, E., Gilbey, S. G., & Bloom, S. R. (1993). A role for neuropeptide-Y, dynorphin, and noradrenaline in the central control of food intake after food deprivation. *Endocrinology, 133,* 29–32.

Langhans, W., Egli, G., & Scharrer, E. (1985). Regulation of food intake by hepatic oxidative metabolism. *Brain Research Bulletin, 15,* 425–428.

Le Magnen, J. (1992). *Neurobiology of feeding and nutrition.* San Diego, CA: Academic Press.

Leibowitz, S. F. (1986). Brain monoamines and peptides: Role in the control of eating behavior. *Federation Proceedings, 45,* 1396–1403.

Leibowitz, S. F. (1988). Hypothalamic paraventricular nucleus: Interaction between a_2-noradrenergic system and circulating hormones and nutrients in relation to energy balance. *Neuroscience and Biobehavioral Reviews, 12,* 101–109.

Levin, M. C., Sawchenko, P. E., Howe, P. R. C., Bloom, S. R., & Polack, J. M. (1987). Organization of galanin-immunoreactive inputs to the paraventricular nucleus with special reference to their relationship to catecholaminergic afferents. *Journal of Comparative Neurology, 261,* 562–582.

Li, B.-H., & Rowland, N. E. (1993). Dexfenfluramine induces fos-like immunoreactivity in discrete brain regions in rats. *Brain Research Bulletin, 31,* 43–48.

Li, B.-H., & Rowland, N. E. (1994). Cholecystokinin- and dexfenfluramine-induced anorexia compared using devazepide and *c-fos* expression in the rat brain. *Regulatory Peptides, 50,* 223–233.

Li, B.-H., & Rowland, N. E. (in press). Peripherally and centrally administered bumbesin induce FOS-like immunoreactivity in different brain regions in rats. *Regulatory Peptides.*

Li, B.-H., Spector, A. C., & Rowland, N. E. (1994). Reversal of dexfenfluramine-induced anorexia and c-Fos/c-Jun expression by lesion in the lateral parabrachial nucleus. *Brain Research, 640,* 255–267.

Li, B.-H., Xu, B., Rowland, N. E., & Kalra, S. P. (1994). *c-fos* expression in the rat brain following central administration of neuropeptide Y and effects of food consumption. *Brain Research, 665,* 277–284.

Lu, D., Willard, D., Patel, I. R., Kadwell, S., Overton, L., Kost, T., Luther, M., Chen, W., Woychik, R. P., Wilkison, W. O., & Cone, R. D. (1994). Agouti protein is an antagonist of the melanocyte-stimulating hormone receptor. *Nature, 371,* 799–802.

Mayer, J. (1953). Glucostatic mechanisms of regulation of food intake. *New England Journal of Medicine, 249,* 13–16.

Menzaghi, F., Heinrichs, S. C., Pich, E. M., Tilders, F. J. H., & Koob, G. F. (1993). Functional impairment of hypothalamic corticotropin-releasing factor neurons with immunotargeted toxins enhances food intake induced by neuropeptide Y. *Brain Research, 618,* 76–82.

Merali, Z., Moody, T. W., & Coy, D. (1993). Blockade of brain bombesin/GRP receptors increases food intake in satiated rats. *American Journal of Physiology, 264,* R1031–R1034.

Moore-Ede, M. C. (1986). Physiology of the circadian timing system: Predictive versus reactive homeostasis. *American Journal of Physiology, 250,* R737–R752.

Moran, T. H., Ameglio, P. J., Schwartz, G. J., & McHugh, P. R. (1992). Blockade of type A, not type B, CCK receptors attenuates satiety actions of exogenous and endogenous CCK. *American Journal of Physiology, 262,* R46–R50.

Morley, J. E. (1987). Neuropeptide regulation of appetite and weight. *Endocrine Reviews, 8,* 256–287.

Mrosovsky, N. (1990). *Rheostasis: The physiology of change.* New York: Oxford University Press.

Nicolaidis, S., & Rowland, N. E. (1976). Metering of intravenous versus oral nutrients and regulation of energy balance. *American Journal of Physiology, 231,* 661–668.

Olson, B. R., Drutarosky, M. D., Stricker, E. M., & Verbalis, J. G. (1991). Brain oxytocin receptors mediate corticotropin-releasing hormone-induced anorexia. *American Journal of Physiology, 260,* R448–R452.

Olson, B. R., Hoffman G. E., Sved, A. F., Stricker, E. M., & Verbalis, J. G. (1992). Cholecystokinin induces *c-fos* expression in hypothalamic oxytocinergic neurons projecting to the dorsal vagal complex. *Brain Research, 569,* 238–248.

Panula, P., Yang, H. Y. T., & Costa, E. (1982). Neuronal location of bombesin-like immunoreactivity in the central nervous system of the rat. *Regulatory Peptides, 4,* 275–283.

Pollock, J. D., & Rowland, N. E. (1981). Peripherally administered serotonin decreases food intake in rats. *Pharmacology, Biochemistry and Behavior, 15,* 179–183.

Ranson, S. W. (1939). Somnolence caused by hypothalamic lesions in the monkey. *Archives of Neurology and Psychiatry, 41,* 1–23.

Rawson, N. E., Blum, H., Osbakken, M. D., & Friedman, M. I. (1994). Hepatic phosphate trapping, decreased ATP, and increased feeding after 2,5-anhydro-D-mannitol. *American Journal of Physiology, 266,* R112–R117.

Ritter, S., & Dinh, T. T. (1994). 2-Mercaptoacetate and 2-deoxy-D-glucose induce Fos-like immunoreactivity in rat brain. *Brain Research, 641,* 111–120.

Ritter, S., Dinh, T. T., & Friedman, M. I. (1994). Induction of Fos-like immunoreactivity (Fos-li) and stimulation of feeding by 2,5-anhydro-D-mannitol (2,5-AM) require the vagus nerve. *Brain Research, 646,* 53–64.

Ritter, S., & Taylor, J. S. (1990). Vagal sensory neurons are required for lipoprivic but not glucoprivic feeding in rats. *American Journal of Physiology, 258,* R1395–R1401.

Romsos, D. R., Gosnell, B. A., Morley, J. E., & Levine, A. S. (1987). Effects of kappa opiate agonists, cholecystokinin and bombesin in intake of diets varying in carbohydrate-to-fat ratio in rats. *Journal of Nutrition, 117,* 976–985.

Rowland, N. E. (1991). Biological factors in eating and its disorders. *Bulletin of the Psychonomic Society, 29,* 244–249.

Rowland, N. E. (1992). Effects of glucose and fat antimetabolites on norepinephrine turnover in rat hypothalamus and brainstem. *Brain Research, 595,* 291–294.

Rowland, N. E. (1995). Interplay of behavioral and physiological mechanisms in adaptation. In M. J. Fregly and C. M. Blatheis (Eds.). *Handbook of Physiology, Section 4, Environmental Physiology.* New York: Oxford University Press.

Rowland, N. E., Bellinger, L. L., Li, B.-H., & Mendel, V. E. (in press). Satietin: For mapping of putative brain sites of action, *Brain Research.*

Rowland, N. E., Bellush, L. L., & Carlton, J. (1985). Metabolic and neurochemical correlates of glucoprivic feeding. *Brain Research Bulletin, 14,* 617–624.

Rowland, N. E., & Carlton, J. (1986). Neurobiology of an anorectic drug: Fenfluramine. *Progress in Neurobiology, 27,* 13–62.

Sahu, A., Kalra, P. S., & Kalra, S. P. (1988). Food deprivation and ingestion induce reciprocal changes in neuropeptide Y concentrations in the paraventricular nucleus. *Peptides, 9*, 83–86.

Sahu, A., White, J. D., Kalra, P. S., & Kalra, S. P. (1992). Hypothalamic neuropeptide Y gene expression in rats on scheduled feeding regimen. *Molecular Brain Research, 15*, 15–18.

Sanacora, G., Kershaw, M., Finkelstein, J. A., & White, J. D. (1990). Increased hypothalamic content of preproneuropeptide Y messenger ribonucleic acid in genetically obese Zucker rats and its regulation by food deprivation. *Endocrinology, 127*, 730–737.

Schwartz, G. J., Netterville L. A., McHugh, P. R., & Moran, T. H. (1991). Gastric loads potentiate inhibition of food intake produced by a cholecystokinin analogue. *American Journal of Physiology, 261*, R1141–R1146.

Schwartz, M. W., Figlewicz, D. P., Baskin, D. G., Woods, S. C., & Porte, D., Jr. (1992). Insulin in the brain: A hormonal regulator of energy balance. *Endocrine Reviews, 13*, 387–414.

Sharp, F. R., Sagar, S. M., & Swanson, R. A. (1993). Metabolic mapping with cellular resolution: c-fos vs. 2-deoxyglucose. *Critical Reviews in Neurobiology, 7*, 205–228.

Shibasaki, T., Oda, T., Imaki, T., Ling, N., & Demura, H. (1993). Injection of anti-neuropeptide Y g-globulin into the hypothalamic paraventricular nucleus decreases food intake in rats. *Brain Research, 601*, 313–316.

Smith, B. K., York, D. A., & Bray, G. (1994). Chronic cerebro-ventricular galanin does not induce sustained hyperphagia or obesity. *Peptides, 15*, 1267–1272.

Smith, G. P., & Gibbs, J. (1979). Postprandial satiety. *Progress in Psychobiology and Physiological Psychology, 8*, 179–242.

Smith, G. P., Jerome, C., Cushin, B. J., Eterno, R., & Simansky, K. J. (1981). Abdominal vagotomy blocks the satiety effect of cholecystokinin in the rat. *Science, 213*, 1036–1037.

Stanley, B. G., Kyrkouli, S. E., Lampert, S., & Leibowitz, S. F. (1986). Neuropeptide Y chronically injected into the hypothalamus: A powerful neurochemical inducer of hyperphagia and obesity. *Peptides, 7*, 1189–1192.

Stanley, B. G., Magdalin, W., Seirafi, A., Thomas, W. J., & Leibowitz, S. F. (1993). The perifornical area: The major focus of a patchily-distributed hypothalamic neuropeptide Y feeding system(s). *Brain Research, 604*, 304–317.

Stanley, B. G., Schwartz, D. H., Hernandez, L., Hoebel, B. G., & Leibowitz, S. F. (1989). Patterns of extracellular norepinephrine in the paraventricular hypothalamus: Relationship to circadian rhythm and deprivation-induced eating behavior. *Life Sciences, 45,* 275–282.

Stellar, E. (1954). The physiology of motivation. *Psychological Review, 61,* 5–22.

Stricker, E. M. (1983). Brain neurochemistry and the control of food intake. In E. Satinoff & P. Teitelbaum (Eds.), *Handbook of behavioral neurobiology: Vol. 6. Motivation* (pp. 329–366). New York: Plenum Press.

Stricker, E. M., & Verbalis, J. G. (1991). Caloric and noncaloric controls of food intake. *Brain Research Bulletin, 27,* 299–303.

Stuckey, J. A., Gibbs, J., & Smith, G. P. (1985). Neural disconnection of gut from brain blocks bombesin-induced satiety. *Peptides, 6,* 1249–1252.

Swanson, L. W., & Sawchenko, P. E. (1983). Hypothalamic integration: Organization of the paraventricular and supraoptic nuclei. *Annual Review of Neuroscience, 6,* 269–324.

Tempel, D. L., Leibowitz, K. J., & Leibowitz, S. F. (1988). Effects of PVN galanin on macronutrient selection. *Peptides, 9,* 309–314.

Tordoff, M. G., Rawson, N., & Friedman, M. I. (1991). 2,5-Anhydro-D-mannitol acts in liver to initiate feeding. *American Journal of Physiology, 254,* R283–R288.

Van Essen, D. C., & Deyoe, E. A. (1995). Concurrent processing in the primate visual cortex. In M. S. Gazzaniga (Ed.), *The cognitive neurosciences* (pp. 383–400). Cambridge, MA: MIT Press.

Verbalis, J. G., McCann, M. J., McHale, C. M., & Stricker, E. M. (1986). Oxytocin secretion in response to cholecystokinin and food intake: Differentiation of nausea from satiety. *Science, 232,* 1417–1419.

Verbalis, J. G., Stricker, E. M., Robinson, A. G., & Hoffman, G. E. (1991). Cholecystokinin activates C-Fos expression in hypothalamic oxytocin and corticotropin-releasing hormone neurons. *Journal of Neuroendocrinology, 3,* 205–213.

Weigle, D. S. (1994). Appetite and the regulation of body composition. *FASEB Journal, 8,* 302–310.

Weingarten H. (1990). Learning, homeostasis, and the control of feeding behavior. In E. D. Capaldi & T. R. Powley (Eds.), *Taste, experience and feeding* (pp. 14–27). Washington DC: American Psychological Association.

Woods, S. C., Taborsky, G. J., Jr., & Porte, D., Jr., (1986). Central nervous system control of nutrient homeostasis. In F. E. Bloom (Ed.), *Handbook of physiology,* (Sec. 1, Vol. 4, pp. 365–411). American Physiological Society.

Zhang, Y., Proenca, R., Maffei, M., Barone, M., Leopold, L., & Friedman, J. M. (1994). Positional cloning of the mouse *obese* gene and its human homologue. *Nature, 372,* 425–432.

PART FIVE

How the Social Context Influences Eating

8

Social Influences on Food Preferences and Feeding Behaviors of Vertebrates

Bennett G. Galef, Jr.

T o survive and reproduce in natural environments, animals not only must eat foods that provide all of the various nutrients necessary for self-maintenance and reproduction, they also must avoid eating lethal amounts of any toxic plants or animals that they encounter. Selecting a nutritionally adequate diet is no simple task, and physiologists, biologists, and psychologists have spent decades trying to understand how animals manage to discriminate foods containing needed nutrients from ingestible substances that are either valueless or dangerous to eat.

At first, interest focused on the fundamental question of whether animals are, in fact, able to select a nutritionally balanced diet when choosing foods from a cafeteria of items that vary in nutritional content (Crichton-Browne, 1910; Jordan, 1906). Once that question appeared to have been resolved (Richter, 1942–43; but see Galef, 1991a), interest shifted, first, to the question of how animals learn to select foods containing needed nutrients (Harris, Clay, Hargreaves, & Ward, 1933; Rozin, 1967), and then to the issue of how animals learn to avoid ingesting deleterious quantities of any toxins they might encounter while sampling unfamiliar potential foods in the search for nutrients (Garcia & Hankins, 1977; Rozin & Kalat, 1971).

Given the immense contribution of social interactions to the development of patterns of food selection by members of our own species, it is surprising that early students of food selection never looked for social influences on the ingestive behavior of the animals they studied. Perhaps the emphasis throughout the present century on understanding adaptive rather than maladaptive patterns of food selection (Galef, 1991a; Richter, 1942–43) and on describing neural and physiological substrates of ingestive behavior diverted attention from investigation of social influences on feeding.

Whether they are in the theoretical mainstream or not, social influences on food choice could not be ignored forever. The last 2 decades have seen a striking increase in the number of studies of the role of social interactions in shaping not only food selection but also a range of behaviors from predator avoidance (Cook, Mineka, Wolkenstein, & Laitsch, 1985); Curio, Ernst, &, Vieth, 1978) to choice of breeding site (Warner, 1988, 1990a, 1990b) and sexual partner (Dugatkin, 1992; Dugatkin & Godin, 1992, 1993; Schlupp, Marler, & Ryan, 1994). Studies of social influence on the food choices of animals have been particularly fruitful, at least in part because such studies have been able to take advantage of decades of earlier research describing nonsocial factors that influence food selection by animals.

In this chapter, I review research, almost all completed during the last 20 years, on the role of social factors in the development of food preferences, food aversions, and feeding behaviors in vertebrates. The evidence clearly demonstrates the importance of socially acquired information, particularly information extracted from adults by juveniles, in shaping the development of food preferences and feeding behaviors of both birds and mammals.

SOCIAL FACTORS IN THE ACQUISITION OF FOOD PREFERENCES

Prenatal Effects

Even before birth, a young mammal can acquire information from its female parent about at least some of the foods that she has eaten. Hepper (1988) fed garlic to pregnant rats late in gestation. Within an hour of birth of each of their litters, he gave the young to foster mothers that had never eaten garlic to rear. When the foster-reared pups were 12 days old, each was offered a choice between two dishes, one containing garlic, the other onion.

Hepper found that rat pups that had been delivered by mothers that ate garlic while pregnant stayed near the dish containing garlic, whereas pups from control litters (whose mothers had not eaten garlic during pregnancy) did not exhibit any preference between garlic and onion.

Although Hepper's data demonstrate only that young rats can become familiar with the taste or odor of a food that their mother has eaten during pregnancy, it seems likely that pups with an enhanced preference for the odor of garlic when 12 days of age would have exhibited enhanced intake of either garlic or garlic-flavored food if their food preferences had been examined at weaning. Clearly, a potentially informative experiment remains to be done.

Effects While Nursing

Direct evidence is available that (a) flavors of foods that a dam eats while lactating can affect the flavor of her milk and (b) exposure to milk flavored by foods a lactating dam has eaten can affect food preferences of her nurslings at weaning. For example, at weaning, infant rat pups that had been made ill immediately after they were fed milk expressed manually from a lactating rat eating a distinctively flavored diet exhibited an aversion to the diet eaten by the lactating rat whose milk they had received (Galef & Sherry, 1973). Similarly, weaning rat pups exhibited enhanced preferences for foods eaten by a lactating female from whom the pups had suckled for several hours, but not for the same food if it had been eaten by a female rat that acted in a maternal way but did not give milk during the hours the pups spent with her (Bronstein, Levine, & Marcus, 1975; Galef & Henderson, 1972; Martin & Alberts, 1979).

Effects During Weaning

Presence of an Adult at a Feeding Site

Galef and Clark (1971b) used closed-circuit television and time-lapse video recorders to observe nine wild rat pups from three different litters each take its very first meal of solid food. All nine pups were observed to eat for the first time under exactly the same circumstances: Each ate while an adult was eating, and each ate at the site where the adult was eating, not at a nearby feeding site where no adult was feeding. Weaning mice also exhibit a strong tendency both to approach an adult feeding at a distance from the nest and to initiate their first bouts of feeding on solid food near the place where the adult is eating (Valsecchi, Mainardi, Sgoifo, & Taticcchi, 1989).

In fact, simply anesthetizing a rat and placing it near a feeding site makes that site significantly more attractive to weaning rat pups than alternative sites that have no rat placed near them (Galef, 1981). Apparently, the simple physical presence of an adult rat at a feeding site makes that site attractive to young rats and markedly increases the probability that they will wean to whatever food is to be found there (Galef & Clark, 1971b).

In a methodologically innovative series of experiments on the role of maternal interaction on the development of food preferences in kittens, Wyrwicka (1978; 1981) used rewarding electrical stimulation of the hypothalamus to train mother cats to eat unusual foods such as banana. She then let weanling kittens (4–10 weeks of age) interact with their dam while she was eating the unusual food. After a few test sessions during which the kittens became habituated to the experimental setting, most started to lick and eat the food their mother was eating, often attempting to eat from exactly the same spot in the food dish where she had been feeding. Four months after eating banana with their mothers, many kittens continued to accept banana, whereas almost no kittens of the same age that had never before eaten bananas would do so.

Sheep can also induce their young to begin feeding on unfamiliar foods. Weaning lambs offered wheat for the first time ate much less wheat if exposed to wheat while alone than if offered wheat in the presence of their respective mothers, who had been trained to eat wheat (Lynch, Keogh, Elwin, Green, & Mottershead, 1983). In a similar experiment, Thorhallsdottir, Provenza, and Balph (1990) found that lambs exposed to a novel food while alone ate far less of that food than did lambs exposed to the same novel food while in the presence of their feeding dam.

It is not clear in either of the studies in which sheep served as subjects whether presence of a ewe simply provided an environment in which the probability of a lamb eating was enhanced (a social facilitation effect; Clayton, 1978) or the adult sheep were in some way directly influencing their young to eat the foods that they were eating. However, regardless of the mechanism involved, lambs exposed to an unfamiliar food while their mothers ate it were more likely to eat and learn to accept that food than were lambs offered the same unfamiliar food while alone.

In sheep, as in kittens, the effects of eating a food on its later acceptance were long lasting. Lambs that ate wheat with their dams when 12 weeks of age ate considerably more wheat when 3 years old than did sheep of a like age that had never before eaten wheat (Green Elwin, Mottershead, Keogh, & Lynch, 1984).

Feeding hens (*Gallus gallus*) can also influence choices of foods and feeding sites of their chicks. Observation of a mechanical pointer "pecking" at a visually distinctive foodlike object caused newly hatched chicks to peck at matching objects (Suboski, 1989; Turner, 1964). Such social orientation of pecking may be a means for transmission of food preferences from hen to chick, allowing a hen to designate edible objects for her young (Suboski & Bartashunas, 1984).

In more natural circumstances, when a mother hen finds food, she emits a special "food call," which attracts her chicks. The hen then pecks at the food, picking up bits of it in her beak and then dropping them in front of her chicks. The hen's activity causes the chicks to eat the food she has been manipulating (Roper, 1986; Stokes, 1971). Presumably, the experiments of Suboski and of Turner described here tapped into these species-typical behaviors of mother hens and their young.

Older chickens are also able to learn to select particular feeding sites by observing the behavior of conspecifics. The sight of either an adolescent chicken or its television image feeding from a visually distinctive feeding site caused observing birds to feed from similar feeding sites when tested 2 days later (McQuoid & Galef, 1992, 1993).

Residual Olfactory Cues

In the examples described in the preceding section, the presence or activities of adults at a feeding site affected the feeding behavior of younger individuals. However, adults need not be physically present at a feeding site to guide their young to that site. While eating, adult rats deposit residual olfactory cues both in the vicinity of a food source (Galef & Heiber, 1976; Laland & Plotkin, 1990, 1993) and on any food that they are eating (Galef & Beck, 1985). These odorants are attractive to rat pups and cause them to feed at marked sites in preference to unmarked ones (Galef & Heiber, 1976; Laland & Plotkin, 1990, 1993).

Exposure to Foods and Food Related Cues

The young of many species seem particularly attentive to the food objects that they see adults manipulating. For example, infant chimpanzees actively solicit food from their mothers, and chimpanzee mothers share the food items they are eating with their offspring (Silk, 1978). The young of other primate species, although often less active in soliciting scraps from adults than are young chimpanzees, still manage to focus their ingestion on the same items of food that adults of their troop are eating (e.g., chacma baboon [Hall, 1962, 1963a, 1963b], ringtailed lemur [Sussman, 1977], anubis baboon [Ransom & Rowell, 1972], Japanese macaque, [Kawai, 1965]). Hall's account of feeding interactions between adult baboons and their young is typical: "Dark-phase [chacma baboon] infants, prior to their actually eating food-plants, watch the feeding of their mothers or of other mature animals near them, and tend to direct their exploratory movements upon the same plants, chewing them or putting parts of them in their mouths (1963a, p. 220)."

In a systematic study of the interaction of infant monkeys and adults in feeding situations in the wild, Whitehead (1986) observed the feeding interactions of 4- to 12-month-old infant mantled howler monkeys (*Alouatta palliata*) and their mothers in the forests of western Costa Rica. Infants ate leaves only from species of plant on which they had observed adult group members feed, and the infants often fed from the same branch from which their mother was eating. On the other hand, infants frequently began to ingest unfamiliar fruits before adult group members did and, when eating fruit, seldom attempted to feed from the same branch from which an adult was feeding.

Although there is presently no direct evidence that such social introduction of young primates to food items that adults are eating shapes the later dietary repertoire of the young, it is difficult to imagine that eating foods that adults are eating has no effect on development of food preferences of young primates.

Primates are not the only animals that attend closely to foods that adults eat. McFadyen-Ketchum and Porter (1989) reported frequent investigations of the nose and mouth of lactating female spiny mice (*Acomys cahirinus*) by their weanling young. After weanling spiny mice were returned to their mother (who, in their absence, had been given an unfamiliar food to eat), these young spent more than twice as long in nose-to-mouth and nose-to-head interactions with their dam as did pups assigned to a control condition and returned to a home cage containing a dam that had eaten a familiar food. In a subsequent choice test, weanlings that interacted with a mother that was fed a new food ate significantly more of that food than did pups whose mothers had not eaten it.

Other investigators (Ewer, 1963, 1969; Leyhausen, 1956; Liers, 1951; Schaller, 1967) have described a multitude of ways in which mothers of several predatory species (meerkat, otter, domestic cats, tiger; see Ewer, 1968, for a review) bring prey to their weaning young, which may either facilitate development of predatory behavior in their offspring or cause their young to prefer certain types of prey. For example, in an anecdotal report, Ewer (1963) described a maternal meerkat (*Suricata suricata*) inducing her young to eat banana, a food that they would not normally eat, by holding a piece of banana in her mouth and running to and fro in front of her offspring. Again, such informal observations are not sufficient to establish that the exposure to prey that a mother gives to her young either facilitates development of their predatory behavior or affects their later food preferences (Galef, 1990).

In a formal experiment, Caro (1980a, 1980b) found that kittens that had been exposed to a mother that killed mice in their presence were more likely to become mouse killers as adults than were cats that, as kittens, had been exposed to mice without their mother present. Unfortunately, Baerends-van Roon and Baerends (1979) found precisely the reverse. In several early experiments in which adult cats or rats that were not spontaneous killers of vertebrate prey were given repeated opportunities to observe conspecifics kill, the observers' probabilities of starting to kill were significantly enhanced (Johnson, DeSisto, & Koenig, 1972; Kuo, 1930; Pion, 1969). Clearly, effects of observation of predatory behavior on its expression are complex and have not yet been fully explored. Because of the change in public attitude toward experiments involving staged predatory encounters, however, studies of development of predatory behavior in vertebrates are no longer pursued, and many questions concerning the role of social learning in the development of predatory behavior remain unanswered.

Effects After Weaning

Transmission of Flavor Preferences in Rats

During the last decade, considerable attention has been focused on the ability of rats of all ages to determine which foods others of their species have been eating and on the surprising effectiveness of such socially acquired information in guiding its recipients' future food choices (Galef & Wigmore, 1983; Posadas-Andrews & Roper, 1983; Strupp & Levitsky, 1984).

Both olfactory cues escaping from the digestive tract of a recently fed rat and the smell of bits of food clinging to its fur and vibrissae allow other rats to identify foods eaten by an individual with whom they interact (Galef, Kennett, & Stein, 1985). Experience of the odor of a food together with rat-produced odors results in substantial enhancement of preferences for foods smelled on conspecifics. House mice show a similar (and probably homologous) enhancement of their preferences for foods experienced in contiguity with another of their species (Valsecchi & Galef, 1989).

Such socially enhanced preferences for foods experienced by a rat on the body or breath of a conspecific are not the result of simple exposure to the smell of a food that happens to be carried on a conspecific (Galef & Stein, 1985; Heyes & Durlach, 1990). For example, rats exposed to pieces of cotton batting dusted with an unfamiliar food do not develop a preference for it, whereas rats exposed to an anesthetized rat dusted with the same food exhibit a markedly increased preference for the food (Galef, Kennett, & Stein, 1985; Galef & Stein, 1985).

Surprisingly, changes in odor preference that result from exposure to the scent of a diet on the breath or fur of a conspecific are relatively specific to food odors. Rats that interact with a conspecific that has eaten cinnamon-flavored food subsequently show an enhanced preference for cinnamon-flavored food but not for cinnamon-scented nesting materials or cinnamon-scented nesting sites (Galef, Iliffe, & Whiskin, 1994).

Investigations of the nature of the rat-produced odor that increases preference for food odors experienced together with it indicate that the relevant chemical is carried on the breath of rats (Galef & Stein, 1985). Mass-spectrographic analyses of rat breath reveal the presence of carbon disulfide in the air taken from the noses but not from the mouths of rats. (Rats breathe only through their noses, not through their mouths.) Also, rats exposed to pieces of cotton batting both dusted with a novel food and moistened with a dilute carbon disulfide solution subsequently exhibited an enhanced preference for that food, whereas rats exposed to pieces of cotton batting dusted with the same food and moistened with water did not (Galef, Mason, Pretti, & Bean, 1988).

Effects of exposure to a recently fed rat on the food choices of its fellows are surprisingly robust (Galef, Kennett, & Wigmore, 1985; Richard, Grover, & Davis, 1987). For example, rats that learned a profound aversion to an unfamiliar palatable diet and subsequently, interacted with other rats that had eaten that diet frequently abandoned their aversion (Galef, 1986; for similar data in hyena, see Yoerg, 1991). Many rats that had interacted with others that were eating a base diet to which cayenne pepper, a highly unpalatable adulterant, had been added exhibited a durable preference for the adulterated form of the diet (Galef, 1989).

Rats' olfactory communications about foods are also quite sophisticated. Individuals are able to exchange useful information with conspecifics about three or four different foods that each has eaten (Galef & Whiskin, 1992) and to use socially acquired information to determine which potential food sites to visit when foraging in an environment where several different foods are intermittently available at specific locations (Galef & Wigmore, 1983).

Social Transmission of Flavor Aversions in Rats

There is one way in which rats do not seem to be able to use socially acquired information about foods when such information would appear to be potentially useful. Unexpectedly, after a naive rat interacts with a conspecific that has eaten a novel food and become either violently ill or unconscious, the naive individual subsequently exhibits a preference for the food that the sick individual ate, not an aversion to it (Galef, McQuoid, & Whiskin, 1990; Galef, Wigmore & Kennett, 1983; Grover, Kixmiller, Erickson, Becker, & Davis, 1988). The finding that rats are not capable of direct social transmission of avoidance of toxins was completely unexpected.

After the fact, it could be argued that because wild Norway rats are exceedingly hesitant to eat any foods they have not previously eaten, biasing a rat to eat one food effectively prevents that rat from eating other foods (Galef & Clark, 1971a). A wild rat may wait for as long as 5 days before sampling a novel food available to it, even if it does not have access to any familiar foods and hesitancy to eat the unfamiliar food results in several days of self-starvation (Barnett, 1958; Galef, 1970). Consequently, any behavioral processes that direct rats to a safe food would result in their avoiding ingestion of any toxic alternatives; therefore, avoidance of poisons may be transmitted among rats indirectly rather than directly (Galef, 1985).

Social Transmission of Flavor Preferences and Aversions in Other Animals

Compelling evidence of direct transmission of poison avoidance, as well as of food preference, has been reported in species other than Norway rats. Mason, Arzt, and Reidinger (1984) trained "model" red-winged blackbirds either to eat or to avoid food presented in a yellow cup while "observer" conspecifics watched the training of the models. After training was completed, both models and observers were given a choice between yellow and green cups containing the same food. Observer birds that had watched conspecifics learn to eat from a yellow cup preferred the food in the yellow cup, whereas observer birds that had watched conspecifics become ill after feeding from a yellow cup avoided the yellow cup almost completely.

It is not clear why blackbirds should be able to learn to avoid a toxic food by watching their fellows eat the food and become ill, whereas rats are unable to learn the same thing; however, that seems to be the case.

In an early laboratory experiment on social learning of food preference, adult baboons (*Mandrillus sphinx*) were offered slices of banana that had been both colored blue and adulterated with quinine to make them unpalatable as well as slices of banana that had simply been colored red. Five infant baboons that watched an experienced adult select palatable, red slices of banana and ignore unpalatable, blue ones were then offered a choice between equal numbers of red, palatable slices and blue, unpalatable slices of banana. Four of the five infants readily ate red slices of banana and hesitated before tasting blue ones (Jouventin, Pasteur, & Cambeferd, 1976). Jouventin and his coworkers interpreted these data as providing evidence of an ability of young baboons to learn to avoid a food that they had seen adults avoid, although their data are equally consistent with the hypothesis that young baboons learn to eat the foods that they see adults eat.

Local Enhancement

A review of social influences on feeding behavior in adult vertebrates would surely be incomplete without explicit mention of the important role of local enhancement (Thorpe, 1963) in the foraging behavior of a wide range of species; for example, the sight of vultures descending on a carcass draws others of their kind to a recent kill (Houston, 1979; Schaller, 1972). The distinctive rasping sound made by an agouti gnawing on a fallen nut carries dozens of meters through the rain forest and attracts other agouti to a newly discovered feeding site (Smythe, 1970). The "feeding buzzes" made by bats (*Lasiurus borealis*) as they home in on their insect prey informs others of their species both of the location of a potentially rich source of food and of possible opportunities to steal food from successful foragers (Balcombe & Fenton, 1988). There are many such examples in the literature describing situations in which the activities of an individual at a food source attract others of its species to the location where it is eating and biases them to begin eating there. The work of Krebs and his colleagues on social foraging by flocks of small birds (Krebs, 1973; Krebs, MacRoberts, & Cullen, 1972) is prototypical of the more informative of such studies.

Krebs et al. (1972) established small flocks, each consisting of four birds, in an indoor aviary and compared the success of these flocks in finding seed concealed in one of many food cups scattered about the branches of treelike constructions in the aviary with the success of both individual birds and pairs of birds foraging in the same enclosure. Krebs and his colleagues found that an individual bird foraging in a flock of four was significantly more likely to find concealed food during a 15-minute test period than it was when foraging either alone or as a member of a pair. The greater success in finding food exhibited by flocks of four birds than by individual or paired birds was the result of two factors. First, the greater the number of birds searching for the concealed food, the more likely one of the searchers was to find food during a 15-minute test period. Second, once one bird in a flock found food, the other members of the flock took advantage of the find by flying to and searching in the place where food had been found. In a later experiment in the same series, Krebs et al. (1972) examined the effects on foraging by flock members of observing one of their fellows find food in one of four different types of food container. When one bird found food in a particular type of food cup, others in its flock increased their frequency of searching for food in other containers of that type.

Such local, or stimulus, enhancement (Galef, 1988; Spence, 1937) of one potential feeding site at the expense of others can, at least in principle, have important effects on the food choices of individuals that use social information to select locations in which to forage. By attracting conspecifics to one food source rather than another, local enhancement can indirectly determine which prey species foragers will encounter; the experience of feeding on one prey species or of foraging success in one microhabitat could have important effects on subsequent food choices (Galef, 1988).

SOCIAL FACTORS IN THE ACQUISITION OF FEEDING BEHAVIORS

Although great progress has been made in analyzing social interactions that affect food preferences, less is known about the ways in which social learning influences acquisition of motor patterns used in feeding.

Field Observations

In recent years, field workers have described a number of behaviors that are used to acquire food by only some of the many social groups that make up a species. Chimpanzees seem particularly likely to exhibit such population-specific patterns of behavior (Galef, 1992; McGrew, 1992). For example, chimps at Gombe National Park in Tanzania use twigs as probes to fish for termites (Goodall, 1986); their fellows in Tai National Park in Ivory Coast do not (McGrew, 1992). Chimpanzees in Tai National Park use hammers and anvils to crack open kola nuts (Boesch, 1991; Boesch & Boesch, 1990); chimps in East Africa do not (McGrew, 1992). Four chimpanzees at Bossou in the Republic of Guinea extracted sap from palm oil trees by using a palm stalk as a pestle to pound at the center of the top of the trees and a wad of vegetable fiber as a sponge to absorb sap. No other chimpanzees have ever been reported to be engaging in the behavior (Sugiyama, 1994).

Although essentially nothing is known either about how such idiosyncratic feeding behaviors develop in individuals or why they are found in some populations but not in others, it is not improbable (even if not proven) that social learning plays an important role in the development and diffusion of population-specific patterns of feeding behavior.

Some observations by Hauser (1988) of a free-ranging troop of vervet monkeys at Amboseli National Park in Kenya that, like chimps at Tai National Park (Sugiyama, 1994) and at Gombe (Goodall, 1986), learned to use plant material as sponges to acquire liquids that were otherwise inaccessible; the report may provide some hint as to how such behaviors originate and spread. Vervets' use of a dry pod as a sponge to extract exudate from a tree during a period of drought was first seen when only one troop member was engaging in the behavior. Over a period of 22 days, diffusion of the behavior from its inventor to six other troop members was observed. Details of the conditions under which transmission of the behavior occurred are consistent with the hypothesis that some of the animals learned to use dry pods to acquire exudate by imitating a troop mate, though in uncontrolled environments it is impossible to know with certainty how any individual acquired the behavior.

Laboratory Analyses

There are only a few cases in which it has been clearly demonstrated, under controlled conditions, that social interactions contribute directly to the development of the kinds of idiosyncratic feeding behaviors that are exhibited by free-living animals.

Roof rats in the pine forests of Israel

Aisner discovered some years ago that the pine forests of Israel were inhabited by roof rats (*Rattus rattus*) that subsisted on a diet consisting solely of pine seeds and water (Aisner & Terkel, 1992). Extraction of pine seeds has been a stable tradition in these forest-dwelling rodents for many generations, and there is every reason to expect persistence of this unique feeding behavior, enabling rats to survive in an otherwise sterile habitat where pine seeds are the sole food available in sufficient quantity to sustain a population of mammals.

Laboratory studies have revealed that there is only one energetically efficient way for rats to remove the tough scales from pine cones and gain access to the energy-rich seeds they conceal. If rats are to realize a net energy gain while feeding on pine cones, they must take advantage of the structure of the cone, first removing scales from the base of the cone and then removing, one after another, the spiral of scales running around the cone's shaft to its apex. Laboratory investigations of development of the energetically efficient spiral pattern of scale removal (necessary if rats are to realize a net energy gain while feeding from pine cones) have shown that only 6 of 222 adult rats maintained in the presence of pine cones for several weeks at 85% of normal body weight were able to learn the efficient pattern of pine cone opening by individual, trial-and-error learning. The remaining 216 subjects either ignored the pine cones or gnawed at them randomly in a way that did not lead to acquisition of more energy from pine seeds than was expended in their extraction and ingestion. On the other hand, essentially all young rats came to exhibit the efficient method of opening pine cones if they were reared by a dam that, in the presence of her young, stripped scales from pine cones efficiently. Rats learned to be efficient strippers of pine cones even if they were gestated and delivered by mothers that did not strip pine cones efficiently but were reared by a foster mother that exhibited the efficient means of cone stripping in the presence of her adopted young. Rat pups failed to learn to strip cones efficiently if they were born to mothers that stripped pine cones efficiently but were foster-reared by dams that didn't exhibit the behavior. Clearly, some aspect of the postnatal interaction between mothers that strip pine cones and the young they rear is necessary for the transmission of the behavior from one generation to another (Aisner & Terkel, 1992; Zohar & Terkel, 1992).

Further experiments demonstrated that the experience of young rats in completing the stripping of pine cones that had been started appropriately by an experienced adult rat (or by an experimenter using a pair of pliers to imitate the pattern of scale removal used by experienced cone-stripping rats) enabled more than 70% of young rats to become efficient strippers (Aisner & Terkel, 1992).

The behavior needed to strip pine cones efficiently is transmitted from one generation of roof rats living in Israel's forests to the next, but that tradition does not appear to be transmitted or maintained either by imitation or by any other complex social learning process. Rather, practitioners of the tradition of cone stripping alter the environment in which their young develop by allowing them access to partially stripped pine cones and thus markedly increase the probability that the young rats will acquire the traditional pattern of behavior.

Milk-Bottle Opening by British Birds

A similar social learning process is implicated in the spread of the traditional habit exhibited by several species of British birds that open the foil covers of milk bottles and feed on the bottles' contents. In a laboratory study of the processes responsible for the spread of milk-bottle opening in populations of wild birds (first described by Fisher & Hinde, 1949), Sherry and Galef (1984) took into account the fact that the presence in an area of a bird that opened milk bottles and fed from them provided naive birds not only with demonstrations of opening behavior to imitate, but also with open milk bottles from which the naive birds could feed.

In the laboratory, wild-caught black-capped chickadees (*Parus atricapillus*) that had experience feeding from milk bottles that were opened by a human experimenter were likely to open closed milk bottles, as were chickadees that had the opportunity to observe other chickadees opening milk bottles (Sherry & Galef, 1984, 1990). However, a chickadee that watched a conspecific opening milk bottles was no more likely to open a closed milk bottle in its own cage than was a chickadee that had a closed milk bottle in its cage and a view of a conspecific in a cage with no milk bottle. Apparently, the simple presence of a conspecific facilitates exploration in chickadees (birds that in natural circumstances often feed as members of flocks) and thus increases the probability that they will open milk bottles for themselves.

Hickory-Nut Opening by Red Squirrels

Weigl and Hanson (1980) measured both the time required and energy expended by two groups of red squirrels (*Tamiasciurus hudsonicus*) opening hickory nuts for the first time. One group of squirrels had been allowed to observe an experienced squirrel feeding on hickory nuts; the other had not. In a subsequent test, members of the group that had observed an experienced conspecific opening hickory nuts took only half as long and used only half as much energy to open hickory nuts as did members of the group that had not observed a model open hickory nuts. Again, social learning of some kind had a major impact on the acquisition of a behavior of importance in the acquisition of food.

SOCIAL INFLUENCES ON HUMAN FEEDING BEHAVIOR

The experimental literature on social effects on human eating (for examples see Birch, 1980a, 1980b; Pliner & Pelchat, 1986; Rozin, Fallon & Mandell, 1984) is relatively sparse (for review, see Rozin, 1988a, 1988b). Much remains to be done before researchers can speak with authority about the various roles that social interaction actually plays in development of both adaptive and maladaptive patterns of food choice in members of our own species. There can be little question that social influences on human food selection can be immense; response to reports in the media of a possible link between human disease and ingestion of British beef (a front-page story as I write the final draft of this manuscript), is but one of many examples bearing witness to the great impact that socially acquired information can have on human food choices. Whether understanding mechanisms of social influence on diet selection in our vertebrate cousins will eventually provide experimental paradigms and theoretical positions of real use in understanding analogous processes in *Homo sapiens* remains to be seen. I am optimistic.

CONCLUSION

Two decades of study of social influences on ingestive behavior have repeatedly demonstrated profound impacts of social interactions on the development of both the food preferences and feeding behaviors of animals. In simple cases of social influence on development of food preferences, the physical presence of one individual at a location attracts others and increases the probability that they will eat whatever food is to be found there. In more complex instances, one animal learns either to eat or to avoid eating some food by observing the behavior of another of its species when it eats the food and either does or does not become ill.

Like social learning of food preferences, social learning of feeding behaviors can proceed along routes of varying complexity. In simple cases, the feeding behavior of one member of a population alters the physical environment in a way that increases the probability that its fellows will acquire that behavior. In more complex instances, a naive individual might learn a complex feeding behavior by observing and then imitating a knowledgeable conspecific, or a knowledgeable animal might actively teach one of its fellows to engage in some feeding behavior, although convincing evidence of either imitation learning or teaching by animals is not yet available (Galef, 1990, 1992; but see Boesch, 1991; Caro & Hauser, 1992).

Even the simplest of social processes known to contribute to establishment and maintenance of traditional patterns of either food preference or feeding behavior should facilitate naive young animals' acquisition of those responses to environmental challenges that others of their social group have found rewarding. Social learning can reduce the time, energy, and risk associated with acquiring food preferences and feeding behaviors that are useful in the specific locale where each juvenile must overcome impressive odds if it is to achieve metabolic independence. The same processes that allow juveniles to exploit the knowledge their elders have acquired as a result of extensive experience in a particular area can also help adult animals to monitor the ebb and flow of resources in changing environments (Galef, 1993).

Members of our own species are not unique in exhibiting profound effects of social interactions on the development of their feeding habits and food preferences. The tardiness of scientists in starting to investigate social influences on feeding behavior is unfortunate, but the relatively brief history of such investigations should not interfere with our recognition of the importance of social learning in the development of feeding behavior in animals. Social interactions play a major role in facilitating development of patterns of ingestive behavior that allow animals to overcome the multitude of metabolic challenges provided by natural environments.

REFERENCES

Aisner, R., & Terkel, J. (1992). Ontogeny of pine-cone opening behaviour in the black rat (*Rattus rattus*). *Animal Behaviour, 44,* 327–336.

Baerends-van Roon, J. M. & Baerends, G. P. (1979). *The morphogenesis of the behaviour of the domestic cat with special emphasis on the development of prey catching.* Amsterdam: North Holland.

Balcombe, J. P., & Fenton, M. B. (1988). Eavesdropping by bats: The influence of echolocation call design and foraging strategy. *Ethology, 79,* 158–166.

Barnett, S. A. (1958). Experiments on "neophobia" in wild and laboratory rats. *British Journal of Psychology, 49,* 195–201.

Birch, L. L. (1980a). Effects of peer models' food choices and eating behaviors on preschoolers' food preferences. *Child Development, 51,* 486–496.

Birch, L. L. (1980b). The relationship between childrens' food preferences and those of their parents. *Journal of Nutrition Education, 12,* 14–18.

Boesch, C. (1991). Teaching among chimpanzees. *Animal Behaviour, 41,* 530–532.

Boesch, C., & Boesch, H. (1990). Tool use and tool making in wild chimpanzees. *Folia Primatologica, 54,* 86–99.

Bronstein, P. M., Levine, M. J., & Marcus, M. (1975). A rat's first bite: The nongenetic, cross-generational transfer of information. *Journal of Comparative and Physiological Psychology, 89,* 295–298.

Caro, T. M. (1980a). Predatory behaviour in domestic cat mothers. *Behaviour, 74,* 128–147.

Caro, T. M. (1980b). Effects of the mother, object play and adult experience on predation in cats. *Behavioral and Neural Biology, 29,* 29–51.

Caro, T. M., & Hauser, M. D. (1992). Is there teaching in nonhuman animals? *Quarterly Review of Biology, 67,* 151–174.

Clayton, D. A. (1978). Socially facilitated behavior. *Quarterly Review of Biology, 53,* 373–391.

Cook, M., Mineka, S., Wolkenstein, B., & Laitsch, K. (1985). Observational conditioning of snake fear in unrelated rhesus monkeys. *Journal of Abnormal Psychology, 94,* 591–610.

Crichton-Browne, J. (1910). *Delusions in diet.* London: Funk & Wagnalls.

Curio, E., Ernst, U., & Vieth, W. (1978). Cultural transmission of enemy recognition: One function of mobbing. *Science, 202,* 899–901.

Dugatkin, L. A. (1992). Sexual selection and imitation: Females copy the mate choice of others. *American Naturalist, 139,* 1384–1489.

Dugatkin, L. A., & Godin, J. G. (1992). Reversal of female mate choice by copying in the guppy (*Poecilia reticulata*). *Proceedings of the Royal Society of London, Series B, 249,* 179–184.

Dugatkin, L. A., & Godin, J. G. (1993). Female mate copying in the guppy (*Poecilia reticulata*): Age dependent effects. *Behavioral Ecology, 4,* 289–292.

Ewer, R. F. (1963). The behaviour of the meerkat, *Suricata suricata* (Schreber). *Zeitschrift fur Tierpsychologie, 20,* 570–607.

Ewer, R. F. (1968). *Ethology of mammals.* New York: Plenum Press.

Ewer, R. F. (1969). The "instinct to teach." *Nature, 222,* 698.

Fisher, J., & Hinde, R. A. (1949). The opening of milk bottles by birds. *British Birds, 42,* 347–357.

Galef, B. G., Jr. (1970). Aggression and timidity: Responses to novelty in feral Norway rats. *Journal of Comparative and Physiological Psychology, 70,* 370–381.

Galef, B. G., Jr. (1981). The development of olfactory control of feeding site selection in rat pups. *Journal of Comparative Psychology, 95,* 615–662.

Galef, B. G., Jr. (1985). Direct and indirect behavioral pathways to the social transmission of food avoidance. In P. Bronstein & N. S. Braveman (Eds.), *Experimental assessments and clinical applications of conditioned food aversions.* (pp. 203–215). New York: New York Academy of Sciences.

Galef, B. G., Jr. (1986). Social interaction modifies learned aversions, sodium appetite, and both palatability and handling-time induced dietary preference in rats (*Rattus norvegicus*). *Journal of Comparative Psychology, 100,* 432–439.

Galef, B. G., Jr. (1988). Imitation in animals: History, definition and interpretation of data from the psychological laboratory. In T. R. Zentall & B. G. Galef, Jr. (Eds.), *Social Learning: Psychological and biological perspectives.* (pp. 3–28). Hillsdale, NJ: Lawrence Erlbaum Associates.

Galef, B. G., Jr. (1989). Enduring social enhancement of rats' preferences for the palatable and the piquant. *Appetite, 13,* 81–92.

Galef, B. G., Jr. (1990). Tradition in animals: Field observations and laboratory analyses. In M. Bekoff & D. Jamieson (Eds.), *Interpretation and explanation in the study of behavior: Comparative perspectives.* (pp. 74–95). Boulder: Westview Press.

Galef, B. G., Jr. (1991a). A contrarian view of the wisdom of the body as it relates to food selection. *Psychological Review, 98,* 218–224.

Galef, B. G., Jr. (1991b). Information centres of Norway rats: Sites for information parasitism and information exchange. *Animal Behaviour, 41,* 295–301.

Galef, B. G., Jr. (1992). The question of animal culture. *Human Nature, 3,* 157–178.

Galef, B. G., Jr. (1993). Functions of social learning about food: a causal analysis of effects of diet novelty on preference transmission. *Animal Behaviour, 46,* 257–265.

Galef, B. G., Jr., & Beck, M. (1985). Aversive and attractive marking of toxic and safe foods by Norway rats. *Behavioral and Neural Biology, 43,* 298–310.

Galef, B. G., Jr., & Clark, M. M. (1971a). Social factors in the poison avoidance and feeding behavior of wild and domesticated rat pups. *Journal of Comparative and Physiological Psychology, 25,* 341–357.

Galef, B. G., Jr., & Clark, M. M. (1971b). Parent-offspring interactions determine time and place of first ingestion of solid food by wild rat pups. *Psychonomic Science, 25,* 15–16.

Galef, B. G. Jr., & Heiber, L. (1976). Role of residual olfactory cues in the determination of feeding site selection and exploration patterns of domestic rats. *Journal of Comparative and Physiological Psychology, 90,* 727–739.

Galef, B. G., Jr., & Henderson, P. W. (1972). Mother's milk: A determinant of feeding preferences of weaning rat pups. *Journal of Comparative and Physiological Psychology, 78,* 213–219.

Galef, B. G., Jr., Iliffe, C. P., & Whiskin, E. E. (1994). Social influences on rats' (*Rattus norvegicus*) preferences for flavored foods, scented nest materials, and odors associated with harborage sites: Are flavored foods special? *Journal of Comparative Psychology, 108,* 266–273.

Galef, B. G., Jr., Kennett, D. J., & Stein, M. (1985). Demonstrator influence on observer diet preference: Effects of simple exposure and presence of a demonstrator. *Animal Learning & Behaviour, 13,* 25–30.

Galef, B. G., Jr., Kennett, D. J., & Wigmore, S. W. (1984). Transfer of information concerning distant food in rats: A robust phenomenon. *Animal Learning & Behavior, 12,* 292–296.

Galef, B. G., Jr., Mason, J. R., Preti, G., & Bean, N. J. (1988). Carbon disulfide: A semiochemical mediating socially-induced diet choice in rats. *Physiology & Behaviour, 42,* 119–124.

Galef, B. G., Jr., McQuoid, L. M., & Whiskin, E. E. (1990). Further evidence that Norway rats do not socially transmit learned aversions to toxic baits. *Animal Learning & Behavior, 18,* 199–205.

Galef, B. G., Jr., & Sherry, D. F. (1973). Mother's milk: A medium for the transmission of cues reflecting the flavor of mother's diet. *Journal of Comparative and Physiological Psychology, 83,* 374–378.

Galef, B. G., Jr., & Stein, M. (1985). Demonstrator influence on observer diet preference: Analyses of critical social interactions and olfactory signals. *Animal Learning & Behavior, 13,* 131–138.

226

Galef, B. G., Jr., & Whiskin, E. E. (1992). Social transmission of information about multiflavored foods. *Animal Learning & Behavior, 20,* 56–62.

Galef, B. G., Jr., & Wigmore, S. W. (1983). Transfer of information concerning distant foods: A laboratory investigation of the "information-centre" hypothesis. *Animal Behaviour, 31,* 748–758.

Galef, B. G., Jr., Wigmore, S. W., & Kennett, D. J. (1983). A failure to find socially mediated taste aversion learning in Norway rats (*R. norvegicus*). *Journal of Comparative Psychology, 97,* 458–463.

Garcia, J., & Hankins, W. G. (1977). On the origin of food aversion paradigms. In L. M. Barker, M. R. Best, & M. Domjan (Eds.), *Learning mechanisms in food selection.* (pp. 3–22), Waco, Texas: Baylor University Press.

Goodall, J. (1986). *The chimpanzees of Gombe: Patterns of behavior.* Cambridge MA: Belknap Press.

Green, G. C., Elwin, R. L., Mottershead, B. E., Keogh, R. G., & Lynch, J. J. (1984). Longterm effects of early experience to supplementary feeding in sheep. *Proceedings of the Australian Society of Animal Production, 15,* 373–375.

Grover, C. A., Kixmiller, J. S., Erickson, C. A., Becker, A. H., & Davis, S. F. (1988). The social transmission of information concerning aversively conditioned liquids. *Psychological Record, 38,* 557–566.

Hall, K. R. L. (1962). Numerical data, maintenance activities and locomotion of the wild chacma baboon, *Papio ursinus. Proceedings of the Zoological Society of London, 139,* 181–220.

Hall, K. R. L. (1963a). Observational learning in monkeys and apes. *British Journal of Psychology, 54,* 201–226.

Hall, K. R. L. (1963b). Social learning in monkeys. In P. Dolhinow (Ed.), *Primate patterns* (pp. 261–275). New York: Holt, Rinehart & Winston.

Harris, L. J., Clay J., Hargreaves, F., & Ward, A. (1933). Appetite and choice of diet: The ability of the vitamin B deficient rat to discriminate between diets containing and lacking the vitamin. *Proceedings of the Royal Society of London, Series B, 113,* 161–190.

Hauser, M. D. (1988). Invention and social transmission a case study with wild vervet monkeys. In R. W. Byrne & A. Whiten (Eds.), *Machiavellian intelligence: Social expertise and the evolution of intellect in monkeys, apes and humans.* (pp. 327–344). Oxford: Oxford University Press.

Hepper, P. G. (1988). Adaptive fetal learning: Prenatal exposure to garlic affects postnatal preference. *Animal Behaviour, 36,* 935–936.

Heyes, C. M., & Durlach, P. J. (1990). Social blockade of taste-aversion learning in Norway rats (*Rattus norvegicus*): Is it a social phenomenon. *Journal of Comparative Psychology, 104,* 82–87.

Houston, D. C. (1979). The adaptations of scavengers. In A. R. E. Sinclair & M. Norton-Griffiths (Eds.), *Serengeti: Dynamics of an ecosystem* (pp. 263–286). Chicago: University of Chicago Press.

Johnson, R. N., DeSisto, M. J., & Koenig, A. B. (1972). Social and developmental experience and interspecific aggression in rats. *Journal of Comparative and Physiological Psychology, 79,* 237–242.

Jordan, W. H. (1906). *The feeding of animals.* New York: Macmillan.

Jouventin, P., Pasteur, G., & Cambefort, J. P. (1977). Observational learning of baboons and avoidance of mimics: Exploratory tests. *Evolution, 31,* 214–219.

Kawai, M. (1965). Newly acquired pre-cultural behavior of the natural troop of monkeys on Koshima islet. *Primates, 6,* 1–30.

Kline, L. W. (1898). Methods in animal psychology. *American Journal of Psychology, 10,* 256–279.

Krebs, J. R. (1973). Social learning and the significance of mixed species flocks of chickadees (*Parus* spp.). *Canadian Journal of Zoology, 51,* 1275–1288.

Krebs, J. R., MacRoberts, M. H., & Cullen, J. M. (1972). Flocking and feeding in the great tit *Parus major:* An experimental study. *Ibis, 114,* 507–530.

Kuo, Z. Y. (1930). The genesis of the cat's response to the rat. *Journal of Comparative Psychology, 11,* 1–35.

Laland, K. R., & Plotkin, H. C. (1990). Social learning and social transmission of digging for buried food in Norway rats. *Animal Learning & Behavior, 18,* 246–251.

Laland, K. N., & Plotkin, H. C. (1993). Social transmission of food preferences among Norway rats by marking of food sites and by gustatory contact. *Animal Learning & Behavior, 21,* 35–41.

Leyhausen, P. (1956). Verhaltensstudien an Katzen. *Zeitschrift fur Tierpsychologie Bieheft 2,* 1–120.

Liers, E. E. (1951). Notes on the River Otter (*Lutra canadensis*). *Journal of Mammalogy, 32,* 1–9.

Lynch, J. J., Keogh, R. G., Elwin, R. L., Green, G. C., & Mottershead, B. E. (1983). Effects of early experience on the post-weaning acceptance of whole grain wheat by fine-wool merino lambs. *Animal Production, 36,* 175–183.

Martin, L. T., & Alberts, J. R. (1979). Taste aversions to mother's milk: The age-related role of nursing in acquisition and expression of a learned association. *Journal of Comparative and Physiological Psychology, 93,* 430–445.

Mason, J. R., Arzt, A. H., & Reidinger, R. F. (1984). Comparative assessment of food preferences and aversions acquired by blackbirds via observational learning. *Auk, 101,* 796–803.

McFadyen-Ketchum, S. A., & Porter, R. H. (1989). *Behavioral Ecology and Sociobiology, 24,* 59–62.

McGrew, W. C. (1992). *Chimpanzee material culture.* Cambridge, MA: Cambridge University press.

McQuoid, L. M., & Galef, B. G., Jr. (1992). Social influences on feeding site selection by Burmese fowl. *Journal of Comparative Psychology, 106,* 137–141.

McQuoid, L. M., & Galef, B. G., Jr. (1993). Social stimuli influencing feeding behaviour of Burmese fowl: A video analysis. *Animal Behaviour, 46,* 13–22.

Pion, L. V. (1969). Early experience, social contact and the incidence of mouse killing behavior in Norway rats. *American Zoologist, 9,* 10.

Pliner, P. & Pelchat, M. L. (1986). Similarities in food preferences between children and their siblings and parents. *Appetite, 7,* 333–342.

Posadas-Andrews, A., & Roper, T. J. (1983). Social transmission of food preferences in adult rats. *Animal Behaviour, 31,* 265–271.

Ransom, T. W., & Rowell, T. E. (1972). Early social development of feral baboons. In F. E. Poirier (Ed.), *Primate socialization.* (pp. 104–144). New York: Random House.

Richard, M. M., Grover, C. A., & Davis, S. F. (1987). Galef's transfer-of-information effect occurs in a free-foraging situation. *Psychological Record, 37,* 79–87.

Richter, C. P. (1942–43) Total self-regulatory functions in animals and human beings. *Harvey Lecture Series, 38,* 63–103.

Roper, T. J. (1986). Cultural evolution of feeding behaviour in animals. *Science Progress, 70,* 571–583.

Rozin, P. (1967). Thiamine specific hunger. In C. F. Code (Ed.), *Handbook of physiology, Vol. 1. Alimentary canal* (pp. 411–431). Washington, D.C.: American Physiological Society.

Rozin, P. (1988a). Cultural approaches to human food preference. In J. Morley, M. B. Sterman, & M. B. Walsh (Eds.), *Nutritional modulation of neural function* (pp. 137–153). New York: Academic Press.

Rozin, P. (1988b). Social learning about foods by humans. In T. Zentall & B. G. Galef, Jr. (Eds.), *Social learning: Psychological and biological perspectives* (pp. 165–188). Hillsdale: Lawrence Erlbaum.

Rozin, P., & Kalat, J. (1971). Specific hungers and poison avoidance as adaptive specializations of learning. *Psychological Review, 78,* 459–486.

Rozin, P., Fallon, A. & Mandell, R. (1984). Family resemblance in attitudes to foods. *Developmental Psychology, 20,* 309–314.

Schaller, G. B. (1967). *The deer and the tiger.* Chicago: University of Chicago Press.

Schaller, G. B. (1972). *The Serengeti lion.* Chicago, University of Chicago Press.

Schlupp, I., Marler, C. & Ryan, M. J. (1994). Benefit to male sailfin mollies of mating with heterospecific females. *Science, 263,* 373–374.

Sherry, D. F., & Galef, B. G., Jr. (1984). Cultural transmission without imitation: Milk bottle opening by birds. *Animal Behaviour, 32,* 937–938.

Sherry, D. F., & Galef, B. G., Jr. (1990). Social learning without imitation: More about milk bottle opening by birds. *Animal Behaviour, 40,* 987–989.

Silk, J. P. (1978). Patterns of food sharing among mother and infant chimpanzees at Gombe National Park, Tanzania. *Folia Primatoligica, 29,* 129–141.

Smythe, N. (1970). *Ecology and related behavior of the agouti (Dasyprocta punctata) and related species on Barro Colorado Island, Panama.* Doctoral thesis, University of Maryland, College Park, Maryland.

Spence, K. W. (1937). Experimental studies of learning and higher mental processes in intra human primates. *Psychological Bulletin, 34,* 806–850.

Stokes, A. W. (1971). Parental and courtship feeding in red jungle fowl. *Auk, 88,* 21–29.

Strupp, B. & Levitsky, D. A. (1984). Social transmission of food preferences in adult hooded rats (Rattus norvegicus). *Journal of Comparative Psychology, 98,* 257–266.

Suboski, M. (1989). The acquisition of stimulus control over released pecking by hatchling chicks. *Canadian Journal of Psychology, 43,* 431–443.

Suboski, M. D. & Bartashunas, C. (1984). Mechanisms for social transmission of pecking preferences to neonatal chicks. *Journal of Experimental Psychology: Animal Behavior Processes, 10,* 182–194.

Sugiyama, Y. (1994). Tool use by wild chimpanzees, *Nature, 367,* 327.

Sussman, R. W. (1977). Socialization, social structure, and ecology of two sympatric species of Lemur. In S. Chevalier-Skolnikoff and F. E. Poirier (Eds.), *Primate biosocial development* (pp. 515–528). New York: Garland Press

Thorhallsdottir, A. G., Provenza, F. D., & Balph, D. F. (1990). Ability of lambs to learn about novel foods while observing or participating with social models. *Applied Animal Behaviour Science, 25,* 25–33.

Thorpe, W. H. (1963). *Learning and instinct in animals.* London: Methuen.

Turner, E. R. A. (1964). Social feeding in birds. *Behaviour, 24,* 1–46.

Valsecchi, P., & Galef, B. G., Jr. (1989). Social influences on the food preferences of house mice (*Mus Musculus*): A comparative analysis of behavioural processes. *International Journal of Comparative Psychology, 2,* 245–256.

Valsecchi, P., Mainardi, M., Sgoifo, A., & Taticchi, A. (1989). Maternal influences on food preferences in weanling mice (*Mus domesticus*). *Behavioural Processes, 19,* 155–166.

Warner, R. R. (1988). Traditionality of mating-site preferences in a coral reef fish. *Nature, 335,* 719–721.

Warner, R. R. (1990a). Male versus female influences on mating-site determination in a coral reef fish. *Animal Behaviour, 39,* 540–548.

Warner, R. R. (1990b). Resource assessment versus tradition in mating-site determination. *American Naturalist, 135,* 205–217.

Weigl, P. D., & Hanson, E. V. (1980). Observational learning and the feeding behavior of the red squirrel *Tamiasciurus hudsonicus:* The ontogeny of optimization. *Ecology, 61,* 213–218.

Whitehead, J. M. (1986). Development of feeding selectivity in mantled howling monkeys, (*Alouatta palliata*). In J. G. Else & P. C. Lee (Eds.), *Primate ontogeny, cognition and social behaviour* (pp. 105–117). Cambridge, England: Cambridge University Press.

Wyrwicka, W. (1981). *The development of food preferences.* Springfield, IL: Charles C Thomas.

Wyrwicka, W. (1978). Imitation of mother's inappropriate food preference in weanling kittens. *Pavlovian Journal Of Biological Science, 13,* 55–72.

Yoerg, S. I. (1991). Social feeding reverses learned flavor aversions in spotted hyenas (*Crocuta crocuta*). *Journal of Comparative Psychology, 105,* 185–189.

Zohar, O., & Terkel, J. (1992). Acquisition of pine cone stripping behaviour in black rats (*Rattus rattus*). *International Journal of Comparative Psychology, 5,* 1–6.

Sociocultural Influences on Human Food Selection

Paul Rozin

At first glance, eating may appear to be a nonsocial activity. This is so for some solitary animal species, such as clams, koalas, and tigers, but for most species, and especially for humans, almost all instances of eating can be fully understood only in a social context. The diverse and unelaborated food habits of feral humans speak to the looseness of genetic determination of food selection and hence the power of cultural forces (Zingg, 1940).

Almost all of the literature in psychology and physiology that relates to eating in animals or humans is concerned with *how much* is eaten (the regulation of food intake) rather than *what* is eaten. Introductory psychology textbooks typically devote a section to hunger (regulation of food intake) and usually do not even mention the determinants of food selection. Sociocultural factors surely play a role in determining how much is eaten. For example, Americans tend to eat more when in the company of others (deCastro, 1990). Culturally acquired standards for a desirable body image operate as a substantial part of the control of how much is eaten, especially in American women. Cultural forces are the principal determinants of the

This paper is an updated, modified version of a paper entitled "The importance of social factors in understanding the acquisition of food habits" in *Taste, Experience and Feeding*, edited by E. D. Capaldi and T. L. Powley, American Psychological Association, Washington, DC, 1990. Adapted with permission of the publisher.

This chapter was prepared with the assistance of funding from the John D. and Catherine T. MacArthur Foundation Network for the Study of Health-Related Behaviors and from the Whitehall Foundation.

serving of meals at an appropriate time of day, and this occurrence, by itself, can induce people to begin eating. A major reason for meal termination is that one knows one has already eaten an amount that constitutes an appropriate meal as defined by the culture, for example, soup, a sandwich, and a beverage for lunch. My colleagues and I recently showed that amnesic patients who had no recall of what happened more then a few minutes before consumed a second full lunch and began a third, when each was served a few minutes after the prior meal was cleared away (P. Rozin, Dow, Moscovitch, & Rajaram, 1996). The lack of memory for having just eaten a culturally appropriate, full meal, along with the presence of food, is sufficient to maintain eating.

Sociocultural factors are even more important in food selection than in intake control. Cultural differences in food preferences and choices are enormous. Consider an apparently solitary act of food choice to illustrate the layers of social context that are involved: Sylvia, an 18-year-old American woman, has a desire for something good to eat and goes into a convenience store. She is faced with, among hundreds of other things, a choice between a chocolate bar and a package of sugar-free chewing gum. The convenience store is itself a product of culture, and of course it is operated by people other than Sylvia. How did the chocolate get to be a choice for Sylvia, as it glistens temptingly on the shelf? It originated in a tropical cacao plantation and was grown, extracted, and processed by a wide variety of people, including farmers, transporters, and workers at the manufacturing plant.

But that is only part of the story. Chocolate comes from Mexico and was unknown in Europe until after the colonization of the Americas. It was brought back to Spain, and eventually, with the availability of cheap sugar, chocolate became one of the most highly desired foods in Europe. Chocolate returns to the United States as an import from Europe, not from Mexico. All of these pathways are inherently social; that is, they involve other human beings and the cultural institutions created by those human beings. The same is true for chewing gum and the development of artificial sweeteners. Sylvia does not know all of this and does not think about it much, but a rich and complex set of social forces has made it possible for her to have the chocolate–gum choice at this place and time.

What Sylvia is keenly aware of is that she would love to eat the luscious chocolate, but she thinks of the chocolate as sinful and fattening and is worried about her figure. Her attitude toward her figure is a consequence of her enculturation; it is characteristic of women in her culture. Her knowledge of chocolate as a high-calorie food is also something that she has learned from others, either directly or through the media. She also knows, from the experience of others, that sugar-free gum has virtually no calories, and after checking that the gum in question does not contain saccharin, which she has heard can cause cancer, she takes out her dollar and buys it. The purchase itself, the money, and the interaction with the salesperson are also, of course, deeply social.

It is seen from this example that social factors enter into an act of eating or food choice in many ways, at many levels. Of course, if Sylvia had a friend with her at the time, more overt social events would have occurred, including perhaps urgings for restraint from her thinner friend and Sylvia's discomfort about choosing chocolate in front of her friend.

Suppose one wishes to know as much as possible about the foods another person likes and eats and can ask that person only one question. What should that question be? There is no doubt about it, the question should be, What is your culture or ethnic group? There is no other single question that would even approach the informativeness of the answer to this question.

For humans, the search and preparation of food and its ingestion at meals are social occasions, and food is a very social entity. Ingestion of food means taking something of the world into the body, and that something typically has a social history: It was procured, prepared, and presented by other humans. Food is a form of social exchange and is imbued with meanings in many cultures. The earliest significant events in the lives of mammals include food at their center: the processes of nursing and, later, weaning. From the very first, the taking of food is exquisitely social.

For more detailed information about human food selection, see books by Logue (1991), Booth (1994), and Fischler (1990) and the volumes edited by Barker (1982) and Shepherd (1989). See also the work of P. Rozin (1982), P. Rozin (1988, 1990a, 1990d), and Zellner (1991).

Galef (1976, 1985), Birch (1986, 1987), and P. Rozin (1988, 1990c, 1994) have catalogued and discussed the various ways in which social factors influence eating and food choice. A major source of social influence is *indirect;* that is, indirect social influences set the stage for or modulate the interpretation of food encounters. The presence of a conspecific is not necessary for this route of influence. Indirect social factors include beliefs, culinary traditions, and occasions that are established as part of the acquisition of culture.

Other social influences are *direct;* that is, they require the mediation of another organism who is present on the occasion. In *inadvertent social agency,* the direct social presence is necessary, but it is not specifically oriented to producing an effect. In *active social agency,* the social agent participates in the learning task as an active teacher. Both indirect and direct social influences are discussed in this chapter.

INDIRECT SOCIAL INFLUENCES

Culture, Biology, and Cuisine

A major part of the cultural influence on food selection can be summarized with reference to the term *cuisine.* There are two aspects of cuisine. In the narrower sense, it refers to specific dishes and how they are prepared. According to the taxonomy that has been developed by Elisabeth Rozin (1982, 1983), cuisines are defined by the basic ingredients they employ (e.g., rice, potatoes, fish), the characteristic flavors (flavor principles) employed (e.g., a combination of chili pepper with either tomato or lime for Mexico; a varied mixture of spices called "curry" for India), and particular modes of food preparation (e.g., stir-frying for China). These three components describe, with considerable success, the properties of the main-course foods in most of the world's cuisines. In addition, there are culinary rules about the ordering of dishes within a meal, what can be served with what, and what is to be served at particular times or occasions. All of these important features of food are, to some extent, culture-specific.

Over and above the aspect of cuisine that concerns specific dishes, there are many culture-based attitudes toward foods and toward the role of foods in daily life. Cultures and individuals vary in the importance they attribute to food in their lives, the ritual and moral significance of food, and the role of food as a social vehicle. In varying degrees depending on the culture, food serves to establish social linkages through sharing or to maintain social distance through food taboos.

Cuisines and food attitudes, although features of cultures, have their own evolutionary histories, and they may ultimately be accounted for in terms of the characteristics of the individual humans who cumulatively gave rise to cultures. This framework allows for the possibility of the explanation of sociocultural rules about food in terms of biological features of the human omnivore. Such an enterprise has been promoted, in different ways, by scholars such as Marvin Harris (1985), Solomon Katz (1982), and Frederick Simoons (1961, 1982). Any discussion of social influences on food selection should consider the origin of these influences.

There are two pathways through which biological aspects of humans influence cuisine. The *behavioral path* originates with biologically determined aspects of human food-selection behaviors that guide the evolution of cuisine. The *metabolic path* originates in biologically determined features of metabolism and nutritional needs. These establish constraints on food choice and guide behavior (and hence cuisine) indirectly, by strengthening those behaviors or traditions that ensure health and minimize illness and weakening those that do not.

Pathway From Genetically Determined Behaviors to Cuisine

The behavioral path is bound to be minimal, as a consequence of humans' omnivorous nature. Omnivores, (more broadly, food generalists) are biologically open to a wide variety of potential foods; hence, their genes do not provide a lot of guidance. Rather, experience, either direct or socially transmitted, determines food choice (see P. Rozin, 1976; P. Rozin & Schulkin, 1990, for more elaborate discussions). However, there are some genetically determined predispositions. Omnivore–generalists, such as rats and humans, have a suspicion of new foods (neophobia) and, at the same time, an attraction to them (neophilia;) (P. Rozin, 1976). This is presumably because new foods are potentially toxic but also potential sources of nourishment. Omnivores have a general ability to learn about the consequences of eating particular foods, mediated by a special learning ability. This ability facilitates learning about the relation between a food ingested at one time and metabolic effects that occur as long as hours later. Perhaps most critically for the understanding of cuisine, humans (and rats) have built-in taste biases, which serve as adaptive, general rules of thumb in dealing with the food world. There is an innate attraction to sweet tastes (associated in the natural environment primarily with fruits) and an avoidance of bitter tastes (associated in the natural environment with the presence of toxins). Although it is less well documented, there is probably also an innate preference for fatty textures (associated with fat, protein, and in particular, meat) and an innate avoidance of irritating sensations (such as generated by hot peppers or tobacco).

A few general features of cuisines can be derived from these genetic biases. The widespread use and popularity of sweeteners, including the massive development of a sugar-growing and processing industry in Western cultures, can be traced to the biological desire for sweets (P. Rozin, 1982). Harris (1985) argued for the existence of a strong motivation in humans to seek and develop sources of protein and fat. This may be mediated by a biological desire for the fatty texture. E. Rozin and P. Rozin (1981) suggested that the consistent flavoring traditions, or flavor principles, of individual cuisines may be a way of dealing with the conflict between neophobia (flavor all foods in a similar way, to make them familiar) and neophilia (allow acceptance of a new food by using the familiar flavorings on it). However, because the generalist has few genetically based behavioral biases, there are severe limitations on the explanatory power of this approach.

Metabolic–Nutritional Pathway to Cuisine

The potential for explaining culinary practices in terms of adaptive combinations of foods or food-processing technologies is much greater than that of genetically determined behavior; adaptive nutritional explanations account for the bulk of the literature in this area. The major contributors to this view (e.g., Harris, Katz, and Simoons) are less concerned with how humans discovered particular foods or combinations than they are with demonstrating that cuisines represent adaptive choices. The basic approach assumes that if there are substantial nutritional advantages to particular types of food processing, selection, or combinations, people will discover them. For a psychology of eating, however, it is of particular interest to develop scenarios that can reasonably account for the discovery of adaptive food relations. Following are three examples of adaptive human practices; for two of the three, a reasonable discovery scenario can be constructed (see P. Rozin, 1982, for further details).

Milk Drinking and Lactose Intolerance

Simoons (1970, 1982) demonstrated that the great majority of humans are lactose-intolerant after infancy; that is, they cannot digest milk sugar, or lactose, which is a major constituent of milk. The enzyme lactase, which all human infants necessarily have for digestion of mother's milk, is deprogrammed in the period around and after weaning. Simoons has shown that a small segment of humanity, primarily people of northern European origin, have genes that block the deprogramming of lactase production.

For most people in the world, including almost all natives of Asia, Africa, and the Americas, consumption of moderate amounts of raw milk leads to fermentation in the hindgut, caused by bacteria that break down the lactose. This leads to gas, cramps, and diarrhea. Not only is the carbohydrate component of milk not usable, but there is attendant discomfort, and the diarrhea reduces the ability of the system to absorb other components of milk and other foods. Although some of the lactose-intolerant cultures, particularly China, have rejected all dairy products, most have "discovered" a way to digest lactose externally and thus render dairy products edible in susbtantial amounts. If milk is simply left around for a few days, at normal temperatures, bacterial action cleaves the lactose into its two digestible components, glucose and galactose. Hence, by a process appropriately called *culturing*, fermented products such as cheese and yogurt are created. Yogurt is an important staple for the second largest country in the world, India. It is easy to imagine how people would have discovered (a) that modest amounts of raw milk cause adults gastrointestinal distress and (b) that spoiled milk, a product that is extremely easy to come by in the absence of refrigeration, does not produce such distress. The rest is history.

Manioc Detoxification

Manioc is a basic staple food in parts of Brazil and was discovered and imported to Europe and Africa by the early explorers (reviewed in Jones, 1959; P. Rozin, 1982). Manioc grows well in the tropics, is resistant to predation, and is easy to maintain. The problem is that the principal form, sometimes referred to as *bitter manioc*, contains toxic levels of cyanide. The traditional, pre-Columbian Brazilian processing of manioc eliminates the water-soluble cyanide by grinding the manioc and rinsing it many times with water. It is known that unrinsed manioc powder was used by Brazilians to poison fish as a means of capturing them in fresh water; it was clearly evident that consumption of manioc produced rapid and severe illness or death. The effects of rinsing in water, a common culinary technique, would have been easily discovered. The beneficial effect of this practice, like that of removing lactose from milk, would have been readily apparent, within minutes, to those who tried it. The path to discovery is clear. Manioc became an important staple in parts of Africa; the detoxification technique was exported with the manioc from Brazil.

Corn and the Tortilla Technology

The third and more problematic example has to do with corn and the tortilla technology. Corn is native to the Americas and was exported to Europe and the rest of the world in the post-Columbian period, along with manioc, chocolate, peanuts, potatoes, chili peppers, and other important foods. Corn is a staple product in many traditional American cultures and constitutes a major part of the caloric intake. This presents a problem because corn is not an adequate, complete nutrient; it is low in niacin (one of the B vitamins), has an inadequate pattern of essential amino acids, and is low in calcium. Analyses by Katz and his colleagues (Katz, 1982; Katz, Hediger & Valleroy, 1974) demonstrated that the complex tortilla technology, including the soaking of corn kernels in an alkaline medium has the effect of (a) increasing the level of niacin (by freeing bound niacin), (b) markedly improving the amino acid pattern, and (c) adding calcium.

The technology consists of soaking the corn in a solution with the mineral lime, which contains high levels of calcium hydroxide. The corn is then ground and fashioned into flat cakes that are grilled. The tortilla is usually consumed with beans and chili pepper. Both corn and beans have inadequate amounts of particular essential amino acids, but the amino acids in short supply are complementary. Together, corn and beans make an adequate protein source.

Neither the corn–bean combination nor the tortilla technology were imported to Europe with the corn. The cooking technique probably was not imported for the simple reason that the Spanish exploratory parties (Cortez's group and others) did not include European women, and none of the men had learned the cooking technique (P. Rozin, 1982). This may be part of the explanation for the fact that, unlike potatoes and bell peppers, corn never became a major staple food in most of Europe. Additionally, it is unlikely that the Europeans would have rediscovered the tortilla technology; it includes a number of steps, quite a bit of processing, and the unlikely addition of lime (actually, ash or powdered shells).

It is hard to imagine how the early Americans discovered the tortilla technology; the improved nutritional properties of the resulting corn are subtle and would not show up in a matter of hours. Indeed, it may be that the evolution of the technique had a culinary motivation: making the corn tastier and easier to roll out. I surveyed some residents in a traditional Mexican village and asked them why they added "cal" (lime) to the tortillas. Men had no idea (not knowing how to make tortillas), and women reliably responded that it made the tortilla easier to roll out. Some brief experiments with these women confirmed this; the soaking in lime softens the corn husk and makes it easier to pulverize it when rolling out the tortillas (P. Rozin, 1982).

Learning About Relatively Subtle Nutritional Effects

The problem that the corn tortilla raises is to understand the process through which humans learn elaborate culinary techniques that have subtle nutritional consequences. There are many important examples of this, including the elaborate and complex preparation of soy sauce. One question is whether their origin is directly guided by the nutritional advantages or is indirectly guided, as the case of the tortilla suggests. A second question is whether most culinary practices can be explained in terms of nutritional value, because food serves also as a major source of pleasure, a major social vehicle, and a moral instrument in many cultures. For example, Harris (1985) explained the prohibition on eating beef in Hindu India in nutritional–adaptive terms; The cow is more useful as a dairy source than as a meat source. However, an alternative view traces beef avoidance to deep Hindu commitments to the sacredness of animal life, specifically, the principle of *ahimsa* (the principle of causing no harm to living things), which may be linked to the belief in reincarnation (Simoons, 1961). Although Harris is inclined to see culinary practices as shaped primarily by optimization of diet, Simoons is more inclined to account for culinary practices in terms of social forces, such as the prohibition against eating the foods of despised neighboring groups.

There are many culinary practices that seem to defy explanation in biological–adaptive terms (although Harris has suggested adaptive accounts). These include elaborate traditions such as the dietary rules for keeping kosher, the widespread use of spices and innately unpalatable foods such as coffee and chili pepper, and the revulsion shown in almost all cultures to most forms of animal food. These customs seem driven by issues of pleasure maximization, social meanings, and moral principles rather than adaptation.

Finally, in focusing on routes through which human omnivore biology or metabolic needs might shape food-related cultural institutions, one should not ignore the inverse process. Culture can affect biology and, in particular, genes. The other side of the lactose-intolerance story (Simoons, 1970, 1982; P. Rozin, 1982) is that the domestication of animals made milk available for the first time as a food for noninfant humans. The usefulness of raw milk was limited by lactose intolerance. This presumably set up a selection pressure, in cultures (principally northern European) where milk was abundantly available, for the ability to digest milk. Genes that blocked the deprogramming of lactose at about the time of weaning were selected for, with the result that some populations became lactose-tolerant. For that very special human food, milk, therefore, there have been two pathways to acceptance: culturing, involving changing the product before it enters the human body, and selection of genes that make the body able to handle raw milk.

Beliefs and Attitudes

A small percentage of human beliefs and attitudes about food result directly from our interaction with specific foods. Most beliefs and attitudes (e.g., beliefs that fat foods are unhealthy and natural foods are healthy and attitudes favoring shellfish and shunning worms as food) derive from socially transmitted information. Most critically, the meaning of food (source of nutrition, source of pleasure, social–moral statement) is laid down by culture. The great concern that Western women have about eating too much and their preoccupation with dieting surely relate to the cultural ideal body image. There is a striking correspondence between the occurrence of anorexia and bulimia and the presence of a thin female ideal (McCarthy, 1990).

Availability, Price, and the Setting of Occasions

Exposure is a recurrent and necessary, if not sufficient, cause for food preferences (Pliner, 1982; Zajonc, 1968). Exposure itself is largely a product of culture. One is exposed to that subset of all possible foods that one's ecology and culture supports. The lack of exposure of White rural Midwestern Americans to bean curd or pork kidneys is accounted for by the fact that local mores regard such things as "not food," not because the sources are ecologically unavailable. Cost is another major determinant of degree of exposure.

Cultural valuation of a food may increase its price in the short term, but in the long term, it leads to improved methods of harvesting and processing such that the food becomes more available. Many foods have moved from luxury to commonplace at the table, two of the most striking examples being coffee and sugar. Technological advances, motivated by high demand, led to enormous increases in availability (with concurrent price drop) for sugar and to its availability for mixture with a wide variety of foods for almost all people (Mintz, 1985). This availability led to its widespread use as a sweetener for items like coffee and chocolate that were too bitter for wide acceptance without such treatment.

The context within which a food is presented also affects the attitudes to it. Lolli, Serianni, Golder, and Luzz atto-Fegiz (1958) called attention to the fact that although alcohol consumption is quite high in Italy, there is relatively little alcohol abuse. They traced this to deeply rooted Italian attitudes to alcohol, which is considered a food and served as part of meals. It is introduced to children early, in the context of a meal and a family event. This role for alcohol (wine in this case) places it in a situation in which its absorption is slower: it becomes a part of normal life rather than a focus for rebellion from family values.

The acceptability of any food is determined, in large part, by context (P. Rozin & Tuorila, 1993). Most Americans readily accept foods such as bacon and eggs or hot cereal as breakfast foods, but consider them relatively undesirable in other meal contexts. Most Americans like both chocolate and French fried potatoes, but not the combination of the two. Within any cuisine, there are many "rules" about what goes with what and about the order of eating foods within a meal. Most laboratory research on food selection in humans conducted before 1990 employed pure nutrients outside their normal context. Participants were offered different concentrations of sugar water or salt water. Unfortunately, responses to these unusual, decontextualized nutrients are not highly predictive of responses to the same nutrients in normal food contexts, such as in the form of lemonade, for sugar, or potato chips, for salt (see Pangborn, 1980, for a description of the line of research that brought context to center stage in the study of food acceptance).

Universal Cultural Themes Linking Food and Social Life

Food is a social instrument for humans by virtue of the fact that more than one person is almost always involved with any food, from harvesting to ingestion. This social "passage" takes on added significance because of the existence of three, probably universal, patterns of thought.

The Mouth as Gateway to the Body

The first principle concerns the special position of the mouth as the dominant entry point to the body. People are sensitive to the status of their body and cannot help but be concerned about what goes into it. Beause the mouth is the gateway, there is great concern and strong feeling about what goes into the mouth (P. Rozin & Fallon, 1987; P. Rozin, Nemeroff, Horowitz, Gordon, & Voet, 1995).

"You Are What You Eat"

Concern about what goes into the body becomes engaged in a more social sense when coupled with the second principle, "you are what you eat." The view that persons take on the physical, behavioral, and intentional properties of the food they eat is widespread in traditional cultures (e.g., Frazer, 1890/1959; reviewed in Nemeroff & Rozin, 1989). The idea seems entirely reasonable, in the absence of knowledge of the theory of digestion and the common small set of molecules that result after digestion of all foods. In general experience, when two things combine, the product takes on the properties of both.

In a more subtle and unacknowledged form, "you are what you eat" seems to be held as a belief by educated Westerners. American undergraduates who read a cultural vignette about a group that consumes boar rated members of this culture as more boarlike and less turtlelike than did other students who read an equivalent vignette in which turtle was mentioned as part of the diet in place of boar (Nemeroff & Rozin, 1989). "You are what you eat" accounts, in part, for resistance to ingesting things that are offensive or that have other undesirable characteristics. With the exception of cannibals, however, the principle does not directly link humans to other humans through food.

Contagion

The linkage among humans through food is provided by a third, more general principle, the "sympathetic magical law of contagion." This idea was explicated at the turn of the century by the anthropologists Frazer (1890/1959) and Mauss (1902/1972) (see P. Rozin & Nemeroff, 1990, for a detailed exposition of this law). The law of contagion holds that "once in contact, always in contact"; that is, when two objects come into contact, properties are permanently exchanged. Although it was originally expounded as a characteristic of "primitive" thinking, contagion operates clearly among Western, educated adults (reviewed in P. Rozin & Nemeroff, 1990). For example, almost all people surveyed rejected wearing a sweater that had been worn by a disliked or unsavory person and rejected eating an apple bitten by one of these persons. On the positive side, a minority of people said clothing or food was enhanced if it had been worn or tasted, respectively, by a loved or admired person.

The critical importance of contagion is that it links the human preparers or handlers of food to the eaters (P. Rozin, 1990d). According to this principle, "you are what you eat" holds not only for the food eaten, but also for the previous contacts of that food. Food becomes a loaded interpersonal message: Grandma's soup can be better because it was made by Grandma, and an enemy or a disliked person can convey bad fortune by contacting one's food. The importance of these ideas in the food domain is illustrated by food attitudes in two non-Western cultures, the Hua of Papua New Guinea and the Hindu Indians (see P. Rozin, 1990d, for a more detailed exposition of these two cultural examples).

Among the Hua of Papua New Guinea (Meigs, 1984), food is the bearer of vital essence, or "nu," which is both a life force and a carrier of individual properties. It is good to eat food procured or prepared by those in a positive relation to ego; it both improves character and personality and increases good fortune. For example, it is desirable to consume food that an appropriate relative has spat on. On the other hand, food from someone in a competitive or other undesirable relation can cause harm. The Hua had been cannibalistic within the memory of the older current villagers, at the time of Meigs's report, and had consumed their parents, after death; they would never consume killed warriors from another group because of the hostile intent that would be conveyed. From before puberty to a few years postpuberty, Hua males are segregated and not allowed any contact with fertile females, for fear that the nu of these fertile females will feminize the young males. They are not allowed to consume any food procured or prepared by a fertile female. Meigs stated that food and food transactions form the center of Hua conversation; indeed it was this fact that steered her ethnographic study in the direction of food.

Among Hindu Indians, a food's personal history carries social status and moral significance (Appadurai, 1981). Sharing food, or eating food made by a common third person, has a binding or homogenizing significance. Refusal to share establishes distance, or "heterogenizes." Marriott (1968) showed that the complex Hindu caste structure can be reconstructed simply from information on who can eat whose foods. Even within the family, the order of serving and rules about who can eat whose leftovers serve to maintain the family hierarchy and reaffirm proper social relations among family members. The body is viewed as the temple for the soul, and eating is seen as a moral transaction in which food can serve as a fundamental link between humans and the gods. For example, Brahmin children rate the statement "one of your family members eats beef regularly" as reflective of a more serious moral offense than the statement "there was a rule in a hotel; invalids and disfigured persons are not allowed in the dining hall" (Shweder, Mahapatra, & Miller, 1987).

In both India and New Guinea, contagion and "you are what you eat" play important roles in establishing food–person linkages. Although these feelings also exist in the United States, they are muted. To a large extent, we Americans have decontextualized food. Americans buy food in plastic wrapped parcels, often frozen, with no record of or information about the other people who have been involved in the harvesting and preparation of the food. Because food has been made impersonal, it has lost much of its moral–social significance. Even in the United States, food has some social significance, however. It is the center of social occasions, such as evening dinner and holiday feasts. Dinner is the center of social life for many families. Among Americans, the principle of contagion is seen primarily in the emotion of disgust in response to animal products (e.g., insects, reptiles, and for many Americans viscera and raw meat), whereas in India and New Guinea, the emotion of disgust is evoked primarily by human interactions (P. Rozin, Haidt, & McCauley, 1993).

Disgust and Social Ideation: The Human–Animal Distinction

Fallon and I have identified the emotion of disgust as oriented to food rejection, at its core. The derivation of the word means "bad taste"; facial expressions of disgust center around the nose and mouth; and nausea, a gastrointestinal sensation, is its most characteristic physiological feature (P. Rozin & Fallon, 1987). Contagion is a critical feature of disgust; when a disgusting entity (e.g., a cockroach in the United States) touches an otherwise acceptable food, it renders that food inedible. The expression of disgust does not depend on the presence of another person, but the entire emotion, and particularly the stimuli that elicit it, are culturally conditioned. Feces may be the only universal object of disgust, and even this strong aversion does not appear until after 1.5–2 years of age (P. Rozin, Hammer, Oster, Horowitz, & Marmara, 1986).

The stimuli that elcit disgust cross-culturally are almost all animal products (Angyal, 1941; P. Rozin & Fallon, 1987). There is a common cultural "theme" that "humans are not animals" and are to be clearly distinguished from animals. This theme, together with the "you are what you eat" principle, leads to an avoidance of animal foods to prevent becoming animal-like (P. Rozin & Fallon, 1987). Such a sequence of thought is explicit in the account of Hebrew animal prohibitions dating from the Old Testament (Grunfeld, 1982). The interesting question concerns when and how certain animals or their parts become exempt, in specific cultures, from this prohibition. In the case of the Hebrews, one principle that seems to be involved is that animals that are exceptions are not particularly "animal-like" (e.g., slow-moving plant-eating animals versus more "animal-like," fast-moving predators; Grunfeld, 1982). The point is that the powerful response humans have to food, disgust, is conditioned in multiple and complex ways by cultural forces, although disgust may be manifested under solitary conditions.

Food and the Moral Domain: Moral–Physical Confusion

The "moral" status of food and a confounding of physical–health issues and moral thinking even among Westerners is illustrated by a simple example. When one asks Americans why they reject drinking a glass of juice that just had a cockroach dipped into it, they almost invariably refer to the health risk: that cockroaches are dirty and disease vectors. If one repeats this question but stipulates that the cockroach involved is dead and sterilized, the degree of aversion remains very high, and persons ultimately resort to the fact that "it's a cockroach!" That is, it is "cockroachness," not health, that now accounts for their strong aversion. This illustrates, in a sense, a switch from a physical to a moral explanation. Among Hindus, the moral aspect is more salient, so that a health explanation of attitudes to pollution is not felt to be necessary. If one were worried primarily about health issues in consuming foods contacted by lower castes, one would avoid raw as opposed to cooked foods. In fact, one can purchase raw foods from lower-class people, but one cannot eat their cooked (microbially safe) food, because the cooked food has a lot of the lower-caste persona, or essence, in it.

The tendency for Westerners to rely (superficially) on physical explanations and shun moral explanations extends to scholars. A popular explanation for the Hebrew pork taboo had to do with the avoidance of trichinosis, although the danger seems minimal because the trichina is killed by cooking. Similarly, the common justification for modern table manners in Europe (e.g., not eating from a common pot, not spitting at the table) has to do with hygiene. According to the social–historical analysis of Elias (1978), however, the driving force for these changes was social: the desire to be less animal-like and more like the upper classes.

DIRECT SOCIAL INFLUENCES
Inadvertent Social Action
Preference and Liking

Analysis of the acquisition of preferences in humans and animals depends on a fundamental distinction between preference and liking. An animal or a person can prefer A to B on two very different grounds. The preference may be based on expectations about the consequences of ingestion; "this food will make me feel better" or "this food will make me sick." Foods that are preferred or avoided on these grounds are called *beneficial* or *dangerous* foods, respectively (P. Rozin, 1984). Other preferences are based on reactions to the sensory properties of the food. When one says one likes (or dislikes) lima beans, one is referring to the sensory properties, not the postingestive consequences. This distinction is neatly illustrated by the taste aversion phenomenon. When a person gets nauseated after eating a food, the food becomes disliked; that is, it now tastes bad. On the other hand, when lower gut cramps, pains in other organs, respiratory distress, or skin rashes develop after eating a food, it is typically avoided as dangerous, but it does not become disliked (Pelchat & Rozin, 1982). A parallel distinction has been shown with rats, using facial expression as a measure of disliking (as opposed to avoidance because of anticipated consequences) (Pelchat, Grill, Rozin, & Jacobs, 1983).

Animal studies. There is an extensive literature on animal food preferences, dating back to Curt Richter (1943) and P. T. Young (1948); the literature is reviewed in Booth (1982), P. Rozin (1976), and P. Rozin and Schulkin (1990), and it is discussed at length in other chapters in this volume. The most rapid and robust effect is that of conditioned taste aversions, a phenomenon that does not engage social factors at all (see chapter 2, this volume). The acquisition of preferences by rats has been demonstrated many times (see chapter 3, this volume). Sclafani and Nissenbaum (1988) reported striking effects in terms of rapidity and robustness, but there remains no effect as robust and rapid (reliable conversion of a preference to an aversion in one trial) as conditioned taste aversions. This has led to the suggestion (e.g., P. Rozin, 1976, P. Rozin & Kalat, 1971) that there is a bias to learn about negative events, in food and in other domains. Adaptively, the cost of errors in learning to avoid toxins is very high in comparison to errors in identifying a possible new source of nutrients.

Although this generalization still has merit, the introduction of the idea of inadvertent social agency has added a powerful new force for explaining the creation of positive preferences. Galef and colleagues (reviewed in Galef, 1988; Galef & Beck, 1990; see chapter 8, this volume) have produced robust effects in the direction of increasing preference simply by exposing a target rat to a "demonstrator" rat that has already consumed a novel, target food. The positive effects seem to be produced primarily by an olfactory route; carbon disulfide on the breath of the demonstrator functions to enhance the value of food residues or odorants associated with that chemical (Galef, Mason, Preti, & Bean, 1988). These striking effects are observable only on the "positive" side. Galef has sought but not found evidence of aversions induced by social factors. The absence of such effects is puzzling from an adaptive point of view.

Few of the animal studies in the literature have attempted to distinguish between liked and beneficial foods or between dangerous and disliked foods.

Human studies. The modest-sized literature on social factors in human food choice has concentrated on the positive (preference creation) side. These studies are reviewed by Birch (1986, 1987) and P. Rozin (1988). (See also chapter 5, this volume). Briefly, early studies by Duncker (1938) showed that children preferred a food if it was chosen by admired others, and Duncker (1938) and Marinho (1942) showed that children preferred a food that was preferred by a fictional hero.

These suggestions that children's preferences were changeable by the intermediation of admired others were extended and confirmed in a series of studies by Leann Birch and colleagues (reviewed in Birch, 1986, 1987). Preschoolers preferred a food that their peers selected (Birch, 1980a). Approval by a significant adult (nursery school teacher) also caused an enhancement of preference that endured for weeks (Birch, Zimmerman, & Hind, 1980). Birch interpreted these findings as indicating the importance of a positive social–affective context in preference (liking) acquisition. Although most of these studies did not carefully distinguish between liked and beneficial foods, the results suggest that changes in liking have been produced. Although social factors surely play a dominant role in the formation of both adults' and children's food preferences, it is surprising that the experimental literature on this subject consists of the few studies mentioned.

The importance of social factors is also suggested by research on the acquisition of liking for innately unpalatable foods. Humans develop strong likings for such foods, including bitter foods like coffee, burnt food, quinine water, and some vegetables, and irritant foods such as tobacco, alcohol, chili pepper, ginger, and raw garlic or onion. My colleagues and I have studied the acquisition of a liking for chili pepper, as an exemplar of foods in this category (reviewed in P. Rozin, 1990b). It is clear that when people come to prefer chili pepper, the preference is based on a liking for the sensory properties; the same properties of the "burn" that are innately negative at first become positive. People eat chili pepper because they like the taste, not because they think it is good for them.

Interviews as well as observations in a traditional Mexican village point to an important role for social factors. In the traditional setting, young children are regularly exposed to older siblings and their parents eating and enjoying hot peppers, usually in the form of a hot sauce. This positive affective context seems to encourage liking for the burn of the peppers (P. Rozin, 1990b). It is interesting in this regard that attempts to establish chili preferences in rats have generally failed. The only exception is recent work by Galef (1989), whose powerful rat social transmission mechanism can induce a preference for mildly irritating diets. The only clear cases of nonhuman, mammalian preferences for piquant foods involve social mediation. P. Rozin and Kennel (1983) reported that two captive chimpanzees were trained to like chili pepper in a social situation in which they were fed chili crackers regularly by their trainer. Cases of two rhesus monkeys (Dua-Sharma & Sharma, 1980) and one dog (P. Rozin & Kennel, 1983) also involved delivery of the food in the social context of a family meal. Hence, the animal literature on chili pepper strongly supports a social mediation model. With the exception of Galef's (1989) finding, the literature suggests direct involvement with humans in a positive social context as a condition for reversing innate aversions, and even Galef's finding implicates social processes in animals. It is notable that Mexican dogs do not develop a preference for chili pepper even though they eat it regularly mixed in with other discarded foods. Dogs in a rural Mexican setting are not treated as "pets" and do not consume chili pepper in a positive social affective context in association with humans.

Mechanisms of Inadvertent Social Effects

There is no strong evidence supporting a particular mechanism of action for the effects of social factors on preferences. More generally, the internalization or socialization process is not well understood. One account, which

involves the nonsocial acquisition of preferences, invokes Pavlovian conditioning. In this view, evaluations of objects can change, in animals and
humans, as a result of pairing of an event (e.g., a flavor) with an already
positive or negative event. This process has been termed *evaluative conditioning* (Baeyens, Eelen, van den Bergh, & Crombez, 1990; Martin & Levey,
1978; P. Rozin & Zellner, 1985). Conditioned taste aversions are an example
of evaluative conditioning; a food (conditioned stimulus) is paired with a
negative internal event, nausea (unconditioned stimulus), resulting in a
change in liking for the food. Such pairings are themselves nonsocial, but
they may be socially engineered. For example, a possible route to the liking
of unsweetened black coffee is earlier experiences of coffee with cream and
sugar. The coffee can be considered the conditioned stimulus, and the sugar,
the unconditioned (positive) stimulus. The contingent pairing of coffee and
sweetness increases the liking for the coffee flavor. Coffee sweetening is
made possible by cultural innovation and is often staged by friends or
parents as a means of making coffee more attractive. Hence, the pairings
are scheduled in a social context.

A direct social effect may be produced within the framework of evaluative conditioning. Baeyens, Kaes, Eelen, and Silverans (1996) recently demonstrated an increase in preference for an object (a wine glass of a particular
shape) when it was contingently paired with positive (as opposed to negative)
facial expressions. Such a paradigm fits well both with Galef's social effects
in animals (carbon disulfide on the rat's breath, paired with the food odor)
and with Birch's results with preschoolers (using social approval as the
unconditioned stimulus). Tomkins (1963) suggested particular pathways,
including the idea that the facial expression in the "demonstrator" or
"model" is the unconditioned stimulus and that this expression is induced
in the "subject." It is surprising how little is known at present about such
an important process.

The Pavlovian perspective offers only one way of conceptualizing inadvertent social effects. Lefebvre and Palameta (1988) distinguished three
modes of social influence involving inadvertent social agency: social facilitation, local enhancement, and observational learning. They provided criteria
for observational learning, the most elaborate of the three, and demonstrated
evidence for it in food-finding behavior of feral pigeons. It seems likely
that many of the examples of inadvertent social agency in humans involve

observational learning, whether or not one wishes to place a Pavlovian interpretation on this observation.

Active Social Agency: Teaching

In an extensive review of "tradition" and the effects of social factors on feeding in animals, Galef (1990) concluded that there is no evidence for active teaching in animals (see also chapter 8, this volume). This is clearly not the case for humans. Parents, among others, are active forces in teaching children about foods, and at least in the United States, parents attempt to shape children's food preferences.

Parents seem to have some insight into the process. A survey of feeding practices of American parents suggested that they are aware of the central importance of social factors in inducing preferences in their children; the two most popular techniques were engaging the child in the preparation of the food and exposing the child to displays of positive affect in association with the food (Casey & Rozin, 1989). However, parent educative efforts may not always have the intended effect. Birch, Birch, Marlin, and Kramer (1982) showed that rewarding ingestion of a target food has the long-term effect of decreasing the preference for that food. The interpretation is that although social approval indicates the valuation of the food in question by elders, rewarding the ingestion of the food indicates a lack of adult valuation of the food. A parent survey indicated that, in contrast to these findings, parents are more optimistic about the value of rewarding ingestion of a target food than about the efficacy of using the target food as a reward (Casey & Rozin, 1989).

The Family Paradox

In light of the (mostly circumstantial) evidence suggesting a major role for social factors in human food preferences and in recognition of the fact that, in the earlier years of life, the family is the dominant influence on the child, one would predict (a) strong family (particularly parent–child) resemblances (correlations) in food preferences; (b) higher correlations with the mother's preferences, given her much more substantial traditional role in food preparation and feeding; and (c) greater resemblance among same-sex child–parent pairs, on the grounds of modeling. None of these three predictions seem to hold, a pattern of results that I call the 'family paradox' (P. Rozin, 1991).

Across about six studies (reviewed in P. Rozin, 1991, including Birch, 1980b; Pliner, 1983), the results are mixed for all three claims. A weakly positive parent–child correlation (usually between 0 and .30) has been reported in family resemblance studies. This compares with much higher values (of the order of .5) for resemblance in disgust sensitivity or in values (e.g., attitudes to abortion) in parent–child correlations (P. Rozin, 1991). One cause for the low correlations might be that parents may be discordant on a particular preference. If so, there is no reason to predict that a child would fall on the midparent value; it is not clear how one would expect a child to respond to a mixed message about a particular food. P. Rozin (1991) separately analyzed parent–child food preference correlations for cases in which parents were concordant or discordant for the particular preference. Parent concordance did have a slight effect, but the correlations between parents who were concordant and their children were still quite modest (mean correlation of .18 across 12 foods).

One reason for the lack of a mother effect may be that, at least at the level of selection of foods, mothers may be more influenced by their husbands' preferences than by their own (Burt & Hertzler, 1978; Weidner, Archer, Healy, & Matarazzo, 1985).

There is no simple explanation for this set of results, which is why I label them a paradox. It is possible that parent–child correlations would improve if they were established between fully mature children (e.g., 30-year-olds) and their parents. It is also the case that there are other social routes besides that of parents' preferences. Pliner and Pelchat (1986) reported much larger food preference correlations between siblings, and there are also probably major peer influences, influences of adults other than parents, and media influences. However, it remains a puzzle that culture-wide food preferences must be, in substantial part, communicated by parents, who seem at the same time quite ineffective at communicating their own, more unique preferences.

It is widely believed, at least in the United States, that food preferences and attitudes, along with other preferences, attitudes, and basic features of personality, are formed in the first 6 years of life. This is the period in life in which parents have the greatest amount of contact with their children.

There is, in fact, virtually no evidence in any domain that there is *special* importance to the first 6 years of life. For food, in particular, there are reasons to think that the first few years of life should be of little importance. Like other mammals, humans in traditional societies spend the first few years of life on a diet dominated by mother's milk. It is associated with warmth, touch, a nurturing mother, and relief of hunger. Yet before the origin of dairying, milk was unavailable after the first few years of life. It would be maladaptive for young children to develop powerful milk preferences in such a setting. A number of features of mammals, including the development of lactose intolerance, the relative unpalatability of milk sugar, and a resistance to food imprinting, conspire to reduce the ultimate importance of early food experiences (P. Rozin & Pelchat, 1988).

Values and Preferences: Moralization

Two studies (Cavalli-Sforza, Feldman, Chen, & Dornbusch, 1982; P. Rozin, 1991) have suggested that values are transmitted from parent to child much more effectively than are preferences. This finding is of particular significance in the food domain, because, even in the United States, food selection can engage issues of values and morals. For example, in a recent study, Stein and Nemeroff (1995) presented college students with vignettes describing a college student. Students read one of two versions of the vignette, which were identical except that one described the student as regularly eating fruit, salad, homemade whole-wheat bread, chicken, and potatoes, and the other as regularly eating steak, hamburgers, French fries, doughnuts, and double-fudge ice cream sundaes. After reading the vignette, participants were asked to rate the student on a number of dimensions. The salad eater was rated as significantly more moral on a checklist of moral attributes (e.g., the person is either immoral or virtuous, considerate or inconsiderate). In subtle and not so subtle ways, therefore, food has moral implications in the United States, although the moral implications are much more overt and meaningful in other cultures, such as Hindu India.

Vegetarianism is increasing in the United States. There are two major strands of motivation for this practice, moral–ecological and health. Some vegetarians can be clearly classified as one of the two types (Amato & Partridge, 1989; Rozin, Markwith, & Stoess, 1996). Moral–ecological vegetarians are motivated by concern about causing pain or death to animals and by concern about the ecosystem. Health vegetarians are concerned primarily about the reported ill effects of animal foods on health. For moral vegetarians, meat represents a negative value, whereas for most health vegetarians, it is a matter of preference. There is evidence that moral vegetarians are more likely to find meat disgusting than are health vegetarians (P. Rozin, Markwith, & Stoess, 1996).

As moral vegetarianism increases, meat eating becomes more an issue of values and less one of mere preference. As a consequence, societal attitudes concerning meat consumption, and presumably, the transmission of attitudes toward meat from parents to children becomes more substantial. In the late 20th century, in the United States, one can see the beginning of the moralization of meat eating (P. Rozin, in press). The same process can be seen, at a more advanced stage, in the change in Americans' attitudes toward cigarette smoking.

CONCLUSION

The main thrust of this chapter has been to establish the importance of sociocultural factors in the understanding of food in general and of the acquisition of preferences in particular. The chapter has been short on mechanisms, because not much is known in that realm. The main research agenda in this area is to establish how sociocultural forces act and why they are ineffective in some cases, as in the case of low parent–child resemblance. At the moment, I cannot be of much help to the many parents who want their kids to like broccoli better than chocolate.

REFERENCES

Amato, P. R., & Partridge, S. A. (1989). *The new vegetarians: Promoting health and protecting life.* New York: Plenum Press.

Angyal, A. (1941). Disgust and related aversions. *Journal of Abnormal and Social Psychology, 36,* 393–412.

Appadurai, A. (1981). Gastro-politics in Hindu South Asia. *American Ethnologist, 8,* 494–511.

Baeyens, F., Eelen, P., van den Bergh, O., & Crombez, G. (1990). Flavor-flavor and color-flavor conditioning in humans. *Learning & Motivation, 21,* 434–455.

Baeyens, F., Kaes, B., Eelen, P., & Silverans, P. (1996). *Observational evaluative conditioning of an embedded stimulus element.* Manuscript submitted for publication.

Barker, L. M. (Ed.). (1982). *The psychobiology of human food selection.* Westport, CT: AVI.

Birch, L. L. (1980a). Effect of peer model's food choices and eating behaviors on pre-schoolers' food preferences. *Child Development, 51,* 489–496.

Birch, L. L. (1980b). The relationship between children's food preferences and those of their parents. *Journal of Nutrition Education, 12,* 14–18.

Birch, L. L. (1986). Children's food preferences: Developmental patterns and environmental influences. In G. Whitehurst & R. Vasta (Eds.), *Annals of Child Development (Vol. 4.)* Greenwich, CT: JAI Press.

Birch, L. L. (1987). The acquisition of food acceptance patterns in children. In R. Boakes, D. Popplewell, & M. Burton (Eds.), *Eating habits* (pp. 107–130). Chichester, England: Wiley.

Birch, L. L., Birch, D., Marlin, D. W., & Kramer, L. (1982). Effects of instrumental eating on children's food preferences. *Appetite, 3,* 125–134.

Birch, L. L., Zimmerman, S. I., & Hind, H. (1980). The influence of social-affective context on the formation of children's food preferences. *Child Development, 51,* 856–861.

Booth, D. A. (1982). Normal control of omnivore intake by taste and smell. In J. Steiner & J. Ganchrow (Eds.), *The determination of behavior by chemical stimuli: ECRO symposium* (pp. 233–243). London: Information Retrieval.

Booth, D. A. (1994). *Psychology of nutrition.* London: Taylor & Francis.

Burt, J. V., & Hertzler, A. A. (1978). Parental influence on the child's food preference. *Journal of Nutrition Education, 10,* 127–128.

Casey, R., & Rozin, P. (1989). Changing children's food preferences: Parent opinions. *Appetite, 12,* 171–182.

Cavalli-Sforza, L. L., Feldman, M. W., Chen, K. H., & Dornbusch, S. M. (1982). Theory and observation in cultural transmission. *Science, 218,* 19–27.

de Castro, J. M. (1990). Social facilitation of duration and size but not rate of the spontaneous meal intake of humans. *Physiology & Behavior, 47,* 1129–1135.

Dua-Sharma, S., & Sharma, K. N. (1980). Capsaicin and feeding responses in *Macaca mulata:* A longitudinal study [Abstract]. *International Conference on the Regulation of Food and Water Intake, Warsaw.*

Duncker, K. (1938). Experimental modifications of children's food preferences through social suggestion. *Journal of Abnormal and Social Psychology, 33,* 489–507.

Elias, N. (1978/1939). *The history of manners: Vol. I. The civilizing process.* New York: Pantheon.

Fischler, C. (1990). *L'Homnivore.* Paris: Editions Odile Jacob.

Frazer, J. G. (1890/1959). *The golden bough: A study in magic and religion.* New York: Macmillan. (Reprint of 1922 abridged edition, edited by T. H. Gaster; original work published 1890).

Galef, B. G., Jr. (1976). Social transmission of acquired behavior: A discussion of tradition and social learning in vertebrates. In J. S. Rosenblatt, R. A. Hinde, E. Shaw, & C. Beer (Eds.), *Advances in the study of behavior* (Vol. 6, pp. 77–100). San Diego, CA: Academic Press.

Galef, B. G., Jr. (1985). Direct and indirect pathways to the social transmission of food avoidance. *Annals of the New York Academy of Sciences, 443,* 203–215.

Galef, B. G., Jr. (1988). Communication of information concerning distant diets in a social central-place foraging species: *Rattus norvegicus.* In T. Zentall & B. G. Galef, Jr. (Eds.), *Social learning: A comparative approach* (pp. 119–140). Hillsdale, NJ: Erlbaum.

Galef, B. G., Jr. (1989). Enduring social enhancement of rats' preferences for the palatable and the piquant. *Appetite, 13,* 81–92.

Galef, B. G., Jr. (1990). Tradition in animals: Field observations and laboratory analysis. In M. Bekoff & D. Jamieson (Eds.), *Methods, inference, interpretation and explanation in the study of behavior.* Boulder, CO: Westview Press.

Galef, B. G., Jr., & Beck, M. (1990). Diet selection and poison avoidance by mammals individually and in social groups. In E. M. Stricker (Ed.), *Handbook of behavioral neurobiology: Vol. 10. Food and water intake.* New York: Plenum Press.

Galef, B. G., Jr., Mason, J. R., Preti, G., & Bean, N. J. (1988). Carbon disulfide: A semiochemical mediating socially-induced diet choice in rats. *Physiology & Behavior, 42,* 119–124.

Grunfeld, D. I. (1982). *The Jewish dietary laws: Vol. One. Dietary laws regarding forbidden and permitted foods, with particular reference to meat and meat products* (3rd ed.). London: Soncino Press (Original work published 1972).

Harris, M. (1985). *Good to eat: Riddles of food and culture.* New York: Simon & Schuster.

Jones, W. O. (1959). *Manioc in Africa.* Stanford, CA: Stanford University Press.

Katz, S. H. (1982). Food, behavior and biocultural evolution. In L. M. Barker (Ed.), *The psychobiology of human food selection* (pp. 171–188). Westport, CT: AVI.

Katz, S. H., Hediger, L. A., & Valleroy, L. A. (1974). Traditional maize processing techniques in the new world. *Science, 184,* 765–773.

Lefebvre, L., & Palameta, B. (1988). Mechanisms, ecology, and population diffusion of socially learned, food-finding behavior in feral pigeons. In T. Zentall & B. G. Galef, Jr. (Eds.), *Social learning: A comparative approach* (pp. 141–164). Hillsdale, NJ: Erlbaum.

Logue, A. (1991). *The psychology of eating and drinking* (2nd ed.). New York: Freeman.

Lolli, G., Serianni, E., Golder, G. M., & Luzzatto-Fegiz, P. (1958). *Alcohol in Italian culture.* Glencoe, IL: Free Press.

Marinho, H. (1942). Social influence in the formation of enduring preferences. *Journal of Abnormal and Social Psychology, 37,* 448–468.

Marriott, M. (1968). Caste ranking and food transactions: A matrix analysis. In M. Singer & B. S. Cohn (Eds.), *Structure and change in Indian society* (pp. 133–171). Chicago: Aldine.

Martin, I., & Levey, A. B. (1978). Evaluative conditioning. *Advances in Behavior Research and Therapy, 1,* 57–102.

Mauss, M. (1902/1972). *A general theory of magic* (R. Brain, Trans.). New York: Norton. (Original work published 1902)

McCarthy, M. (1990). The thin ideal, depression and eating disorders in women. *Behaviour Research and Therapy, 28,* 205–215.

Meigs, A. S. (1984). *Food, sex, and pollution: A New Guinea religion.* New Brunswick, NJ: Rutgers University Press.

Mintz, S. W. (1985). *Sweetness and power.* New York: Viking Press.

Nemeroff, C., & Rozin, P. (1989). An unacknowledged belief in "you are what you eat" among college students in the United States: An application of the demand-free "impressions" technique. *Ethos. The Journal of Psychological Anthropology, 17,* 50–69.

Pangborn, R. M. (1980). A critical analysis of sensory responses to sweetness. In P. Koivistoinen & L. Hyvonen (Eds.), *Carbohydrate sweeteners in foods and nutrition* (pp. 87–110). San Diego, CA: Academic Press.

Pelchat, M. L., Grill, H. J., Rozin, P., & Jacobs, J. (1983). Quality of acquired response to taste depends on type of associated discomfort. *Journal of Comparative Psychology, 97,* 140–153.

Pelchat, M. L., & Rozin, P. (1982). The special role of nausea in the acquisition of food dislikes by humans. *Appetite, 3,* 341–351.

Pliner, P. (1982). The effects of mere exposure on liking for edible substances. *Appetite, 3,* 283–290.

Pliner, P. (1983). Family resemblance in food preferences. *Journal of Nutrition Education, 15,* 137–140.

Pliner, P., & Pelchat, M. L. (1986). Similarities in food preferences between children and their siblings and parents. *Appetite, 7,* 333–342.

Richter, C. P. (1943). Total self regulatory functions in animals and human beings. *Harvey Lecture Series, 38,* 63–103.

Rozin, E. (1982). The structure of cuisine. In L. M. Barker (Ed.), *The psychobiology of human food selection* (pp. 189–202). Westport, CT: AVI.

Rozin, E. (1983). *Ethnic cuisine: The flavor principle cookbook.* Brattleboro, VT: Stephen Greene Press.

Rozin, E., & Rozin, P. (1981). Culinary themes and variations. *Natural History, 90* (2), 6–14.

Rozin, P. (1976). The selection of food by rats, humans and other animals. In J. Rosenblatt, R. A. Hinde, C. Beer, & E. Shaw (Eds.), *Advances in the study of behavior* (Vol. 6, pp. 21–76). San Diego, CA: Academic Press.

Rozin, P. (1982). Human food selection: The interaction of biology, culture and individual experience. In L. M. Barker (Ed.), *The psychobiology of human food selection* (pp. 225–254). Westport, CT: AVI.

Rozin, P. (1984). The acquisition of food habits and preferences. In J. D. Matarazzo, S. M. Weiss, J. A. Herd, N. E. Miller, & S. M. Weiss (Eds.), *Behavioral health: A handbook of health enhancement and disease prevention.* (pp. 590–607). New York: Wiley.

Rozin, P. (1988). Social learning about foods by humans. In T. Zentall & B. G. Galef, Jr. (Eds.), *Social learning: A comparative approach* (pp. 165–187). Hillsdale, NJ: Erlbaum.

Rozin, P. (1990a) The acquisition of stable food preferences. *Nutrition Reviews, 48,* 106–113.

Rozin, P. (1990b). Getting to like the burn of chili pepper: Biological, psychological and cultural perspectives. In B. G. Green, J. R. Mason, & M. L. Kare (Eds.), *Chemical irritation in the nose and mouth.* New York: Marcel Dekker.

Rozin, P. (1990c). The importance of social factors in understanding the acquisition of food habits. In E. D. Capaldi & T. L. Powley (Eds.), *Taste, experience and feeding* (pp. 255–269). Washington, DC: American Psychological Association.

Rozin, P. (1990d). Social and moral aspects of eating. In I. Rock (Ed.), *The legacy of Solomon Asch: Essays in cognition and social psychology.* Hillsdale, NJ: Erlbaum.

Rozin, P. (1991). Family resemblance in food and other domains: The family paradox and the role of parental congruence. *Appetite, 16,* 93–102.

Rozin, P. (1994). Food enculturation. In B. G. Galef, Jr., M. Mainardi, & P. Valsecchi (Eds.), *Behavioral aspects of feeding* (pp. 203–228). Chur, Switzerland: Harwood Academic Publishers.

Rozin, P. (in press). Psychological perspectives on the process of moralization. In A. Brandt & P. Rozin (Eds.), *Morality and health.* New York: Routledge.

Rozin, P., Dow, S., Moscovitch, M., & Rajaram, S. (1996). *The role of memory for recent eating experiences in onset and cessation of meals: Evidence from the amnesic syndrome.* Manuscript submitted for publication.

Rozin, P., & Fallon, A. E. (1987). A perspective on disgust. *Psychological Review, 94,* 23–41.

Rozin, P., Haidt, J., & McCauley, C. R. (1993). Disgust. In M. Lewis & J. Haviland (eds.), Handbook of emotions (pp. 575–594). New York: Guilford.

Rozin, P., Hammer, L., Oster, H., Horowitz, T., & Marmara, V. (1986). The child's conception of food: Differentiation of categories of rejected substances in the 1.4 to 5 year age range. *Appetite, 7,* 141–151.

Rozin, P., & Kalat, J. W. (1971). Specific hungers and poison avoidance as adaptive specializations of learning. *Psychological Review, 78,* 459–486.

Rozin, P., & Kennel, K. (1983). Acquired preferences for piquant foods by chimpanzees. *Appetite, 4,* 69–77.

Rozin, P., Markwith, M., & Stoess, C. (1996). *Moralization: Becoming a vegetarian, the conversion of preferences into values and the recruitment of disgust.* Manuscript submitted for publication.

Rozin, P., & Nemeroff, C. J. (1990). The laws of sympathetic magic: A psychological analysis of similarity and contagion. In J. Stigler, G. Herdt, & R. A. Shweder (Eds.), *Cultural psychology: Essays on comparative human development* (pp. 205–232). Cambridge, England: Cambridge University Press.

Rozin, P., Nemeroff, C., Horowitz, M., Gordon, B., & Voet, W. (1995). The borders of the self: Contamination sensitivity and potency of the mouth, other apertures and body parts. *Journal of Personality Research, 29,* 318–340.

Rozin, P., & Pelchat, M. L. (1988). Memories of mammaries: Adaptations to weaning from milk in mammals. In A. N. Epstein & A. Morrison (Eds.), *Advances in psychobiology* (Vol. 13, pp. 1–29). San Diego, CA: Academic Press.

Rozin, P., & Schulkin, J. (1990). Food selection. In E. M. Stricker (Ed.), *Handbook of behavioral neurobiology: Vol. 10. Food and water intake* (pp. 297–328). New York: Plenum Press.

Rozin, P., & Tuorila, H. (1993). Simultaneous and temporal contextual influences on food choice. *Food Quality and Preference, 4,* 11–20.

Rozin, P., & Zellner, D. A. (1985). The role of Pavlovian conditioning in the acquisition of food likes and dislikes. *Annals of the New York Academy of Sciences, 443,* 189–202.

Sclafani, A., & Nissenbaum, J. W. (1988). Robust conditioned flavor preferences produced by intragastric starch infusions in the rat. *American Journal of Physiology (Regulatory, Integrative, Comparative Physiology) 24,* R672–R675.

Shepherd, R. (Ed.). (1989). *Handbook of the psychophysiology of human eating.* Chichester, England: Wiley.

Shweder, R. A., Mahapatra, M., & Miller, J. G. (1987). Culture and moral development. In J. Kagan & S. Lamb (Eds.), *The emergence of moral concepts in young children* (pp. 1–82). Chicago: University of Chicago Press.

Simoons, F. J. (1961). *Eat not this flesh.* Madison: University of Wisconsin Press.

Simoons, F. J. (1970). Primary adult lactose intolerance and the milking habit: A problem in biologic and cultural interrelations. II. A cultural-historical hypothesis. *American Journal of Digestive Diseases, 15,* 695–710.

Simoons, F. J. (1982). Geography and genetics as factors in the psychobiology of human food selection. In L. M. Barker (Ed.), *The psychobiology of human food selection* (pp. 204–225). Westport, CT: AVI.

Stein, R. I., & Nemeroff, C. J. (1995). Moral overtones of food: Judgments of others based on what they eat. *Personality and Social Psychology Bulletin, 21,* 480–490.

Tomkins, S. S. (1963). *Affect, imagery, consciousness: Vol. II. The negative affects.* New York: Springer.

Weidner, G., Archer, S., Healy, B, & Matarazzo, J. D. (1985). Family consumption of low fat foods: Stated preference versus actual consumption. *Journal of Applied Social Psychology, 15,* 773–779.

Young, P. T. (1948). Appetite, palatability and feeding habit: A critical review. *Psychological Bulletin, 45,* 289–320.

Zajonc, R. B. (1968). Attitudinal effects of mere exposure. *Journal of Personality and Social Psychology, 9 (part 2),* 1–27.

Zellner, D. A. (1991). How foods get to be liked: Some general mechanisms and special cases. In R. C. Bolles (Ed.), *The hedonics of taste* (pp. 199–218). Hillsdale, NJ: Erlbaum.

Zingg, R. M. (1940). Feral man and extreme cases of isolation. *American Journal of Psychology, 53,* 487–517.

PART SIX

How Patterns of Eating Are Established

10

Sensory-Specific Satiety: Theoretical Frameworks and Central Characteristics

Marion M. Hetherington and Barbara J. Rolls

All living organisms must feed to survive. However, human eating behavior is further complicated by cultural and social factors. Eating is both necessary for life and a source of considerable pleasure. In a survey of German consumers, the word *eating* was spontaneously associated with pleasure in 44.5% of the sample (Westenhoefer & Pudel, 1993). The pleasure derived from eating is produced by both innate and learned mechanisms. Innate preferences may be expressed for simple tastes at birth; however, in omnivores the process of developing food preferences occurs in stages over time, exploiting the ability to pair certain tastes, smells, flavors, and foods with postingestive consequences. For example, newborn infants respond positively to the taste of sweet solutions and reject sour and bitter solutions (Steiner, 1977). As feeding experiences progress, however, the infant also learns to associate certain tastes with positive or negative postingestive consequences; for example, when liquid formula is provided to infants and then either diluted or enriched, intake of the formula increases or decreases to accommodate energy manipulation (Fomon, 1974). Young children learn to associate the orosensory characteristics of foods with the immediate and later consequences of eating those foods. For example, Kern et al. (1993) provided young children with a flavor paired with a yogurt drink containing either fat or nonfat dry milk. They found that children aged 3–4 years developed preferences for the flavors associated with fat. Although some flavor preferences seem to be present just after birth, most flavor preferences develop as a result of repeated experience with foods.

The pleasure derived from a food is learned and can vary from individual to individual as well as within individuals. A food that was generally liked by an individual may become aversive as a function of a negative experience, such as the classic "sauce béarnaise" phenomenon reported by Martin Seligman in the 1970s. This particular sauce had been a favorite with Seligman until one evening when he became ill following dinner. Although the meal had not been responsible for his illness, Seligman found he could no longer eat sauce béarnaise. This experience illustrates the power of food aversions and highlights the importance of past experience on food choice. (Taste aversions are discussed in detail in chapter 2, this volume.)

Even within a meal, the pleasure derived from a food can change from very positive to less positive. In 1957, Paul S. Siegal, referring to monotony effects, wrote that the palatability of a food declines when it is repeatedly eaten. However, this statement can be applied equally well to the changes that occur in pleasantness as a food is eaten within a single meal.

When a food is approached, sensory systems are engaged, and arousal is heightened by the appearance, smell, texture, and taste of the food. LeMagnen (1990) suggested that the stimulation to eat arises from both internal or metabolic signals, which underlie the state of hunger, and the orosensory features of the food. The appraisal of the orosensory features of the food as positive (i.e., pleasant) depends on energy status, previous experience of eating that food, and the hedonic response to the orosensory features of the food as it is perceived by the organism. When an organism is energy-deprived, the pleasantness of the orosensory experience is greater than when the organism is energy-replete (Cabanac, 1979). This phenomenon of need state influencing the pleasantness of a gustatory stimulus is termed *alliesthesia* (Cabanac, 1971). If previous encounters with a food have been positive, that is, there have been no previous negative consequences such as malaise occurring after ingestion, the food is likely to be approached again (Rozin & Kalat, 1971). Finally, the hedonic response to a particular food begins during the preliminary stages of seeing, smelling, and tasting the food. If the food is not perceived as positive in its appearance, smell, texture, or taste, it is unlikely to be eaten, although this evaluation is dependent on deprivation state and food availability.

Assuming that under certain conditions the food is judged to be pleasant and it is consumed, the pleasure derived from the food decreases as a function of eating (Rolls, 1986). The notion that pleasure is dynamic derives in part from what the individual brings to the eating context before consumption and in part from the current experience the individual has with the food.

Following consumption of a particular food, consumers report a decrease in the subjective pleasantness of the appearance, smell, texture, and taste of the food that lasts for at least 1 hour after eating (Hetherington, Burley, & Rolls, 1989). In addition, during eating, the rate of consuming the food slows (Bellisle, Lucas, Amrani, & Le Magnen, 1984), and the likelihood of the same food being chosen again from an array of different foods is reduced (Rolls & Hetherington, 1989). This dynamic aspect of pleasure as reflected in subjective judgments, rate of eating, and food choice has been named *sensory-specific satiety* (Rolls, 1986). That satiety can be specific to a particular food as it is eaten appears to be a reliable phenomenon; however, the mechanisms that underlie the expression of sensory-specific satiety remain to be elucidated.

There are several theoretical systems that can be explored to identify mechanisms that may underlie sensory-specific satiety, including habituation (Epstein, Rodefer, Wisniewski, & Caggiula, 1992; Swithers & Hall, 1994; Wisniewski, Epstein, & Caggiula, 1992), change in reward value of the food (E. T. Rolls, 1993), alterations in affect generated by the food (Berridge, 1991), opioid mediation (Hetherington, Vervaet, Blass, & Rolls, 1991), and opponent processes (Solomon, 1980).

This chapter explores sensory-specific satiety in detail by examining theoretical issues underlying its expression, its nature and characteristics, and several factors that influence its expression, ranging from characteristics of the food itself (e.g., macronutrient content) to characteristics of the consumer (cognitive influences and eating styles). In addition, some alternative interpretations of sensory-specific satiety are explored and evaluated critically.

POTENTIAL MECHANISMS UNDERLYING SENSORY-SPECIFIC SATIETY

Habituation

A model that has been used to assess changes in the pleasantness of a substance as it is consumed is that developed by Swithers and Hall (see Swithers & Hall, 1994, for a review). In this paradigm, rat pups with no previous exposure to the stimulus and little experience of feeding are prepared with indwelling cannulas. The rat pups are then provided with brief intraoral infusions of various substances including sucrose and saccharin. The pups' response can be either to "reject" the substance by allowing the infusion to spill out or "accept" the substance by actively lapping, licking, and swallowing. It has been demonstrated that responsivity to the intraoral infusions is a reliable index of willingness to ingest and is sensitive to both nutrient and water deprivation. This technique is used to explore the phenomenon of "oral habituation," that is, the decline in oral responsiveness to the stimulus over time. With repeated exposure to the infusion, responsivity declines, yet in the early stages of this experience there is no significant postingestive input; oral habituation occurs before absorption of nutrients takes place. In their studies of this phenomenon, Swithers and colleagues found that oral habituation is long lasting, can be specific to the substance that is infused, and can have a significant impact on subsequent ingestion. Evidence that oral habituation does not merely reflect muscle fatigue is provided by the fact that changing the substance delivered into the oral cavity restores the response rate.

The role of postingestive consequences in the decline of responsivity has been examined by administering gastric loads of sucrose solution before giving the oral infusions. Results suggest that preloading the pups adds to the lowered response rate observed during oral habituation. Postingestive inputs play a role in modifying oral habituation, but oral habituation is nevertheless observed without any significant postingestive input.

The parallels between oral habituation and sensory-specific satiety are clear. In an experiment conducted by E. T. Rolls et al. (cited in Rolls & Rolls, 1982), participants tasted and rated the pleasantness of water after overnight deprivation. One group drank to satiety, whereas a second group tasted but did not swallow the water. The pleasantness of the taste of water declined in both groups. Although this decline was greater in the group that drank to satiety, the finding demonstrates the power of oropharyngeal stimulation alone to reduce the pleasantness of the water stimulus. Similarly, Wooley, Wooley, and Dunham (1972) found that the pleasantness of the taste of sucrose declined to the same extent following ingestion of a noncaloric solution (cyclamate) as it did after a caloric solution (glucose).

In a series of studies exploring changes in pleasantness of foods sweetened with aspartame or sucrose, it was found that the magnitude and time course of changes in pleasantness did not differ between low- and high-calorie versions of Jello gelatin dessert or pudding (Rolls, Hetherington, & Burley, 1988a; Rolls, Laster, & Summerfelt, 1989). Moreover, intake of a test meal offered 60 or 120 minutes after the different versions of the foods were given was not differentially affected by aspartame compared to sucrose.

In the short term, therefore, a reduction in pleasantness ratings has been observed after drinking water, after drinking a low-calorie solution, and following a very low energy load. Before absorption takes place, signals from the mouth relay to the brain the sensory features of the substance. Whether by a process of habituation or a process by which the reward value of the food is altered, there is a decline in the acceptability of the substance, which may contribute to the termination of ingestion. Satiation appears to begin in the oral cavity, which acts as more than a mere sensor of volume; it also provides information for hedonic modulation.

Taste Reactivity

Berridge (1991) used a different model to examine hedonic responses to food. In this paradigm, rats have chronic indwelling cannulas in the oral cavity, and taste reactivity patterns are quantified. This procedure permits investigation of both the appetite (tendency to eat) and the degree of pleasure–displeasure produced by the infusion. Responses that suggest positive affective reactions include tongue protrusions and paw licks, whereas those suggesting negative affective reactions include gapes, chin rubbing, and head shaking. Berridge (1991) found that manipulating hunger by having the animals deprived for either 24 or 48 hours and manipulating satiety by gastric intubation (involuntary satiety) or by allowing 1-hour access to wet mash (voluntary satiety) influenced the taste affect reactions to water and to two sweet solutions. Following 48 hours of deprivation, positive hedonic reactivity was enhanced, and following voluntary or involuntary satiety, positive hedonic reactions were significantly reduced. There is an apparent overlap between these findings and observations of alliesthesia by Cabanac (1979). Thus, the hedonic appraisal of the solution was dependent on biological usefulness, that is, need (hunger) or repletion (satiety).

Moreover, changes in hedonic reactions were specific to the food provided in the oral infusions (sensory-specific satiety). Rats given sucrose solution to satiety demonstrated reduced positive hedonic reactions to the taste of sucrose compared to reactions to milk. It is interesting that only reactions in the positive domain were influenced by these manipulations; there was no increase in aversive responses as a function of sensory-specific satiety or caloric satiety. The response to the stimulus did not change from the positive to the negative hedonic domain.

These experiments provide further evidence of the power of hedonic changes in the development of satiation. Indeed, in his experiments, Berridge demonstrated that sensory-specific satiety produced a greater reduction in hedonic reactivity than that achieved by caloric satiety. This finding emphasizes the difference between alliesthesia and sensory-specific satiety, in that alliesthesia is dependent on caloric input, but sensory-specific satiety develops to the specific ingestant, with or without caloric input, and enhances intake of a different ingestant. Furthermore, as in the studies conducted by Swithers and Hall (1994), the suggestion that changes in hedonic response are merely due to some kind of fatigue is weakened by the observation that in Berridge's experiments, aversive reactions to quinine and sucrose mixtures were maintained. The capacity to respond is not reduced, therefore; rather, the nature of the response changes as a function of exposure to the substance.

Habituation of Salivation

The previous two models used animals; however, phenomena such as habituation have been studied in humans. A potential advantage of using humans is that investigators can ask about pleasure experienced by participants in addition to taking objective measurements of pleasure such as degree of salivation. Although introspection and self-report are problematic (Berridge, 1991), combining self-report with physiological measures increases the reliability of subjective measures. For example, Epstein and colleagues (Epstein, Caggiula, Rodefer, Wisniewski, & Mitchell, 1993; Epstein et al., 1992) measured salivation alongside hedonic judgments in humans. They reported that as the pleasantness of the taste of lemon juice declined with repeated administrations, the amount of saliva produced decreased. Presenting a novel juice after 10 trials with lemon juice or even a nontaste stimulus served to dishabituate the response, and salivation returned to baseline levels.

Similarly, Wisniewski et al. (1992) gave repeated presentations of pizza or cheeseburger and found reductions in salivation, hedonic judgments, and intake of the same food, whereas an increase in salivation, hedonic ratings, and intake was found with a different food.

To assess the influence of postingestive consequences on the habituation effects, Epstein et al. (1993) provided a test meal of either low- or high-calorie lemon gelatin. The magnitude of habituation was equivalent for both conditions, and reductions in hunger ratings, hedonics, and intake were equivalent (Epstein et al., 1993). The authors concluded that habituation of the salivary response was determined by the sensory features of the food to a greater extent than by its energy content.

Central Mechanisms

In a review of the neurophysiological examination of sensory-specific satiety, E. T. Rolls (1993) suggested that changes in hedonic evaluation of a food stimulus can be traced to specific populations of neurons in the lateral hypothalamus. Rolls and colleagues used the alert monkey to conduct neurophysiological recordings of single neurons in various regions of the brain that are involved in the control of feeding. Single cells in the lateral hypothalamus and the substantia innominata responded to the presentation of food only when the animal was hungry. Hunger modulated responsiveness at later stages of sensory processing and was not important for changes in firing rates occurring during visual processing (Rolls, 1993). Modulation of single-cell firing is food-specific; that is, firing rates to the sight, smell, and taste of other foods remained relatively unchanged. It has been proposed that because animals work to obtain self-stimulation of brain regions normally activated during feeding this reflects the reward value of the food (Rolls, 1993). As a specific food is eaten, therefore, the reward value of that food declines relative to other foods.

Rolls and Treves (1990) proposed a neuronal model for the central organization of sensory-specific satiety. They suggested that the early stages of processing of gustatory stimuli are not influenced by satiety, habituation, and adaptation. As the tuning of neurons becomes more specific in the orbitofrontal cortex, however, there is evidence of satiety and habituation affecting responsiveness of these neurons. They suggest, furthermore, that this information-processing system permits differential levels of analysis whereby early on, satiety has no impact on processing because this would attenuate responses to nonfoods and to foods not eaten; at later stages, however there is a motivational interface such that satiety and habituation do influence responsiveness.

Opioid Mediation

The role of opiates in food reward has been reviewed by Le Magnen (1990), who proposed that eating and the accompanying orosensory stimulation produced by foods are associated with hypothalamic release of opioid peptides. It is the release of endogenous opioids that underlies the rewarding aspects of eating, according to Le Magnen. Administration of opioid antagonists influences the hedonic appraisal of sucrose solutions (Fantino, Hosotte, & Apfelbaum, 1986) and judgments of real foods (Yeomans & Wright, 1991).

If sensory-specific satiety is mediated in part by the endogenous opioid system, then by blocking access to opioid receptors at least two outcomes would be predicted: First, sensory-specific satiety might not be demonstrated or might be delayed, and second, the pleasure derived from foods would be weakened, rendering the foods significantly less pleasant relative to placebo. To assess these predictions, we conducted two experiments using the opioid antagonist naltrexone (Hetherington et al., 1991). In the first experiment, naltrexone was administered midmorning, and approximately 1 hour later, a buffet-style test meal was offered to the participants with the instruction to eat as much as they wanted. In this experiment, neither the pleasantness of the taste of the sample foods nor the amount of food consumed was influenced by naltrexone relative to a placebo condition. Because the participants had fasted overnight, and because a wide variety of food choices were available, negative results may have been due to the interference of significant deprivation or to overstimulation by variety. In a second experiment, therefore, we gave a midafternoon snack (chocolate ice cream) after the participants' normal lunch and tracked consumption for the rest of the day using diet records. Naltrexone failed to influence sensory-specific satiety, appetite, and the amount of food consumed overall. Nevertheless, administration of other opioid blockers with different modes of action has yielded positive results. For example, Yeomans and Wright (1991) found that the pleasantness of foods that were rated as highly palatable was significantly reduced by administration of nalmefene. It would be interesting to test the effects of drugs such as nalmefene, which specifically alter palatability, on the development and expression of sensory-specific satiety.

Opponent Processes

Another theoretical avenue that may be explored in connection with sensory-specific satiety is that proposed by Solomon (1980). Solomon's opponent process theory has been applied to a wide variety of behaviors ranging from drug addiction to social attachment. Central to the theory is that when unconditioned stimuli such as pleasant-tasting foods are repeatedly presented, three affective consequences occur. These consequences are, in the following order, (a) affective or hedonic contrast, (b) development of hedonic habituation or tolerance, and (c) a withdrawal effect. In extending his opponent process theory of acquired motivation to food intake, Solomon suggested that the pleasure produced by a highly liked food in the mouth in turn engages an opponent-process, which reduces this pleasure.

The opponent process, which may occur in relation to the changing hedonic response to a food as it is eaten, is not necessarily aversive; that is, the opponent process may not be the absolute opposite of pleasure. Rather, the opponent process may be in the direction of more negative appraisal without entering an aversive zone. Solomon's theory more easily applies to hunger and satiety as opponent processes than to changes in the hedonic evaluation of foods. Because the pleasure derived from food contributes to the development of satiety, however, it is possible that as the food is eaten the pleasure of eating decreases through an opponent process. Solomon (1986) suggested that toward the end of a meal, the affective dynamics of opponent processes are increasingly salient and influence the termination of cating. If a different food is offered that is of a higher preference, eating resumes. This "dessert effect" occurs from introducing a new taste with no opponent process as yet. Although none of these propositions has been tested directly, the opponent process analysis of eating may be a useful theoretical construct in understanding how a food that is initially very pleasant becomes significantly less pleasant relative to other foods as eating progresses.

Along lines similar to the opponent process theory, the notion of dynamic contrast promoting intake was forwarded by Hyde and Witherly (1993). They proposed that intake of a highly liked food such as ice cream is in part due to the sensory properties of the food producing high "motivational contrast," which sustains the pleasure of eating. A food such as ice cream that has properties that may affect both hunger and thirst reward systems could delay opponent processes and, therefore, satiation.

ALTERNATIVE EXPLANATIONS

Pleasant Taste Versus Desire to Eat

Blundell and Rogers (1991) suggested that the pleasantness of the taste of a food does not decline with consumption; rather, the food remains pleasant to taste, but the willingness to eat the food declines with intake. They proposed that participants should be asked to rate the pleasantness of the taste of the food, how pleasant it would be to eat the food, and how much of the food they are willing to eat (Rogers & Blundell, 1990). To test the hypothesis that the pleasantness of the taste of a food remains constant but the pleasure of eating the food declines, a series of experiments was conducted in which both variables were assessed (Hetherington, 1993b).

In one experiment, 78 participants came to the laboratory having eaten nothing in the 3 hours since their breakfast. They rated hunger, appetite, fullness, the pleasantness of the taste, and pleasure of eating two foods: cheese on cracker and chocolate. The instructions asked participants to make a distinction between the pleasure derived from the taste of the food and the pleasure derived from the eating experience. All participants were then given a meal of cheese on cracker and instructed to eat as much as they wanted. They then re-rated hunger, appetite, fullness, pleasantness of the taste, and pleasure of eating the two foods at 2, 20, 40, and 60 minutes after the meal. Subsequently, a second course was offered: either cheese on crackers again (Same Condition) or chocolate (Different Condition). As in previous experiments, the pleasantness of the cheese on cracker (eaten food) decreased significantly more than the pleasantness of the chocolate (uneaten food). However, in this experiment, pleasantness of taste and pleasure of eating were highly correlated and changed to the same extent.

Because participants were asked to rate taste and pleasure of eating together in this experiment, in the next study participants were asked to rate either the pleasantness of the taste or the pleasure of eating the food. In this experiment, 96 participants came to the laboratory having skipped lunch and rated hunger, appetite, fullness, and the pleasantness of cheese crackers and chocolate cookies. Approximately half of the participants rated the pleasure of eating these foods and half rated the pleasantness of the taste of the food. Within both groups, half of the participants received cheese crackers as a test meal to eat to satiety and half received chocolate cookies. Again, ratings were conducted at 2, 20, 40, and 60 minutes after the test meal, and after the 60-minute rating, participants received either the same food again (Same Condition) or the other food (Different Condition). In this design, ratings of pleasure of eating and pleasantness of taste were conducted between groups. However, once again, the correlation between pleasure of eating and pleasantness of taste was highly significant, and both measures declined to the same degree.

Rolls and colleagues also explored this phenomenon using ratings of desire to eat each food and the pleasantness of the taste of the food. These ratings were similar before intake and declined to the same extent as a function of eating (Rolls & McDermott, 1991; Rolls et al., 1992). It seems, therefore, that these two attributes are closely linked and that people find it difficult to tease out the difference between pleasantness of taste and pleasure of eating. Indeed, one might suggest that this is an example of a false dichotomy. Pleasantness of taste contributes to the pleasure of eating, and the pleasure of eating a food is highly dependent on the pleasantness produced by the sensory characteristics of the food, in particular, the taste of the food. Blundell and Rogers (1991) suggested that the food may taste delicious but the person does not desire the food. However, in our experience, participants have been unable to discriminate between the two phenomena. In our results, foods taste less pleasant after eating *and* at the end of the meal, consumers do not want to eat this food again relative to other foods.

Liking Versus Wanting Foods

Berridge (1996) identified two distinguishable components of the pleasure of eating, mostly from work on animals. Liking is measured by pleasure responses in animals and by subjective ratings of pleasantness in humans, and *wanting* is measured by assessment of incentive motivation in animals and by desire to eat (appetite for) a specific food in humans. Findings from neurophysiological studies in animals have indicated that different regions of the brain control these two separable components of pleasure (Berridge, 1996). Similarly, in humans pharmacological manipulations have revealed agents that reduce hunger while sparing the pleasantness of foods (dexfenfluramine; Blundell & Hill, 1988) and agents (opioid blockers) that reduce the pleasantness derived from foods while not influencing hunger (Fantino et al., 1986). Using such agents to separate pleasantness and hunger has been a successful strategy, but the dissociation is much more difficult to find using self-reports. This suggests that in normal eating situations, the two operate together and that there is no subjective awareness of the two different dimensions.

It has been suggested that although hedonic shifts occur, people may be relatively unaware of them or that these shifts are unimportant in terminating food intake (Mook & Votaw, 1992). To test this proposition, a series of studies was conducted by Mook and Votaw (1992) in which consumers were asked to give the main reason for terminating meals. Because most participants selected fullness as the most common reason to stop eating and few selected the hedonic option (i.e., the food stopped tasting as good or the food tastes less good), the authors concluded that hedonic shifts are of little salience or importance in terminating a meal. However, a serious weakness of the three studies was that a meal was not offered to the consumers, so that answers were based on memory rather than on the experience of having just eaten.

A study was devised (Hetherington, 1996) to assess reasons for stopping eating in participants who were given a test meal using a paradigm similar to that of Mook and Votaw (1992). Fifty-seven people were given ad lib access to cheese on crackers and at the end of eating recorded the main reason for stopping from seven possible statements. These statements were modified from the work of Mook and Votaw (1992) and were as follows: Everyone else had finished eating; I had had as much as I am allowed; the food began to taste less pleasant; the food was all gone; I felt full; I got tired of eating the food; some other reason contributed by the participant. They then rank-ordered the importance of each reason. One hour later, participants were offered a second course of the same food or a different food or no second course at all. Again, reasons for stopping were recorded by those who selected a second course. The most common reason given for meal termination in the first course was "I got tired of eating that food" (40%) and for the second course "I felt full" (48%). Because previous studies indicated that getting tired of the food accompanied hedonic changes, participants who rated fatigue as the most important reason for termination and those who rated hedonics the most important were combined. These participants were compared with those who rated fullness as most important. Significant differences in intake between these groups indicated that those who rated fatigue or hedonics as most important consumed significantly fewer calories than those who rated fullness as most important, in the first course.

Fatigue experienced by consumers may reflect sensory fatigue, and this could be a component in the development of sensory-specific satiety. Because participants who rated fullness as the most important reason for terminating the meal consumed more calories, it could be that this index of satiety is less sensitive than sensory or hedonic variables. The participants got tired of the food, reported this reason alongside changes in the hedonic assessment of the eaten food, and after the second course, selected fullness as the most important reason for termination. This pattern sheds some light on the findings by Mook and Votaw (1992) that if people are asked at the end of a large meal (i.e., one containing two courses), the most likely reason given for meal termination is indeed fullness. If they are asked at the end of a first course, however, as satiety is developing, the main reason given for stopping is not fullness but rather that the person is tired of eating that food.

Clearly, different methods yield different results. Relying on memory for the reason a meal was terminated and using currently available information at the end of a meal are likely to reveal different patterns. Even from memory, however, changes in pleasantness (hedonic reasons) and getting tired of the food may be experienced rather more transiently than fullness and then not remembered. Lack of awareness of the contribution of hedonic changes to meal termination may not imply that they are unimportant in the process of satiation. Consumers may not be aware of the process of changing pleasantness normally, but if attention is drawn to the phenomenon by asking for recordings of the pleasantness of food as it is eaten, pleasantness declines reliably and systematically.

Sensory Stimulation Versus Satiety

Another interpretation of sensory-specific satiety is that rather than being a process associated with satiation, variety is a process by which eating is stimulated. For example, in discussing the effects of variety on food intake, Blundell and Rogers (1991) proposed that studies that demonstrate an enhancement of intake through provision of variety reflect a sensory stimulation of appetite. The notion underlying this statement is as follows: If a second food is introduced as a food is eaten, appetite is excited, and eating is reinstated. In two recent experiments, Yeomans has shown that following the first taste of a highly liked food, hunger increases "the appetizer effect" (Yeomans, 1993) and that by adding a strong flavor such as oregano to a pasta base, eating is enhanced relative to consumption of pasta in a plain tomato sauce. The addition of a powerful flavor enhancer that at moderate levels increases intake relative to the plain version has effects that are parallel to those of sensitization, which occurs in habituation; that is, before the decline in responsiveness occurs in habituation processes, there is a temporary increase in response. Despite the appetizer effect or any kind of sensitization effect, a decline inevitably follows. This decline reflects the development of satiation. In other words, initially there appears to be an increased stimulation to eat that occurs as a function of introducing variety into the meal; however, progressively, as the individual becomes sated, the foods decline in pleasantness, and this is accompanied by a decline in the desire to eat that food. Sensory stimulation is an important phenomenon, which explains in part the initiation of eating but not the termination of eating.

The pleasantness of the taste of all foods is likely to decline with consumption, and consumers report sensory-specific satiety to foods however pleasant they are judged initially. For example, chocolate, which is typically considered a well-liked food, is rated as highly pleasant, but as a function of eating it, the pleasantness of the taste declines in a similar way to other foods. Rogers (1994) proposed that some foods are so pleasant that they are resistant to satiation; this phenomenon is termed *moreishness.* However, it is unlikely that any food is inherently resistant to satiation; instead, different foods may take more or less time to produce sensory-specific satiety, and repeatedly eating quantities beyond the typical portion size may alter the amount of food required to produce sensory-specific satiety.

Hetherington and Macdiarmid (1994) found that individuals who overeat chocolate demonstrate significantly smaller changes in the pleasantness of the taste of this food relative to consumers who like chocolate to the same extent but who do not overeat this food. In a laboratory setting, the magnitude of changes in the pleasantness of the taste and pleasure of eating chocolate was compared between overeaters and controls when they had *ad lib* access to a highly liked form of milk chocolate. Although the overeaters consumed significantly more chocolate in this condition relative to controls, changes in pleasantness were significantly smaller (Hetherington & Macdiarmid, 1994). A possible explanation of this finding is that systematic overeating (i.e., increasing intake of a specific food over time) weakens satiety signals including changes in pleasantness of the taste of the food as it is eaten.

These findings go against predictions derived from studies of monotony. For example, Moskowitz (1980) found that foods that had not been eaten for 3 months were highly desired and that foods eaten the day before were less desired. The most frequently eaten foods such as bread, milk, and butter are staple food items, and these foods are rated as less pleasant than less frequently eaten foods. In our work with individuals who overeat foods such as chocolate, however, the items are highly liked and eaten with great frequency (Macdiarmid & Hetherington, 1995). There are circumstances in which consumers can override the normative patterns of intake, therefore, but these are unusual and signify aberrant eating behavior.

CHARACTERIZING SENSORY-SPECIFIC SATIETY

Cognitive Influences

To assess the contribution of cognition to the development of sensory-specific satiety, Tepper (1992) compared restrained and unrestrained eaters on the magnitude of sensory-specific satiety. Restrained eaters share with individuals who have eating disorders a tendency to control food intake on the basis of cognitions, such as eating a certain number of calories each day to lose or maintain weight. Another example of cognitive control of food is to base intake on beliefs about the caloric content of a food rather than relying on the postingestive consequences of eating that food (Polivy, 1976). The prediction made by Tepper (1992) was that individuals who restrict their food intake according to cognitive rather than physiological cues would show a relatively blunted sensory-specific satiety compared to unrestrained eaters. To test this prediction, restrained and unrestrained eaters were given access to either cheese on crackers or cream-filled cookies. Although restrained and unrestrained eaters differed in cephalic phase salivation, the magnitude and expression of sensory-specific satiety were equivalent in the two groups. Although cognition plays a significant role in determining food intake in restrained eaters, cognitive controls did not appear to override or alter hedonic responses.

This finding supports previous work in which unrestrained and restrained eaters were compared to individuals with and without eating disorders (Hetherington & Rolls, 1988). It was found that sensory-specific satiety was equivalent in restrained and unrestrained eaters but was weaker in bulimics compared to controls and exaggerated in anorexics compared to controls.

Subsequent studies of sensory-specific satiety in these different groups have yielded different results. In one study, bulimics demonstrated sensory-specific satiety following a low-calorie salad preload but not following a high-calorie preload. In contrast, anorexics reported sensory-specific satiety following a high-calorie salad and not after the low-calorie preload (Rolls et al., 1992). These results provide some evidence of the significant contribution of cognitive processes to the expression of sensory-specific satiety. For example, a possible interpretation of these results is that for the anorexics, the high-energy preload was considered "dangerous" and therefore they switched off the eaten food rapidly and decisively. The bulimics, on the other hand, experienced the high-energy preload in the same way that they might experience a binge and accordingly recorded no change in response to the eaten food as a function of intake. This observation might explain, in part, why bulimics are capable of consuming very large amounts of food at one sitting (see Hetherington, 1993a for a full review).

That sensory-specific satiety in these groups was dependent on the type of foods given demonstrates the power of cognitive processes over sensory characteristics of the foods in the expression of sensory-specific satiety. Because satiety is specific to certain foods and can be influenced by the type of food and the individual's cognitive appraisal of the food, it has been suggested that a more appropriate term for sensory-specific satiety is *food-specific satiety* (Booth, 1995). Certainly, this term conveys the importance of the features of the food, which are rooted in the sensory domain, but gives due attention to a more cognitive component. The person's appraisal of how safe or dangerous a food is, its inclusion as part of a binge or overeating episode, and expectancy effects of consuming that food may contribute to the development of sensory-specific satiety.

Nutrient Effects Versus Cognitive Inputs

The contribution of both energy density and nutrient content of foods in the development of sensory-specific satiety has been investigated (Rolls et al., 1988a, Rolls, Hetherington, & Burley, 1988b, Rolls et al., 1989). Because humans do not generally consume pure nutrients, however, assessing nutrient-specific satiety or the role of specific nutrients in the development of sensory-specific satiety is subject to the consumer's expectancies and predictions about how satiating a food is.

Early studies of alliesthesia by Cabanac and colleagues did rely on pure nutrients however. Cabanac suggested that changes in the pleasantness of food-related stimuli following ingestion of a nutrient load were dependent on which nutrient had been ingested (Cabanac, 1979). Using peanut oil as the ingestant did not modify judgments of food-related odors and tastes, whereas protein did to a certain extent (Guy-Grand & Sitt, 1976). The clearest and most reliable alliesthesia was found with glucose solutions. The proposal is that fat is less satiating than protein, therefore, and that carbohydrate sources are significantly more potent than fats at producing alliesthesia.

To test the hypothesis that different nutrients influence the development of sensory-specific satiety differentially, we conducted an experiment. We measured lunch intake, changes in subjective ratings of hunger and appetite, and sensory-specific satiety over a 2-hour period following preloads of foods high in fat, simple carbohydrate, complex carbohydrate, protein, and a high fat–high carbohydrate mixture (Rolls et al., 1988b). Lunch intake was significantly smaller following foods high in protein or complex carbohydrate than foods high in simple carbohydrate, fat, and the high fat–high simple carbohydrate mixture. Because the foods also varied along other attributes such as temperature and food type (entree-type food compared to snack), however, it was not possible to attribute differences in intake to nutrient composition alone. Nevertheless, the magnitude of sensory-specific satiety did not differ according to macronutrient composition; thus, foods of different micronutrient content have similar effects on the development of sensory-specific satiety. There is some evidence of a trend toward greater sensory-specific satiety when foods are high in protein (Johnson & Vickers, 1992), but this finding has yet to be confirmed.

Although it is intriguing, it is as yet unclear why foods of different macronutrient content might produce weaker or stronger sensory-specific satiety. Because recent work has shown that fat may be less satiating calorie-for-calorie than carbohydrate (Rolls & Hammer, 1994), it may follow that fats produce weaker sensory-specific satiety than protein or carbohydrate. This proposition has yet to be examined systematically. Moreover, evidence showing that fats are less satiating than other nutrients is still controversial, and the effects are small (Rolls & Hammer, 1994). Finally, because consumers come to the laboratory with beliefs and expectations about the satiating capacity of foods high in different macronutrients, it is possible that these cognitions influence the outcome of experiments testing the effects of nutrients on sensory-specific satiety. Future experimentation must take into account both the nutrient content of foods and cognitive inputs such as beliefs about specific nutrients, attitudes about foods that differ in macronutrient content, and expectations of satiety from foods of different nutrient profiles.

Effects of Age

The pleasantness of a food declines as that food is eaten to satiety. This phenomenon occurs regardless of energy density or nutrient content. As a function of aging, however, the decline in pleasantness is weakened or absent (Rolls, 1992). A study was conducted to compare sensory-specific satiety and sensory perception in adolescents, young adults, older adults, and elderly adults (Rolls & McDermott, 1991). Elderly participants (aged 65–82 years) failed to show a decrease in the pleasantness of the taste of yogurt following either ad-lib access or a 300-g fixed load. Also, desire to eat the yogurt and pleasantness of the texture of the food did not diminish following the fixed load in the elderly participants. Although sensory-specific satiety is observed in young children (Birch & Deysher, 1986) and across different age groups, old age appears to diminish the phenomenon. One possible explanation for this is that sensory processing and acuity decline with age; however, Rolls and McDermott (1991) found no correlation between sensory impairment and loss of sensory-specific satiety. Another explanation is in the cognitive realm: that elderly people are more resistant to changes of any kind. Because elderly individuals are generally less responsive to changes in internal cues such as dehydration (Rolls & Phillips, 1990), however, it may be that aging processes alter appetite regulation including sensory-specific satiety.

IMPLICATIONS AND CONCLUSION

The suggestion that satiation begins as a function of changes in hedonic response to the taste of food before any significant absorption takes place has great intrinsic and heuristic appeal. The most parsimonious explanation for the development of such a system is that it allows satiation to develop to novel foods, before associations are made between specific sensory features and particular postingestive consequences. Moreover, it is both economical and adaptive to have a system that does not depend exclusively on postabsorptive feedback, because postabsorptive cues take a much longer time to be expressed than oral habituation, salivary habituation, or, indeed, sensory-specific satiety.

In summary, pleasure is derived from food rather than a property of the food itself. The pleasure derived is dynamic and changes as a function of consumption. The mechanisms underlying changes in pleasure as a function of ingestion are as yet unknown. Changes in pleasantness of a food stimulus occur before or in the absence of significant postingestive inputs. However, postingestive signals are critical for the development of alliesthesia, and in studies of oral habituation in the rat pup, postingestive signals operated additively to the response decrement. Berridge (1991) assessed changes in hedonic reactivity following both caloric satiety and sensory-specific satiety and showed that both reduce positive hedonic responses and that they act additively. Changes in pleasantness occur before postingestive signals are initiated, therefore but hedonic shifts are, nevertheless, influenced by postingestive events.

It is useful from a theoretical perspective to examine a variety of experimental models from animal and human paradigms that replicate and extend the observation that pleasure declines as a function of consumption. The replicability of these findings across experimental settings underscores the universality and power of the phenomenon. Although a precise theoretical model has not yet been devised to explain phenomena such as sensory-specific satiety, several experimental models have been useful in exploring the broader context of the role of pleasure in eating behavior. For example, studies of habituation of the salivary response in humans, oral habituation in the rat pup, and taste reactivity, as well as the continuing work on single-cell neurophysiology, all contribute to the understanding of pleasure and of the changes in pleasure that accompany ingestion.

In the applied context, studies of sensory-specific satiety contribute to the understanding of how individuals with eating disorders are able to eat very little or to eat to excess (Hetherington, 1993a). Pleasure is important in the eating process, in learning food preferences, in selecting specific foods, in associating flavors with postingestive outcomes, and in determining how much is eaten within a meal; therefore, pleasure is a component of eating that needs to be restored in people who have eating disorders. Those who have anorexia and bulimia have to be taught to respond normally to hunger and satiety cues (Beumont & Touyz, 1995) including sensory-specific satiety.

Pleasure is central to eating. The pleasure of eating and the pleasantness of foods are established through innate and learned mechanisms. The change in pleasantness as a function of eating is adaptive and contributes to normal eating behavior. Sensory-specific satiety is observed across a wide variety of species and within humans across the life span (Rolls, 1986; Rolls & McDermott, 1991). It appears to be a universal and highly replicable phenomenon. However, sensory-specific satiety is influenced by a variety of factors including processes of aging, cognitive mediation, and nutrient content. Future studies that include further investigation of such factors will contribute to the development of theoretical models to explain the phenomenon of sensory-specific satiety.

REFERENCES

Bellisle, F., Lucas, F., Amrani, R., & Le Magnen, J. (1984). Deprivation, palatability and the micro-structure of meals in human subjects. *Appetite, 5,* 85–94.

Berridge, K. C. (1991). Modulation of taste affect by hunger, caloric satiety, and sensory-specific satiety in the rat. *Appetite, 16,* 103–120.

Berridge, K. C. (1996). Food reward: brain substrates of wanting and liking. *Neuroscience and Biobehavioral Reviews, 20,* 1–25.

Beumont, P. J. V., & Touyz, S. W. (1995). The nutritional management of anorexia and bulimia nervosa. In K. D. Brownell & C. G. Fairburn (Eds.), *Eating disorders and obesity: A comprehensive handbook* (pp. 306–312). New York: Guilford.

Birch, L. L. & Deysher, M. (1986). Caloric compensation and sensory-specific satiety: Evidence for self-regulation of food intake by young children. *Appetite, 7,* 323–331.

Blundell, J. E., & Hill, A. J. (1988). On the mechanism of action of dexfenfluramine: Effect on alliesthesia and appetite motivation in lean and obese subjects. *Clinical Neuropharmacology, 11,* S121–S134.

Blundell, J. E., & Rogers, P. J. (1991). Hunger, hedonics, and the control of satiation and satiety. In M. Friedman, M. Tordoff, & M. Kare (Eds.), *Chemical senses, appetite and nutrition* (vol. 4, pp. 127–148). New York: Marcel Dekker.

Booth, D. (1995). *The psychology of nutrition.* London: Tayler and Francis.

Cabanac, M. (1971). Physiological role of pleasure. *Science, 173,* 1103–1107.

Cabanac, M. (1979). Sensory pleasure. *Quarterly Review of Biology, 54,* 1–29.

Epstein, L. H., Caggiula, A. R., Rodefer, J. S., Wisniewski, L., & Mitchell, S. L. (1993). The effects of calories and taste on habituation of the human salivary response. *Addictive Behaviors, 18,* 179–185.

Epstein, L. H., Rodefer, J. S., Wisniewski, L., & Caggiula, A. R. (1992). Habituation and dishabituation of human salivary response. *Physiology & Behavior, 51,* 945–950.

Fantino, M., Hosotte, J., & Apfelbaum, M. (1986). An opioid antagonist, naltrexone, reduces preference for sucrose in humans. *American Journal of Physiology, 251,* R91–R96.

Fomon, S. J. (1974). *Infant nutrition.* Philadephia: Saunders.

Guy-Grand, B., & Sitt, Y. (1976). Origine de l'alliesthésie gustative: Effets comparés de charges orales glucosées ou protido-lipidiques. *Comptes-rendus de l'Académie des Sciences de Paris, 282,* 755–757.

Hetherington, M. M. (1993a). In what way is eating disordered in the eating disorders? *International Review of Psychiatry, 5,* 33–50.

Hetherington, M. M. (1993b). Research on sensory-specific satiety: An update. *Appetite, 21,* 183.

Hetherington, M. M. (1996). Sensory-specific satiety and its importance in meal termination. *Neuroscience & Biobehavioral Reviews, 20,* 113–117.

Hetherington, M., Burley, V. J., & Rolls, B. J. (1989). The time course of sensory-specific satiety. *Appetite, 12,* 57–68.

Hetherington, M. M., & Macdiarmid, J. I. (1994). Pleasure and excess: Liking for and overconsumption of chocolate. *Physiology & Behavior, 57,* 27–35.

Hetherington, M., & Rolls, B. J. (1988). Sensory specific satiety and food intake in eating disorders. In B. T. Walsh (Ed.), *Eating behavior in eating disorders* (pp. 141–160). Washington, DC: American Psychiatric Press.

Hetherington, M. M., Vervaet, N., Blass, E. & Rolls, B. J. (1991). Failure of naltrexone to affect the pleasantness or intake of food. *Physiology & Behavior, 40,* 185–190.

Hyde, R. J., & Witherly, S. A. (1993). Dynamic contrast: A sensory contribution to palatability. *Appetite, 21,* 1–16.

Johnson, J., & Vickers, Z. (1992). Factors influencing sensory-specific satiety. *Appetite, 19,* 15–31.

Kern, D. L., McPhee, L., Fisher, J., & Johnson, S. (1993). The postingestive consequences of fat condition preferences for flavors associated with high dietary fat. *Physiology and Behavior, 54,* 71–76.

LeMagnen, J. (1990). A role for opiates in food reward and food addiction. In E. D. Capaldi & T. L. Powley (Eds.), *Taste, experience and feeding* (pp. 241–252). Washington, DC: American Psychological Association.

Macdiarmid, J. I., & Hetherington, M. M. (1995). Mood modulation by food: An exploration of affect and cravings in "chocolate addicts." *British Journal of Clinical Psychology, 34,* 129–138.

Mook, D. G., & Votaw, M. C. (1992). How important is hedonism? Reasons given by college students for ending a meal. *Appetite, 18,* 69–75.

Moskowitz, H. R. (1980). Psychometric evaluation of food preferences. *Journal of Foodservice Systems, 1,* 149–167.

Polivy, J. (1976). Perception of calories and regulation of intake in restrained and unrestrained subjects. *Addictive Behaviors, 1,* 237–243.

Rogers, P. J. (1994). Mechanisms of moreishness and food craving. In D. M. Warburton (Ed.), *Pleasure: The politics and the reality* (pp. 38–49). Chichester, England: Wiley.

Rogers, P. J., & Blundell, J. E. (1990). Psychobiological bases of food choice. In M. Ashwell (Ed.), *Why we eat what we eat: British Nutrition Foundation Nutrition Bulletin* (Vol. 15, pp. 31–40). London: British Nutrition Foundation.

Rolls, B. J. (1986). Sensory-specific satiety. *Nutrition Reviews, 44,* 93–101.

Rolls, B. J. (1992). Aging and appetite. *Nutrition Reviews, 50,* 422–426.

Rolls, B. J., Andersen, A. E., Moran, T. H., McNelis, A. L., Baier, H. C., & Federoff, I. C. (1992). Food intake, hunger, and satiety after preloads in women with eating disorders. *American Journal of Clinical Nutrition, 55,* 1093–1103.

Rolls, B. J., & Hammer, V. A. (1994). Fat, carbohydrate and the regulation of energy intake. *American Journal of Clinical Nutrition, 62,* 1086s–1095s.

Rolls, B. J., & Hetherington, M. M. (1989). The role of variety in eating and body weight regulation. In R. Shepherd (Ed.), *Handbook of the psychophysiology of human eating* (pp. 57–84). Chichester, England: Wiley.

Rolls, B. J., Hetherington, M., & Burley, V. J. (1988a). Sensory stimulation and energy density in the development of satiety. *Physiology & Behavior, 44,* 727–733.

Rolls, B. J., Hetherington, M., & Burley, V. J. (1988b) The specificity of satiety: The influence of foods of different macronutrient content on the development of satiety. *Physiology & Behavior, 43,* 145–153.

Rolls, B. J. Laster, L. J., & Summerfelt, A. (1989). Hunger and food intake following consumption of low-calorie foods. *Appetite, 13,* 115–127.

Rolls, B. J., & McDermott, T. M. (1991). Effects of age on sensory-specific satiety. *American Journal of Clinical Nutrition, 54,* 988–996.

Rolls, B. J., & Phillips, P. A. (1990). Aging and disturbances of thirst and fluid balance. *Nutrition Reviews, 48,* 137–144.

Rolls, B. J., & Rolls, E. T. (1982). *Thirst.* Cambridge, England: Cambridge University Press.

Rolls, E. T. (1993). The neural control of feeding in primates. In D.A. Booth (Ed.), *Neurophysiology of ingestion* (pp. 137–169). Elmsford, NY: Pergamon Press.

Rolls, E. T., & Treves, A. (1990). The relative advantages of sparse versus distributed encoding for associative neuronal networks in the brain. *Network, 1,* 407–421.

Rozin, P., & Kalat, J. W. (1971). Specific hungers and poison avoidance as adaptive specializations of learning. *Psychological Review, 78,* 459–486.

Siegal, P. S. (1957). The repetitive element in the diet. *American Journal of Clinical Nutrition, 5,* 162–164.

Solomon, R. L. (1980). The opponent-process theory of acquired motivation: The costs of pleasure and the benefits of pain. *American Psychologist, 35,* 691–712.

Solomon, R. L. (1986). *Opponent-processes of motivation in relation to eating.* Paper presented at the Psychology Department, University of Pennsylvania, Philadelphia.

Swithers, S. E., & Hall, W. G. (1994). Does oral experience terminate ingestion? *Appetite, 23,* 113–138.

Tepper, B. J. (1992). Dietary restraint and responsiveness to sensory-based cues as measured by cephalic phase salivation and sensory specific satiety. *Physiology & Behavior, 52,* 305–311.

Westenhoefer, J. & Pudel, V. (1993). Pleasure from food: Importance for food choice and consequences of deliberate restriction. *Appetite, 20,* 246–249.

Wisniewski, L., Epstein, L. H., & Caggiula, A. R. (1992). Effect of food change on consumption, hedonics and salivation. *Physiology & Behavior, 52,* 21–26.

Wooley, O. W., Wooley, S. C., & Dunham, R. B. (1972). Calories and sweet taste: Effects on sucrose preference in the obese and non-obese. *Physiology & Behavior, 9,* 765–768.

Yeomans, M. R. (1993). The appetiser effect: Sensory enhancement of feeding as a measure of reward. *Appetite, 21,* 219.

Yeomans, M. R., & Wright, P. (1991.) Nalmefene reduces the perceived pleasantness of palatable foods in human volunteers. *Appetite, 16,* 249–259.

11

The Behavioral Phenotype in Human Obesity

Adam Drewnowski

H uman obesities represent a complex medical disorder of multiple origin (National Academy of Sciences, 1989; US Department of Health and Human Services 1988). Genetic predisposition, diverse health behaviors, and individual food choices all contribute in varying degrees to the expression of the obese state (Bouchard, 1988; Stunkard et al., 1986). The development of obesity is influenced by familial risk and can be delayed or modulated by changes in energy intake, physical activity, and energy expenditure (Bray, 1988). The degree of overweight can be modified further by dietary choices, including the fat content of the habitual diet (Miller, Lindeman, Wallace, & Niederpruem, 1990; Romieu et al., 1988).

Recent research, conducted with rats and mice, has tended to focus on the genetics of obesity. Studies conducted with one species of obese rodents, the obese ob/ob mice, have succcessfully linked excess body fat with specific genetic loci and with the production of a discrete protein, *leptin* (Halaas et al., 1995). When leptin was administered to genetically obese or diet-induced obese mice, food intake was suppressed and body weights declined. Initially, the hope was that a similar mechanism might operate in humans, with leptin acting as the long sought-after feedback signal regulating body fat stores. However, it now appears that obese humans have sufficient circulating leptin, but are leptin resistant, much as obese diabetics are resistant to circulating insulin. Prospects for leptin therapy appear dim. Although research in genetics can tell us a great deal about the nature of obesity, as a general strategy, linking the obese genotype with its final physiological end point, excess body fat, tells nothing about the intervening physiological or behavioral mechanisms that might have led to gene expression in the first place. One needs to look to the obese phenotype, that is, the outcome of the interaction between the genotype and the environment, for some of the clues regarding the development of obesity in humans.

It must be stressed that gene expression is typically governed by nutrients. Some experts believe that the heritable factor is not excess body weight, but rather a predisposition or a vulnerability to obesity that is expressed under suitable environmental conditions. As a result, dietary behaviors and nutrient selection are likely to play a critical role in obesity development. It is inevitable that the obese phenotype will involve some aspect of behavior: however, few recent studies have seriously explored the potential impact of genetics on food selection or examined the interaction between genetic factors and the dietary environment.

Instead, some scientists have adopted the (admittedly extreme) position that because most, if not all, human obesities are genetic in nature, the study of behavior is superfluous. In this view, the most promising avenue for obesity treatment is either genetic therapy or drugs. This represents a radical departure from the (equally extreme) thinking of the 1970s, when many scientists were firmly convinced that human obesity had a purely behavioral origin and needed to be treated using behavioral therapy or psychoanalysis. At that time, studies on obesity tended to focus on such notions as "externality," "finickiness," or "restraint" to arrive at a purely behavioral explanation for the obese state. Tracing the history of some of these ideas is the purpose of this chapter. This chapter traces the history of some of these approaches, from the behavioral to the genetic. Behavioral, dieting, and central metabolic factors that may influence the expression of human obesity will be considered in turn.

BEHAVIORAL MODELS OF HUMAN OBESITY

The prevailing view among obesity researchers in the 1970s was that human obesity was largely a psychological problem. Overeating was said to be a maladaptive behavior that could be shaped or modified through behavioral therapy (Stuart & Davis, 1972). Eliminating the reinforcing properties of good-tasting foods, it was believed, would shape the behavioral response toward other, equally rewarding, activities. Obese patients or clients were encouraged to become more aware of their eating patterns by keeping food diaries and were taught how to become less susceptible to factors or events that triggered eating behavior (Stunkard & Berthold, 1985). Exerting behavioral control over good-tasting foods was said to be the first step toward successful weight reduction.

One persistent belief was that obese people were more susceptible to external food cues, such as the taste, smell, or even the sight of foods (Cabanac & Duclaux, 1970). As a result, the argument went, obese patients were entirely at the mercy of the external environment and continued eating whether they were hungry or not (Rodin, 1981b; Schachter & Rodin, 1974). Much research was devoted to the absence of internal cues of hunger and satiety among the obese and to the microstructure of eating patterns. Further studies in social psychology addressed issues such as emotional eating among the obese following the playing of sad audiotapes and the fact that the obese rarely used chopsticks in Chinese restaurants (Schachter & Rodin, 1974).

In some studies, external factors were equated with food palatability. The externality hypothesis led some investigators to propose that obese humans (and rats) were "finicky," eating more of good-tasting but less of bad-tasting foods than normal-weight controls (Schachter & Rodin, 1974). Food palatability was in turn wholly equated with sweet taste. Heightened preferences for sweet solutions were thought to be typical of both obese humans and obese rats (Cabanac & Duclaux, 1970). Some researchers proposed that food palatability was the principal determinant of food consumption among obese people, although not among lean individuals. This research focus on the obese "sweet tooth" was not unconnected to the popular wisdom of the time, which regarded carbohydrates as the most fattening foods imaginable. The major weight-loss diets of the time prohibited carbohydrates and sugar in favor of fat and protein. The no-starch but high-meat diets derived up to 72% of energy from fat and provided dieters with a gram and a half of cholesterol per day.

The focus on obesity and sweet taste got further impetus from the presumed connection between sweet taste and physiological need. In this view, the pleasure response to sweet taste reflected the energy needs of the organism. Restrained obese individuals striving to maintain body weight below its predestined level, the physiological set point, were thought to be in a state of chronic caloric need, which was manifested by elevated preferences for sweet taste. Sweet taste preferences were thought to reflect both the concern with dieting and the distance from the physiological set point of body weight.

The externality hypothesis soon outlived its usefulness (Rodin, 1978, 1981a). As later studies showed, the obese as a group were no more external than people of normal weight (Rodin, 1978). Furthermore, although some obese people liked sweet taste, others did not (Drewnowski, 1986). Nor was there evidence that the obese were more sensitive to external cues following weight loss, as the set-point hypothesis would require (Rodin, 1978). Indeed, studies on attitudes, behaviors, food preferences, and eating styles have generally failed to establish consistent differences between obese individuals and lean controls. Of course, one problem was the persistent comparison of obese with lean persons, as though body weight predicted behavior rather than the other way around. Because further obese–lean comparisons were unlikely to provide useful data, subsequent research strategies focused on individual differences and on identifying and contrasting diverse subgroups of obese individuals.

ANIMAL MODELS OF OBESITY

Studies of animal models of obesity provided evidence that some rodent strains, or even individual animals, were differentially susceptible to the effects of diet. Laboratory studies have shown that providing rats or mice *ad lib* with a sufficiently palatable diet led to overeating and weight gain (Sclafani & Springer, 1976). Although some rat strains were highly susceptible to the effects of sweet and high-fat foods, other strains remained resistant (Sclafani, 1985). Furthermore, there was an interaction between the obese genotype and the effects of diet. Whereas the genetically obese ob/ob mice and the obese (fa/fa) Zucker rats gained excess weight on a chow diet, the expression of obesity in other strains of rats strongly depended on diet composition. Intensely sweet (32%) sucrose solutions, oil or lard, and a variety of sweet or high-fat foods all promoted dietary obesity in rats.

Obesity was induced more effectively by high-fat than by high-sugar diets. The best results were obtained with diets containing both sugar and fat. The so-called cafeteria regime used a variety of sweet and high-fat foods, including salami, cookies, marshmallows, cheese wafers, and peanut butter (Sclafani & Springer, 1976). Other diets have included chocolate chip cookies and sweetened condensed milk.

What implications do animal models have for human obesity syndromes? It is unclear how persons with different genetic predispositions to obesity respond to palatable diets, especially diets that are rich in both sugars and fat. One possibility is that genetically transmitted obesities are independent of diet composition and are not associated with altered food preferences or diet choices. Another possibility is that the genetic vulnerability manifests itself as heightened responsiveness to energy-rich or palatable foods. Studies conducted with genetically obese Zucker rats suggested that the rats self-selected a fat-rich diet, given a choice. Studies conducted with ob/ob mice similarly showed that the mice increased their consumption of condensed milk that was sweetened with saccharin. Evidently, even the obese genotype is sensitive to the taste of foods. Because the pleasure response to foods has been used as a predictor of food consumption, taste preferences and food choices may be useful indices of the tendency to gain weight. Studies of the pleasure, or hedonic, response to foods may provide a new insight into the genetic and dietary mechanisms that underlie the expression of obesity.

HUMAN OBESITY AND SWEET TASTE

Studies an animal models of obesity demonstrated that obesity is the outcome of an interaction between a genetic predisposition and exposure to environmental factors such as diet. The most promising strategy for the study of the behavioral phenotype in human obesity might be to focus on dietary behaviors that are most likely to carry a heritable component; however, it is unclear what those behaviors are. Past investigators have variously examined attitudes and beliefs as well as sweet taste preferences, food choices, and eating styles; such studies have almost invariably failed to establish any consistent differences between obese patients and control groups of lean persons. In some cases the relevant behavior was assumed, correctly or not, to be the driving force behind the expression of obesity.

Preferences for the sweet taste of sugar solutions were one case in point.

The conventional view during the 1970s was that excess sugar consumption was the principal cause of human obesity. Since all obese subjects were regarded as "external," it was thought that they would be hyperresponsive to the taste of sweet. Early studies of obesity and palatability were invariably conducted with sugar solutions in water or with sweetened soft drinks (Moskowitz, Kluter, Westerling, & Jacobs, 1974;) Witherly, Pangborn, & Stern, 1980). Such studies reported that obese men and women found sweet solutions difficult to resist (Rodin, Moskowitz, & Bray, 1978). Furthermore, obese persons were insensitive to satiety cues and could not tell if they were hungry or not. Preferences for sweet taste reportedly remained high even after the consumption of a sweet solution containing 50 g of glucose (Cabanac & Duclaux, 1970). No satiety aversion to sucrose or negative alliesthesia was observed among obese respondents, suggesting that the obese were in a continuing state of metabolic need. The obese "sweet tooth" was thought to override satiety signals, leading to overconsumption of sweets and other desserts.

At the time, all obese persons were regarded as a single homogenous group. Eventually, it became clear that not all obese persons were alike. As later studies showed, some obese patients liked the sweet taste of sugar, and others did not. Nor was there evidence that weight loss resulted in increased preferences for sweet taste, as predicted by the set-point hypothesis. In fact, taste response profiles for sweetness appeared to be independent of body weight status (Drewnowski, 1986). Attempts to link sweet taste preferences with body weight also ended in failure. Studies using sucrose solutions, sweetened commercial soft drinks, and chocolate milkshakes found no consistent relationship between sweet taste preferences and overweight. Large-scale consumer studies found no link between body weight and hedonic preferences for increasing concentrations of sugar in such foods as apricot nectar, canned peaches, lemonade, or vanilla ice cream (Drewnowski, 1986). Individual variability was typically far greater than any differences in mean hedonic response between obese participants and lean controls (Witherly et al., 1980).

In retrospect, the observed variability of response is hardly surprising, given that the obese participants in many studies were in fact patients, selected and recruited solely on the basis of their excess body weight. Clinical populations represent different forms of human obesity syndromes and typically include patients with diverse etiologies of the disease and different personal histories of weight loss and regain. If anything, clinical populations overrepresent patients with a past history of treatment failure, and may overrepresent both genetic obesity and the binge-eating syndrome. Segregating subjects on the basis of body weight alone also poses a problem. It is too much to expect that two obese individuals would share common thoughts, attitudes, or dietary behaviors merely because they both weight 210 lb on the day of testing. More recent studies have made more careful distinctions among potential obese subgroups, selecting and comparing participants on the basis of familial risk, age at onset of obesity, past history of weight cycling, or the distribution of body fat.

Some of these factors may be interrelated. At least one study, largely based on female clinic patients, has linked familial risk (increased proportion of obese parents and siblings) with childhood-onset obesity (onset before age 10). In the absence of other biomarkers, familial risk and age at onset have served as potential indices of a genetic predisposition to obesity. At this point, no other markers are readily available.

OBESITY AND THE APPETITE FOR FAT

The development of human obesities is influenced by both diet and behavior. Although the precise role of dietary behaviors is still unclear, clinical studies have suggested that the diet of obese men and women is often rich in fat (Miller et al., 1990; Romieu et al., 1988). In one laboratory study, preferences for fat in foods were directly correlated with the participants' percentage of body fat (Mela & Sacchetti, 1991). Another study showed that obese women consumed more fat energy than did lean women and had a lower carbohydrate to fat ratio (Romieu et al., 1988). A recent study conducted with young children (Fisher & Birch, 1995) showed that the children's preferences for fat in foods were influenced not only by their own body fatness, but also by the fatness of their mother. Given that the fatness of the parent and of the child are said to be genetically linked, that study provided a convincing demonstration that a potential instance of genetic vulnerability might be an increased appetite for energy-dense fat-containing foods.

Fat-containing foods are also highly preferred. Fats supply the characteristic texture, flavor, and aroma of many foods and determine the overall palatability of the diet. Foods that combine sugar and fat are often regarded as uniquely good tasting. Elevated preferences for chocolate, ice cream, pastries, whipped cream, and other sweet desserts are common among obese women and are reported to intensify following caloric restriction and weight loss. Uncontrollable "cravings" for sweet desserts have also been reported among women suffering from the binge-eating disorder or from the eating disorder bulimia nervosa (Paykel, Mueller, & de la Vergne, 1973; Wurtman, 1984). Survey studies have shown further that chocolate was the typical object of food cravings by women (Rozin, Levine, & Stoess, 1991).

Energy-dense foods are also highly rewarding (Drewnowski, 1987). Because dietary fats are the most concentrated source of dietary energy (9 kcal/g), high-fat foods are generally highly preferred by children and adults. Increased appetite for palatable foods, especially those rich in dietary sugars and fats, may provide a behavioral mechanism for the development of obesity in susceptible persons (Drewnowski & Holden-Wiltse, 1992). One possibility might be a mechanism that involves the sensory pleasure response to foods and is mediated by endogenous opiate peptides (Drewnowski, Krahn, Demitrack, Nairn, & Gosnell, 1995). Other researchers have suggested that obese men and women passively overconsume fat-rich foods because they are less sensitive to the satiating qualities of dietary fats.

SENSORY PREFERENCES FOR DIETARY FATS

Although researchers in the areas of obesity and palatability have failed to find a direct link between sweet taste preferences and overweight, such a relationship seemed to hold for dietary fats (Miller et al., 1990; Romieu et al., 1988). Among the complex sensory stimuli used in sensory evaluation studies were milkshakes, soft white cheese ("fromage blanc"), cake frostings, and ice cream (Drewnowski, Brunzell, Sande, Iverius, & Greenwood, 1985; Drewnowski & Greenwood, 1983; Drewnowski, Shrager, Lipsky, Stellar, & Greenwood, 1989). These studies examined the taste response to palatable foods rich in both sugar and fat in obese persons.

In one study, obese women patients and lean controls tasted and rated 20 sweetened dairy products of varying sugar and fat content (Drewnowski et al., 1985). Additional participants were formerly obese women who successfully maintained a lower body weight (Drewnowski et al., 1985). The women tasted each sample in turn and rated its sweetness, creaminess, and perceived fat content. They also rated the acceptability of each sample on a 9-point category scale. The response profile to the sugar–fat mixtures was strongly interactive. Preference ratings for sweetened skim milk or unsweetened dairy products were relatively low. However, combining sugar with fat produced a synergy of hedonic response. Highest ratings were obtained for a mixture containing 8% sugar and 20% fat. Obese women selected stimuli that were rich in fat but relatively low in sugar. In contrast, formerly obese women preferred stimuli that were rich in both sugar and fat. This last observation is consistent with clinical reports that dieting and weight loss may lead to binge-eating episodes involving sweet and high-fat foods. It may also be one reason why maintaining the weight loss is a continuing challenge, even for the successful dieter.

OBESITY AND THE BINGE-EATING SYNDROME

Predisposition to obesity might also be manifested through food "cravings" and episodes of binge eating. Recurrent binge-eating episodes appear to be a common feature of some human obesity syndromes. The binge-eating disorder, a newly proposed *DSM–IV* category (American Psychiatric Association 1994), is said to occur in up to one third of all obese female clinic patients. In contrast, its prevalence outside the clinical setting is reported to be considerably lower. In past studies, the binge-eating disorder has been associated with massive obesity, early age of onset, a history of failed attempts at weight reduction, and weight cycling. All these are potential markers for a genetic predisposition to obesity.

Food "cravings" and eating binges are often thought to be triggered by metabolic events. Much attention has been devoted to the phenomenon of "carbohydrate cravings" among the obese, said to be due to an imbalance of serotonin, a central neurotransmitter (Wurtman, 1984). According to the serotonin hypothesis, selective consumption of carbohydrate-rich snacks in the absence of protein promoted uptake by the brain of a serotonin precursor, the amino acid tryptophan. Obese persons suffering from a serotonin deficiency were assumed to consume carbohydrate-rich snacks as a form of self-medication. Because most obese patients seen in clinics were reported to be "carbohydrate cravers," it was assumed that selective consumption of a single macronutrient, carbohydrate, was linked directly to the development of human obesity.

The serotonin hypothesis provided a convenient molecular explanation for the obese eating patterns. However, food palatability was not taken into account. According to the serotonin hypothesis, any carbohydrate-rich snack that was low in protein should help to redress serotonin imbalance. Yet the typical targets of food "cravings" were not bland carbohydrates but mixtures of sugar and fat, including chocolate candy, chocolate cupcakes, chocolate chip cookies, cakes, and other desserts. Cravings for sweet desserts and other sugar–fat mixtures have been observed among obese patients, bulimic women, and depressed patients, including those suffering from the seasonal affective disorder. In other clinical studies, "carbohydrate cravings" observed as side effects of treatment with antidepressants involved not bread or potatoes but ice cream, frozen pastries with whipped cream, and other desserts (Paykel et al., 1973).

Eating binges, observed in obesity and in bulimia nervosa, also involve sweet and high-fat foods. Chocolate and ice cream figure prominently in clinical descriptions and anecdotal reports of food cravings, food binges, and food addictions (Paykel et al., 1973; Wurtman, 1984). Although sweet desserts are often thought of as carbohydrate-rich foods, they often derive the bulk of their calories from fat.

Food "cravings" are likely to involve the endogenous opiate peptide system. It has long been known that beta-endorphins are associated with overeating in genetically obese (ob/ob) mice and the obese (fa/fa) Zucker rats. Later studies with rats and mice linked intakes of sugar and fat with endorphin release (Blass, 1986). Dietary studies have shown further that morphine-injected animals selectively increased fat intake, whereas the opiate antagonist naltrexone blocked overeating induced by a palatable cafeteria diet (Apfelbaum & Mandenoff, 1981).

To test the hypothesis that the pleasure response to palatable foods is mediated by endogenous opiate peptides, my colleagues and I examined the effects of the opiate antagonist naloxone on taste preferences and food consumption in obese and normal-weight women. Some of the women reported frequent binge-eating episodes involving palatable foods (Drewnowski, Krahn, Demitrack, Nairn, & Gosnell, 1991). During drug infusion, the participants tasted and rated 20 sweetened dairy products and were offered eight snack foods of different sugar and fat content. Naloxone suppressed taste preferences for sugar–fat mixtures in all participants and selectively reduced the consumption of sweet and high-fat snacks in binge eaters but not in nonbingers. Food intakes of obese women were not affected by naloxone.

Naloxone selectively suppressed the consumption of palatable foods that were sweet, rich in fat, or both. The selectivity of naloxone and the limitation to sweet and high-fat foods effects may help explain why chronic treatments with an analogous drug naltrexone have failed to reduce food consumption and induce weight loss in many obese individuals. Although opiate blockade is not a viable strategy for weight reduction in obesity, it may be useful in the clinical management of the binge-eating disorder.

OBESITY AND FOOD CHOICES

Relatively few studies have contrasted food preferences of obese men and women. A large study of U.S. Army personnel showed that overweight people selected red meat dishes rather than desserts (Meiselman, Waterman, & Symington, 1974). Studies conducted with several hundred obese patients confirmed that self-reported food preferences of obese men most often included steaks and roasts, hamburgers, French fries, pizza, and ice cream (Drewnowski, Kurth, Holden-Wiltse, & Saari, 1992). In contrast, obese women tended to list foods that were sweet, rich in fat, or both. Among the most frequent choices were ice cream, chocolate, cake, and other desserts.

As shown in Table 1, obese men and women differed in their food preference profiles. Whereas obese men selected mixtures of fat and protein, obese women selected foods that were mixtures of sugar and fat. The presence of fat, sugar, or salt was critical to food preferences. There was no evidence that preference for bland carbohydrates such as bread and potatoes was a standard feature of human obesity. Although some participants (mostly women) did list bread among their favorite foods, preferences for ice cream were far more frequent. Preferences for dietary fats as opposed to sugars or other carbohydrates appear to be a characteristic feature of obesity syndromes in both humans and rats.

Table 1		

Food Preferences of Obese Men and Women

	Men ($n = 93$)	Women ($n = 386$)
Meats	96.8*	86.0
Carbohydrate–fats	92.5	91.5
Dairy products	50.5	49.2
Fats	16.1	23.8
Starches	44.1	49.2
Sugars	11.8	23.3
High-fat sweets	67.7	80.6*
Vegetables	39.8	48.4
Fruits	29.0	38.9
Low-calorie beverages	3.2	3.4
Alcohol	4.3	4.1

NOTE. The data represent the percentage of men and women who included at least one food item in each category on a list of 10 favorite foods. *Source*: Drewnowski, Kurth, et al., 1992. *$p < .05$.

CLINICAL IMPLICATIONS

Taste responsiveness to sweet and high-fat foods is one index of the individual propensity to consume or reject palatable foods. As a result, taste response profiles may predict the success or failure of dietary intervention for weight loss. One possibility is that elevated preferences for sweet and high-fat foods and the propensity to binge-eat are behavioral manifestations of the obese phenotype. Alternatively, sensory preferences for sugar and fat might be the outcome of past weight cycling, or "yo-yo" dieting. Repeated cycles of weight loss and weight regain in both humans and rats are thought to be associated with improved metabolic efficiency and enhanced fat storage. One study with animals showed that fluctuations in body weight were followed by increased selection of a high-fat diet (Reed, Contreras, Maggio, Greenwood, & Rodin, 1988).

The two hypotheses are not mutually exclusive. In fact, weight cycling might be a symptom of intractable, and potentially familial, obesity. The question arises whether obese weight cyclers have heightened preferences for energy-dense foods relative to other obese persons whose weights are more stable. The participants in one study (Drewnowski, Kurth, & Rahaim, 1991) were divided into subgroups on the basis of age at onset of obesity and past fluctuations in body weight. They tasted five sucrose solutions and nine sugar–fat mixtures resembling cake frostings. The cake frostings contained between 15% and 35% fat and between 20% and 70% sucrose (Drewnowski, Kurth, & Rahaim, 1991).

Chronic dieters, whose weights fluctuated, liked sweet high-fat cake frostings more than did obese participants of stable body weight. Preferences for sucrose solutions in water were the same for both groups. Early age of onset of obesity, thought to be a measure of familial risk, had no effect on taste preferences. Environmental as opposed to familial factors may have a more immediate effect on taste preferences and food choices.

Genetic predisposition and familial obesity syndromes ought to be associated with treatment failure. Obese men and women with an inherited tendency to the obese state might be found among the "intractable" obese characterized by weight cycling and failed attempts at weight loss. There are suggestions that these groups are also characterized by binge eating and by elevated sensory preferences for sugar and fat. However, the potential indices of a genetic predisposition to obesity in humans are so tentative that they have not been used in the classification of obesity syndromes. Instead, the existing classification schemes are largely taxonomic or descriptive, determined on the basis of the amount and distribution of body fat. Although such distinctions are potentially useful, none have been linked so far to treatment success or treatment failure.

What is needed is a more functional scheme for the classification of human obesities, one that is sensitive to dietary behaviors and food choices. Such a scheme is proposed in Table 2. One possibility is that sensory preferences including an appetite for dietary fats constitute one behavioral manifestation of an obese phenotype. Another possibility is that the binge-eating syndrome provides a mechanism for the expression of obesity in vulnerable individuals. These behaviors are characteristic of some obese individuals and have been associated with intractable obesity and failure at weight loss. It remains to be seen whether such diet-related behaviors can be associated with a genetic predisposition to the obese state.

Table 2

Existing and Potential Classifications of Human Obesity Subtypes

Classifications	Corresponding measures or criteria
Existing	
Degree of overweight	Mild (150% IBW), moderate, or massive (> 200% IBW)
Fat distribution	Waist:hip ratio
Health risks	Low, moderate, or high
Proposed	
Familial risk	Proportion of obese parents and siblings
Age of onset	Childhood (<10 years), juvenile (10–20 years), or adult onset (>20 years)
Weight history	Stable or fluctuating
Binge-eating syndrome	Present or absent
Taste responsiveness	Preferences for sugar and fat
Diet composition	Carbohydrate:fat ratio

NOTE.   IBW = ideal body weight.

CONCLUSION

The prevalence of obesity in the United States is rising, and epidemiological studies suggest that one in three American adults is obese. Obesity is a major health problem among ethnic minorities and among newly arrived immigrant groups. The prevalence of obesity among Pima Indians in the Southwest or among Pacific Islanders in American Samoa can exceed 80%. Genetic predisposition clearly is an important factor. However, the expression of obesity can also be tied to nutrition transition and the gradual adoption of a calorie-dense diet that is rich in both sugar and fat. As with animal models, the expression of human obesity genes is strongly influenced by nutrition.

The question of who becomes obese and why remains unsolved. National statistics show that the observed increase in mean body weight or body mass index (kg/m^2) is largely caused by obese persons becoming fatter still. In other words, part of the American population is extremely vulnerable to becoming obese, whereas part of the population remains resistant. It remains to be seen whether the vulnerability to obesity has a genetic, dietary, or sociocultural component, however. Additional research on genetics, diet, and behavior should lead to better prevention and intervention programs targeted at groups of susceptible individuals.

REFERENCES

American Psychiatric Association (1994). *Diagnostic and statistical manual of mental disorders (4th ed.).* Washington, DC: American Psychiatric Association.

Apfelbaum, M., & Mandenoff, A. (1981). Naltrexone suppresses hyperphagia induced in the rat by a highly palatable diet. *Pharmacology, Biochemistry, and Behavior, 15,* 89–91.

Blass, E. M. (1986). Opioids, sugar and the inherent taste of sweet: Broad motivational implications. In J. Dobbing (Ed.), *Sweetness: ILSI-Nutrition Foundation Symposium.* Berlin: Springer-Verlag.

Bouchard, C. (1988). Inheritance of human fat distribution. In C. Bouchard & F. E. Johnston (Eds.), *Fat distribution during growth and later health outcomes: Current topics in nutrition and disease (Vol. 17).* New York: Alan R. Liss.

Bray, G. A. (1988). Controls of food intake and energy expenditure. In G. A. Bray, J. Le Blanc, S. Inover, & M. Suzuki (Eds.), *Diet and obesity* (pp. 17–35). Tokyo: *Japan Scientific Societies Press.*

Cabanac, M., & Duclaux, R. (1970). Obesity: Absence of satiety aversion to sucrose. *Science, 168,* 496–497.

Drewnowski, A. (1986). Obesity and sweet taste. In J. Dobbing (Ed.), *Sweetness: ILSI Nutrition Foundation Symposium.* Berlin: Springer-Verlag.

Drewnowski, A. (1987). Fats and food texture: Sensory and hedonic evaluations. In H.R. Moskowitz (Ed.), *Food texture* (pp. 217–250). New York: Marcel Dekker.

Drewnowski, A., Brunzell, J. D., Sande, K., Iverius, P. H., & Greenwood, M. R. C. (1985). Sweet tooth reconsidered: Taste responsiveness in human obesity. *Physiology of Behavior, 35,* 617–622.

Drewnowski, A., & Greenwood, M. R. C. (1983). Cream and sugar: Human preferences for high-fat foods. *Physiology of Behavior, 30,* 629–633.

Drewnowski, A., & Holden-Wiltse, J. (1992). Taste responses and food preferences in obese women: Effects of weight cycling. *International Journal of Obesity, 16,* 639–648.

Drewnowski, A., Krahn, D.D., Demitrack, M.A., Nairn, K., & Gosnell, B.A. (1991). Taste responses and preferences for sweet high-fat foods: Evidence for opioid involvement. *Physiology of Behavior, 51,* 371–379.

Drewnowski, A., Krahn, D. D., Demitrack, M. A., Nairn, K., & Gosnell, B. A. (1995). Naloxone, an opiate blocker, reduces the consumption of sweet high-fat foods in obese and lean female binge eaters. *American Journal of Clinical Nutrition, 61,* 1206–1212.

Drewnowski, A., Kurth, C., Holden-Wiltse, J., & Saari, J. (1992). Food preferences in human obesity: Carbohydrates versus fats. *Appetite, 18,* 207–221.

Drewnowski, A., Kurth, C. L., & Rahaim, J. E. (1991). Taste preferences in human obesity: Environmental and familial factors. *American Journal of Clinical Nutrition, 54,* 635–641.

Drewnowski, A., Shrager, E. E., Lipsky, C., Stellar, E., & Greenwood, M. R. C. (1989). Sugar and fat: Sensory and hedonic evaluations of liquid and solid foods. *Physiology of Behavior, 45,* 177–183.

Fisher, J. O., & Birch, J. L. (1995). Fat preferences and fat consumption of 3- to 5-year-old children are related to parent adiposity. *Journal of the American Dietetic Association, 95,* 759–764.

Halaas, J. L., Gajiwala, K. S., Maffei, M., Cohen, S. L., Chait, B. T., Rabinowitz, D., Lallone, R. L., Burley, S. K., & Friedman, J. M. (1995). Weight-reducing effects of the plasma protein encoded by the obese gene. *Science, 269,* 543–546.

Meiselman, H. L., Waterman, D., & Symington, L. E. (1974). *Armed Forces food preferences* (Technical Report 75-63-FSL). Natick, MA: U.S. Army Natick Development Center.

Mela, D. J., & Sacchetti, D. A. (1991). Sensory preferences for fats: Relationships with diet and body composition. *American Journal of Clinical Nutrition, 53,* 908–915.

Miller, W. C., Lindeman, A. K., Wallace, J., & Niederpruem, M. (1990). Diet composition, energy intake, and exercise in relation to body fat in men and women. *American Journal of Clinical Nutrition, 52,* 426–430.

Moskowitz, H. R., Kluter, R. A., Westerling, J., & Jacobs, H. L. (1974). Sugar sweetness and pleasantness: Evidence for different psychophysical laws. *Science, 184,* 583–585.

National Academy of Sciences. (1989). *Diet and health: Report of the Food and Nutrition Board.* Washington, DC: National Academy Press.

Paykel, E. S., Mueller, P. S., & de la Vergne, P. M. (1973). Amitryptyline, weight gain and carbohydrate craving: A side effect. *British Journal of Psychiatry, 125*, 501–507.

Reed, D. R., Contreras, R. J., Maggio, C., Greenwood, M. R., & Rodin, J. (1988). Weight cycling in female rats increases dietary fat selection and adiposity. *Physiology of Behavior, 42*, 389–395.

Rodin, J. (1978). Has the internal versus external distinction outlived its usefulness? In G.A. Bray (Ed.), *Recent advances in obesity research II* (pp. 75–85). London: Newman.

Rodin, J. (1981a). The current state of the internal-external hypothesis: What went wrong? *American Psychologist, 36*, 361–372.

Rodin, J. (1981b). Psychological factors in obesity. In P. Bjorntorp, M. Cairella, & A.N. Howard (Eds.), *Recent advances in obesity research III* (pp. 106–123). London: John Libbey.

Rodin, J., Moskowitz, H.R., & Bray, S.A. (1978). Relationship between obesity, weight loss, and taste responsiveness. *Physiology of Behavior, 17*, 391–397.

Romieu, I., Willett, W. C., Stampfer, M., Colditz, G. A., Sampson, L., Rosner, B., Hennekens, C. H., & Speizer, F. E. (1988). Energy intake and other determinants of relative weight. *American Journal of Clinical Nutrition, 47*, 406–412.

Rozin, P., Levine, E., & Stoess, C. (1991). Chocolate craving and liking. *Appetite, 17*, 199–212.

Schachter, S., & Rodin, J. (1974). *Obese humans and rats.* Potomac, MD: LEA.

Sclafani, A. (1985). Animal models of obesity. In R.T. Frankle, J. Dwyer, L. Moragne, & A. Owen (Eds.), *Dietary treatment and prevention of obesity* (pp. 105–123). London: John Libbey.

Sclafani, A., & Springer, D. (1976). Dietary obesity in adult rats: Similarities to hypothalamic and human obesity syndromes. *Physiology of Behavior, 17*, 461–471.

Stuart, R. B., & Davis, B. (1972). *Slim chance in a fat world: Behavioral control of obesity.* Champaign, IL: Research Press.

Stunkard, A. J., & Berthold, H. C. (1985). What is behavior therapy: A very short description of behavioral weight control. *American Journal of Clinical Nutrition, 41*, 821–823.

Stunkard, A. J., Sorensen, T. I. A., Hanis, C., Teasdale, T. W., Chakraborty, R., Schull, W. J., & Schulsinger, F. (1986). An adoption study of human obesity. *New England Journal of Medicine, 314*, 193–198.

US Department of Health and Human Services. (1988). *Surgeon General's report on nutrition and health* (DHHS [PHS] Publication No. 88-50210). Washington, DC: U.S. Government Printing Office.

Witherly, S. A., Pangborn, R. M., & Stern, J. S. (1980). Gustatory responses and eating duration of obese and lean adults. *Appetite, 1,* 52–63.

Wurtman, J. J. (1984). The involvement of brain serotonin in excessive carbohydrate snacking by obese carbohydrate cravers. *Journal of the American Dietetic Association, 84,* 1004–1007.

Author Index

Numbers in italics refer to listings in the reference sections.

Subject Index

About the Editor

Elizabeth D. Capaldi is professor of Psychology at the University of Florida, where she has taught since 1988. She received her BA from the University of Rochester in 1965 and her PhD in experimental psychology from the University of Texas in 1969. Dr. Capaldi's research has focused on animal learning and motivation. She has contributed over 60 chapters, articles, and reviews, and is coeditor (with T. L. Powley) of *Taste, Experience, and Feeding*. She is associate editor of *Psychonomic Bulletin & Review* and a consulting editor for the *Journal of Experimental Psychology: Animal Behavior Processes*. She currently serves on the Governing Board of the Psychonomic Society and on the Board of Directors of the American Psychological Society, of which she is also Secretary.